AF323113

Imaging
of
Urologic Disorders

Edited by

Alexander S. Cass, M.B.B.S., F.R.C.S., F.A.C.S.
Staff Urologist, Hennepin County Medical Center
Associate Professor of Urology
University of Minnesota
Minneapolis, Minnesota

Judith Gunn Bronson, M.S.
Technical Editor

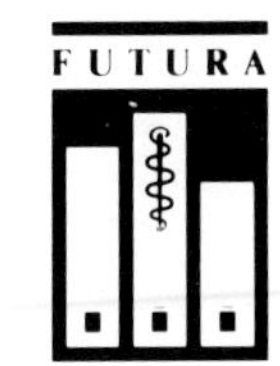

**Futura Publishing
Company, Inc.**
Mount Kisco, NY

Library of Congress Cataloging-in-Publication Data

Imaging of urologic disorders / edited by Alexander S. Cass.
    p.   cm.
    Includes bibliographical references and index.
    ISBN 0-87993-392-5
    1. Genitourinary organs—Imaging.   I. Cass, Alexander.
    [DNLM: 1. Diagnostic Imaging.   2. Urologic Diseases—diagnosis.
WJ 141 I315]
RC874.I43   1992
616.6'0754—dc20
DNLM/DLC
for Library of Congress   91-34814
                                                      CIP

Copyright 1992
Futura Publishing Company, Inc.

Published by
Futura Publishing Company, Inc.
2 Bedford Ridge Road
Mount Kisco, New York 10549

L.C. No.: 91-34814
ISBN No.: 0-87993-392-5

Every effort has been made to ensure that the information in this book is as up to date
and accurate as possible at the time of publication. However, due to the constant
developments in medicine, neither the author, nor the editor, nor the publisher can
accept any legal or any other responsibility for any errors or omissions that may occur.

All rights reserved.
No part of this book may be translated or reproduced in any form without written
permission of the publisher.

Printed in the United States of America

This book has been printed on acid-free paper.

Contributors

Robert Berkseth, M.D.
Assistant Professor of Medicine
University of Minnesota School of Medicine
Hennepin County Medical Center
Minneapolis, Minnesota

Alexander Caciarelli, M.D.
Head, Section of Pediatric Radiology
Department of Diagnostic Radiology
William Beaumont Hospital
Royal Oak, Michigan

John F. Cardella, M.D.
Chief, Cardiovascular/Interventional Radiology
Milton S. Hershey Medical Center
Associate Professor of Radiology
Pennsylvania State University
Hershey, Pennsylvania

Alexander S. Cass, M.B.B.S.
Staff Urologist
Hennepin County Medical Center
Associate Professor of Urology
University of Minnesota
Minneapolis, Minnesota

Jalil Farah, M.D.
Chief, Department of Diagnostic Radiology
William Beaumont Hospital
Royal Oak, Michigan
Clinical Associate Professor of Radiology
University of Michigan
Ann Arbor, Michigan

Michael C. Farah, M.D.
Staff Radiologist, Department of Diagnostic Radiology
William Beaumont Hospital
Royal Oak, Michigan

Jay B. Hollander, M.D.
Staff Urologist, Department of Urology
William Beaumont Hospital
Royal Oak, Michigan

Evan J. Kass, M.D.
Chief, Division of Pediatric Urology
William Beaumont Hospital
Royal Oak, Michigan

Joe Y. Lee, M.D.
Staff Urologist
Hennepin County Medical Center
Minneapolis, Minnesota

Carl S. Smith, M.D.
Chief of Urology
Hennepin County Medical Center
Clinical Instructor, General Surgery
University of Minnesota
Minneapolis, Minnesota

Charles Smith, M.D.
Staff Nephrologist
Hennepin County Medical Center
Assistant Professor of Medicine
University of Minnesota
Minneapolis, Minnesota

Joaquim Vieira, M.D.
Senior Associate Radiologist
Hennepin County Medical Center
Assistant Professor of Radiology
University of Minnesota
Minneapolis, Minnesota

To My Father

Ben

for his Unfailing Support
and
Confidence
in his three Sons

Preface

The rapid advance in high technology used by radiologists to diagnose disease has impinged on the imaging of urologic disorders. This book is intended to be a practical concise volume for the practicing urologist and is aimed at easy understanding and use of the state-of-the-art imaging techniques to diagnose urologic disorders. If more depth of information about an imaging technique is required, or if information is sought on an imaging technique not widely accepted in the diagnosis of the disorder, the reader should consult the radiologic literature.

I thank Barbara McPartlin for typing this manuscript and Mishy Cass for designing the cover.

Table of Contents

Chapter 1

Congenital Anomalies of the Urinary Tract

Evan J. Kass, M.D.

The fetal kidney makes urine between the ninth and twelfth weeks of gestation. After the first trimester, this urine becomes the major constituent of amniotic fluid; therefore, a severe reduction or absence of this fluid (oligohydramnios) suggests the presence of an obstructive uropathy or significant renal abnormality.

It is important to remember that the functional abilities of the kidney in a fetus or a full-term newborn are quite different from those of even a 1-month-old infant. The glomerular filtration rate (GFR) increases dramatically: from 17 to 18 ml/min per 1.73 m^2 at term to 34–35 ml/min per 1.73 m^2 at 2 weeks but does not reach 100 ml/min per 1.73 m^2 until 1 year of age. In addition, a normal term newborn is unable to concentrate urine to more than 700 to 800 mOsm/kg of water, and in a preterm infant, the concentrating capacity is between 600 to 700 mOsm/kg of water.

Knowledge of these physiologic differences influences the selection of imaging modalities. For example, an intravenous urogram (IVU) demands active filtration, excretion, and concentration of a contrast agent and therefore would be expected to produce poorer images of the urinary system in a newborn because of reduced tubular function. For these same reasons, diuretic renography within the first few weeks of life may falsely imply obstruction because the GFR is relatively low and the ability of the kidney to respond to the diuretic challenge is severely reduced. Indeed, when all parameters of renal function increase during the first year of life, it is tempting to attribute this change to the treatment rendered when it may simply reflect a normal developmental process.

Clinical Indications for Imaging the Neonatal Kidney

Prenatal Detection of Fetal Urinary Abnormalities

The fetal kidneys can be imaged by ultrasound at 15 weeks' gestation, and corticomedullary differentiation can be identified at 20 weeks' gestation. By 14 weeks, urine is normally seen in the bladder. The most commonly diagnosed prenatal urinary tract abnormality is hydronephrosis (Fig. 1); unfortunately, the accuracy of ultrasound in determining the precise etiology of the dilated collecting system is only 70% to 80%. When "hydronephrosis" is diagnosed by ultrasound, the differential diagnosis should include ureteropelvic junction (UPJ) obstruction, multicystic dysplastic kidney (MCDK), enlargement of the collecting system secondary to reflux, prune-belly syndrome, primary megaureter, simple renal cysts, urethral valves, duplication of the collecting system with or without a ureterocele,

From *Imaging of Urologic Disorders* edited by Alexander S. Cass, MBBS, © 1992, Futura Publishing Inc., Mount Kisco, NY.

as well as "physiologic," nonobstructive distention of the urinary collecting system. In addition, various intestinal malformations have been mislabeled as prenatal hydronephrosis. In one series of fetuses with "hydronephrosis" whose mothers had normal amniotic fluid volumes, 38% were found to be completely normal postnatally.[1] Differentiation of hydronephrosis resulting from vesicoureteral reflux, obstruction, or physiologic causes is generally not possible prenatally. In addition, the distinction between a multicystic kidney and a kidney with a UPJ obstruction, although generally straightforward, may on occasion be difficult (Fig. 2). Because of this low specificity of prenatal diagnosis, as well as the inability of this modality to detect bilateral "correctable" lesions before 20 weeks, the enthusiasm for in utero surgery has waned.[2,3] Today, in utero surgery is still experimental and is generally limited to those fetuses with severe bilateral hydronephrosis and oligohydramnios.

The primary role of prenatal ultrasonography is the identification of potentially correctable congenital malformations so that prompt postnatal evaluation and treatment may be instituted. The standard postpartum imaging evaluation of the infant with prenatally identified hydronephrosis should include both a renal/bladder ultrasound scan and a voiding cystourethrogram (VCUG). If the initial postpartum examination is normal, it is important to repeat the ultrasound study 1 to 2 weeks after birth because fluid depletion in the first 24 hours may lead to an erroneous "normal" diagnosis (Fig. 3). If the repeat study is normal, one can reasonably conclude that no significant deformity is present.

Failure of Micturition

The most common causes of the failure of micturition are prerenal, that is hemorrhage, shock, or dehydration. The majority of these infants who appear healthy and have a normal physical examination are simply dehydrated and will ultimately void. However, it is important to exclude significant urologic abnormalities whenever an infant has not urinated during the first 12 hours of life. The first study in this setting should be a renal/bladder ultrasound scan. The child should not be catheterized prior to this study because there is a high incidence of normal urine formation with merely a lack of micturition. If urine is present in the bladder, it can be identified atraumatically by ultrasound, and the distended bladder can also serve as an acoustic window for the imaging of surrounding structures. When it is necessary for the bladder to be catheterized, it can be performed just prior to a VCUG.

The renal causes for failure of micturition include congenital anomalies of the kidneys such as polycystic or dysplastic kidneys (Fig. 4), ischemia, and Tamm-Horsfall proteinuria (Fig. 5). It is extremely unusual for postrenal causes such as a posterior urethral valve to result in a failure of the neonate to void unless there is severe renal dysplasia associated with pulmonary hypoplasia and respiratory failure.

The newborn infant with abnormally large cystic or obstructed kidneys may present with oliguria or anuria but more often presents with a mass (Fig. 6). The sonographic appearance of the most common nonobstructive causes of renal failure are as follows. A normal echo pattern may be seen in prerenal azotemia, renal artery thrombosis, or mild renal ischemia. Increased cortical echogenicity with corticomedullary differentiation preserved suggests prerenal azotemia, moderate to severe ischemia, or mild to moderate dysplasia. Loss of corticomedullary differentiation with or without renal enlargement may represent renal vein thrombosis, recessive polycystic renal disease, or cystic renal dysplasia. Increased medullary echogenicity may evidence Tamm-Horsfall proteinuria.

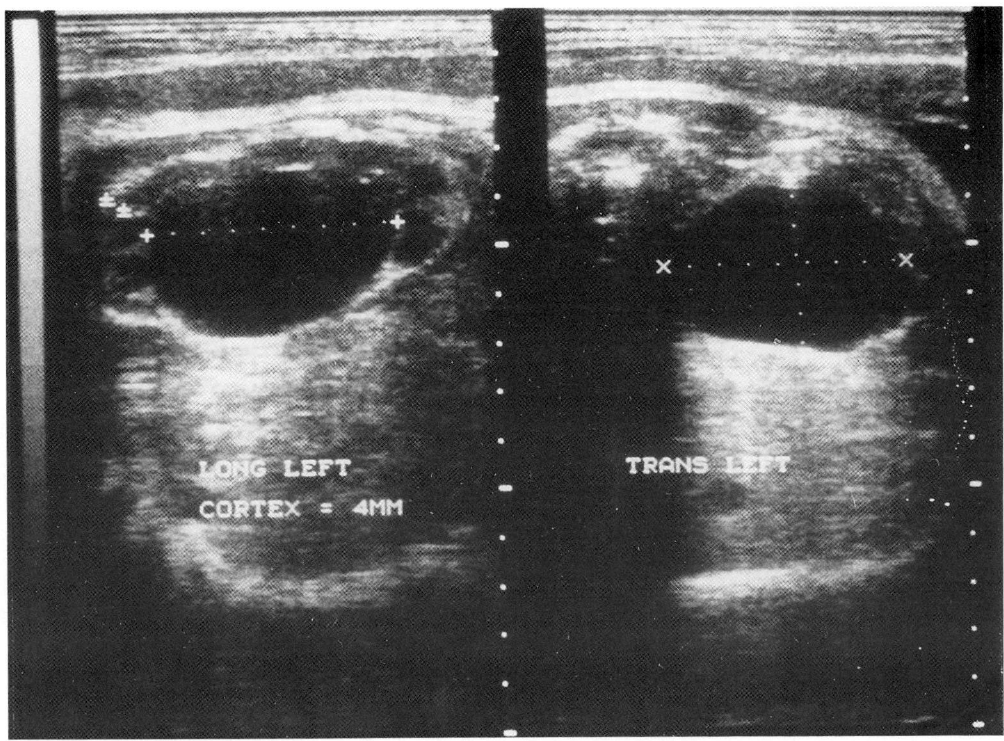

Figure 1.   Prenatal ultrasound scan, (left) demonstrates hydronephrosis suggestive of ureteropelvic junction (UPJ) obstruction. Postnatal evaluation, (right) confirmed such obstruction.

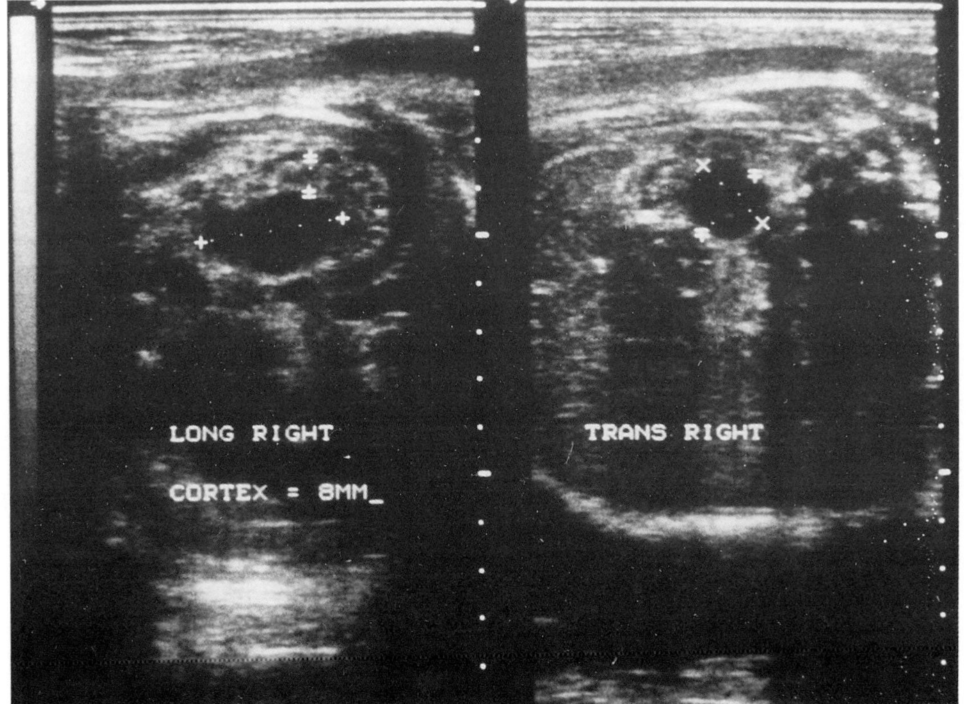

Figure 2.   This prenatal ultrasound scan, (left) is also suggestive of UPJ obstruction. However, postnatal evaluation, (right) demonstrated multicystic dysplastic kidney.

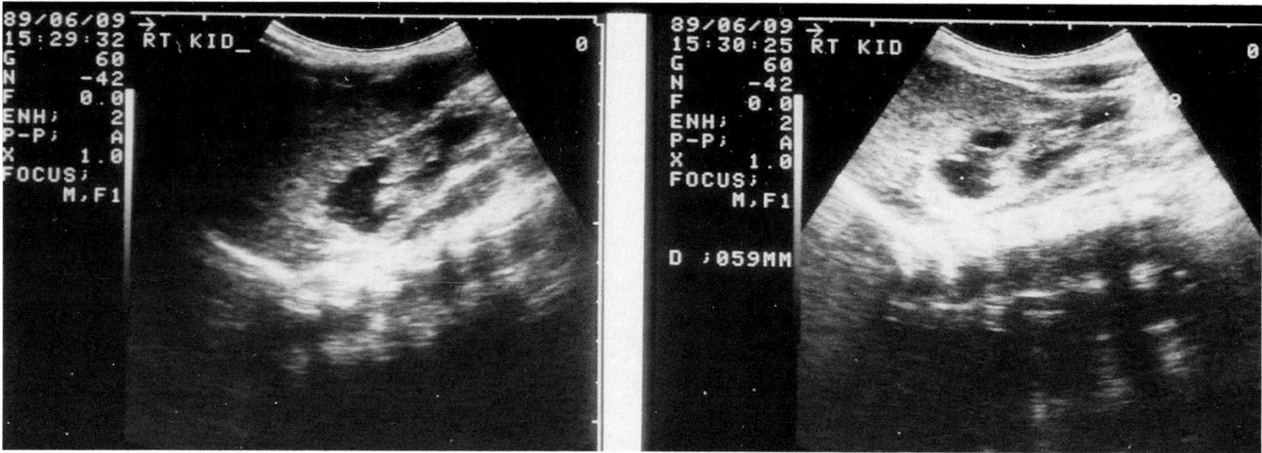

Figure 3A.   This newborn male infant had hydronephrosis detected prenatally. Postnatal ultrasound scans performed on the first day demonstrate only mild dilatation of collecting system.

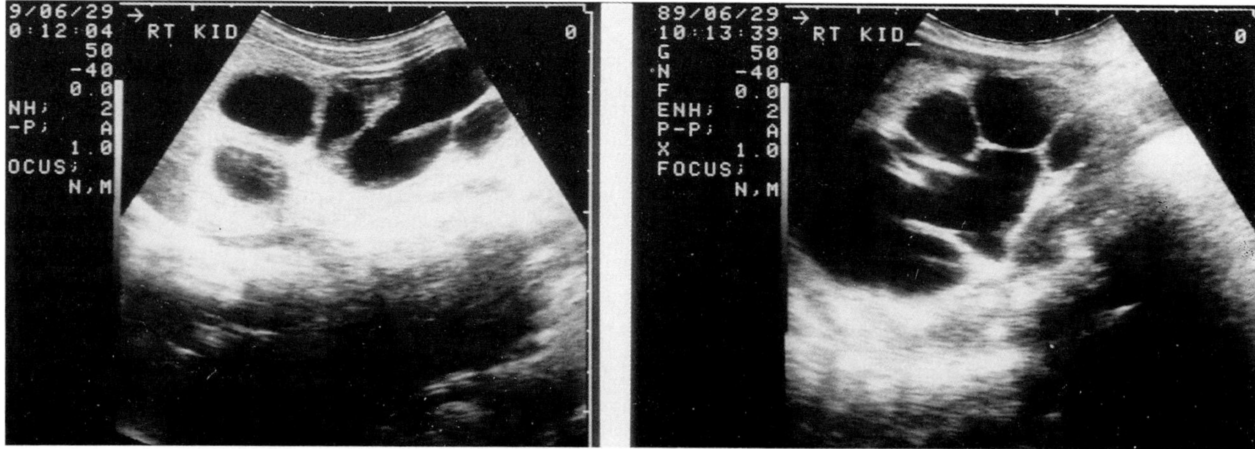

Figure 3B.   Repeat scan 3 weeks later demonstrates substantial dilatation of the collecting system consistent with UPJ obstruction. This case illustrates the importance of repeating the ultrasound scan whenever a scan during the first few days of postnatal life demonstrates minimal or no hydronephrosis.

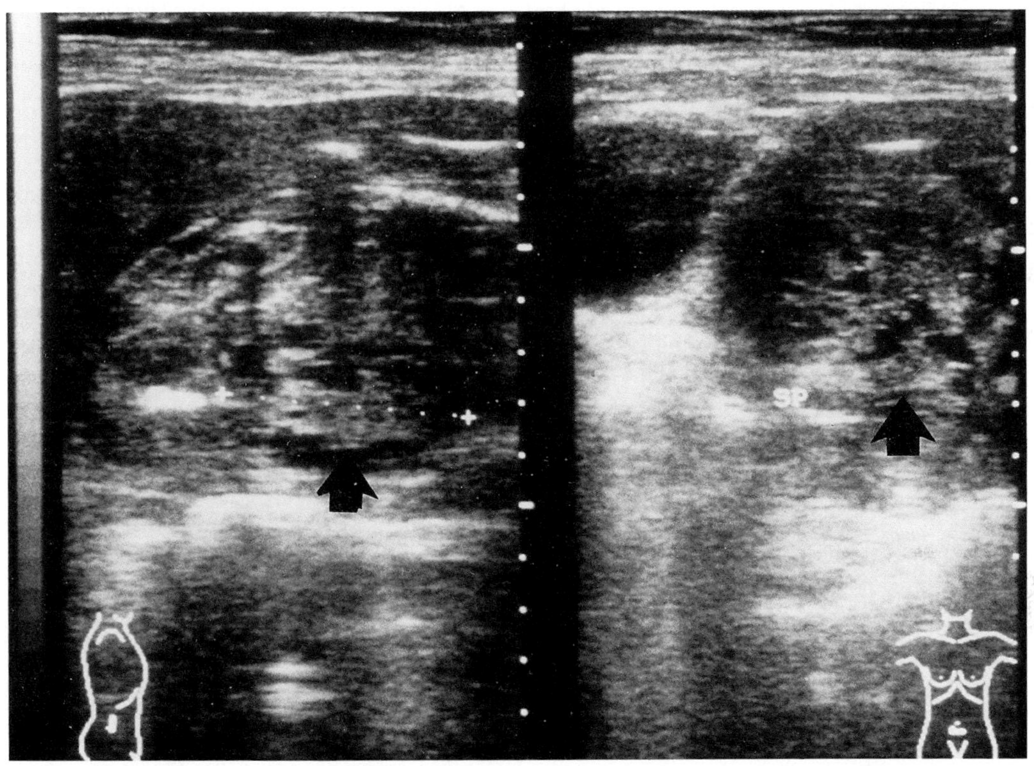

Figure 4. Prenatal ultrasound scan demonstrates bilateral renal cystic dysplasia (arrows). There was no amniotic fluid, and no urine was seen within urinary bladder. Child did not void after birth and rapidly succumbed to respiratory insufficiency.

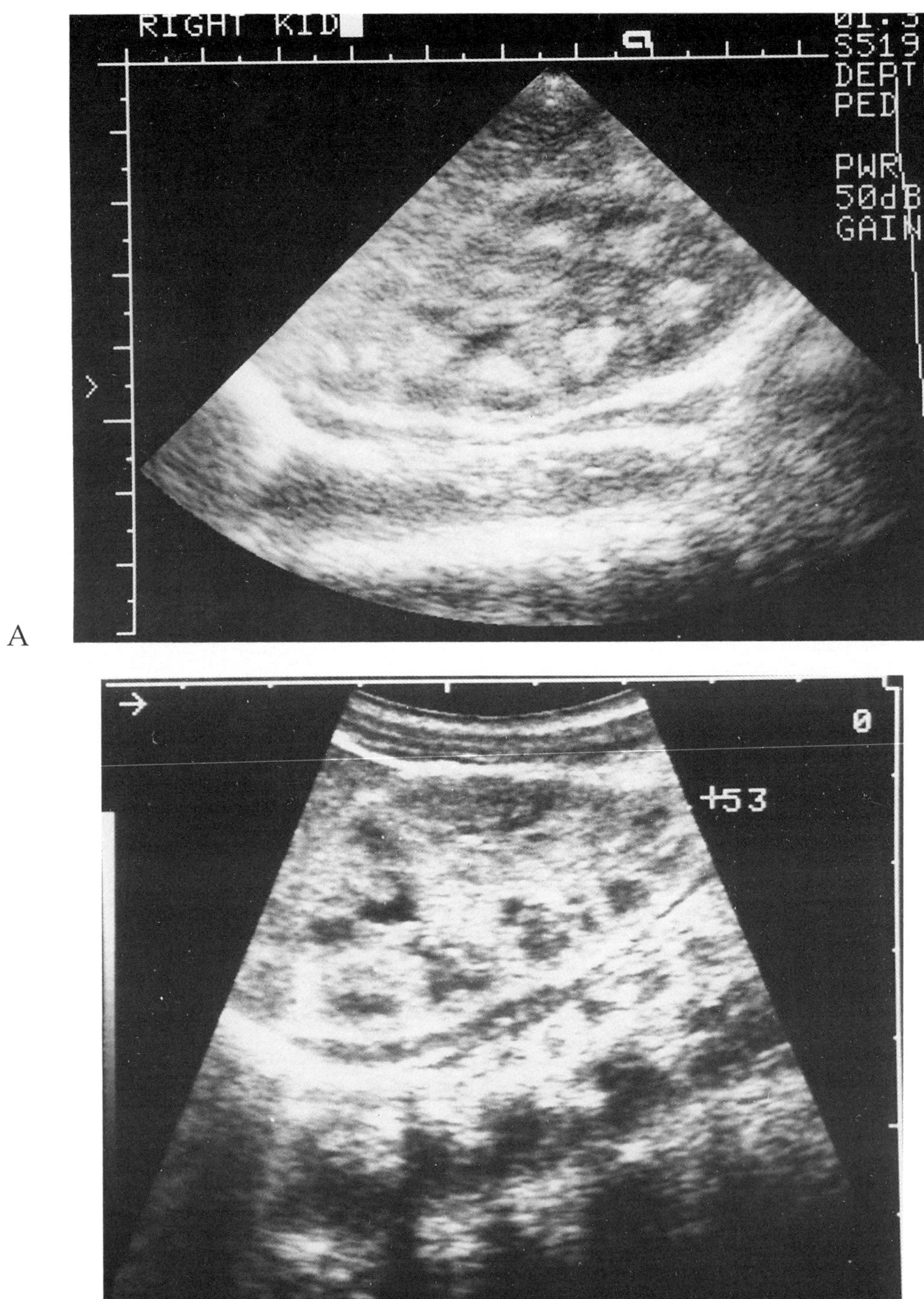

Figure 5.   This child did not void for 24 hours after birth. Serum creatinine concentration was 1.9 mg/dl. (A, top) Urgent renal ultrasound scan demonstrates that renal pyramids have markedly increased echogenicity consistent with the diagnosis of Tamm-Horsfall protein deposition. The child was treated conservatively and over the next week urine output gradually increased, and serum creatinine declined to 0.4 mg/dl. (B, bottom) Repeat ultrasound scan demonstrated hypoechoic renal pyramids, as is normal in the newborn.

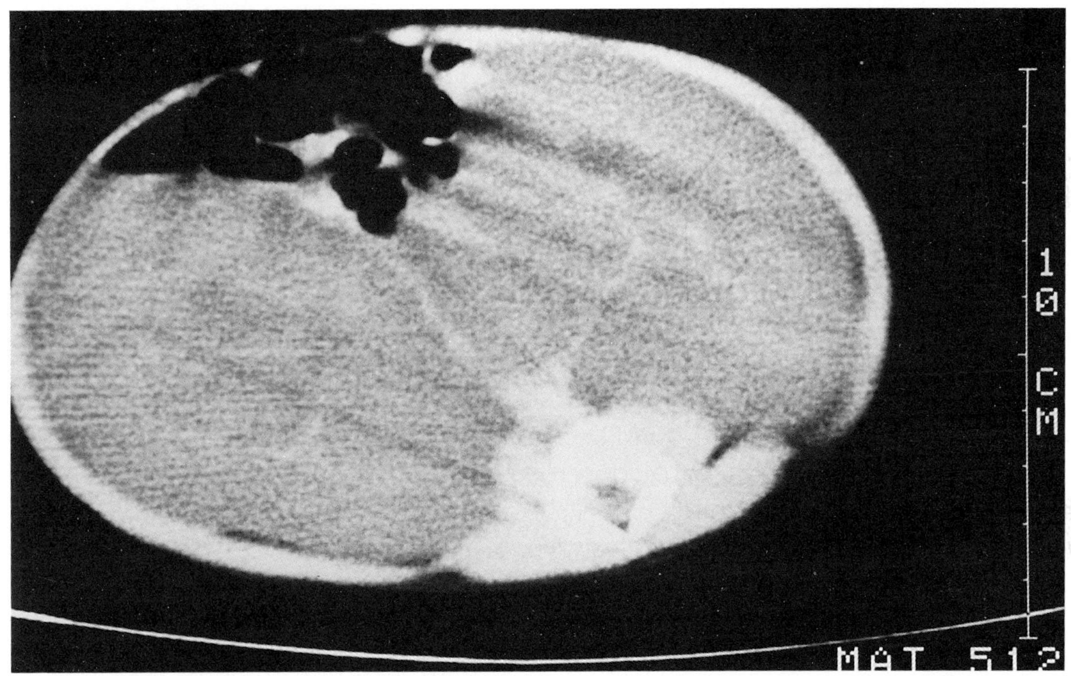

Figure 6.   This newborn presented with bilaterally palpable abdominal masses. He voided normally at birth. Transverse CT scan after administration of intravenous contrast shows massively enlarged kidneys consistent with diagnosis of recessive polycystic kidney disease.

Differential Diagnosis of Neonatal "Hydronephrosis"

The causes of true hydronephrosis are listed in Table 1.

Hydronephrotic Renal Enlargement

Hydronephrosis with or without ureteral dilatation is the most common cause of neonatal renal enlargement. All children with prenatally identified hydronephrosis should have a VCUG to exclude vesicoureteral reflux, which is a common etiology for ureterectasis and pyelectasis (Fig. 7). In addition, these children should have a baseline renal scan, serum creatinine determination, and urine culture. Continuous low-dose antimicrobial prophylaxis should be started, and the children followed as per the standard reflux protocol.

The most common site of obstruction of the urinary tract is the UPJ. This obstruction is congenital and may be secondary to an intrinsic ureteral abnormality such as an aperistaltic segment or intrinsic luminal narrowing; less commonly, it is the result of an extrinsic mechanical compression from bands and aberrant vessels. Today, most newborns with a UPJ obstruction have been identified prenatally, and only a few present with either an asymptomatic abdominal mass or urinary tract infection. However, not all

of these infants with hydronephrosis have a functionally significant obstruction requiring surgical correction. Indeed, a significant proportion have a nonobstructive enlargement of their collecting system that will not progress and may actually improve spontaneously. Unfortunately, the magnitude of the hydronephrosis is not always a reliable guide to therapy (Fig. 8). Therefore, it is essential for all of these individuals to be evaluated in order to determine the presence or absence of mechanical obstruction as well as the degree of functional derangement.

The study most frequently utilized for this purpose is diuretic renography (see discussion in Chapter 6). This test usually is deferred until the child is 1 month old and capable of responding to diuretic stimulation. A radiopharmaceutical (either Tc-99m DTPA or MAG3) is administered intravenously, and when the renal collecting system is maximally filled with the tracer, a diuretic (furosemide) is administered. The relative accumulation of the tracer in each kidney within the first few minutes after injection can be utilized to measure individual renal function, and the clearance half-time ($T\frac{1}{2}$) of the isotope after administration of the diuretic is a measure of whether an obstruction is present.[4] Those children without evidence of obstruction are followed closely with a combination of ultrasound and renal scintigraphy for as long as the hydronephrosis persists. Excretory urography is not a routine part of the evaluation because ultrasonography typically provides equivalent structural renal imaging and nuclear scintigraphy provides superior functional information.

Retrograde pyelography is only occasionally performed in the newborn because of the technical problems involved (particularly in the male), and because it is unusual to find significant abnormalities (Fig. 9). In the rare instance when significant ureteral problems are encountered intraoperatively, antegrade pyelography can be performed.

Table 1. Causes of Hydronephrosis in the Newborn

Pelvicaliceal dilatation—normal ureter
    Ureteropelvic junction obstruction
    Nonobstructive dilatation
    Vesicoureteral reflux
    Duplex collecting system
Pelvicaliceal dilatation—dilated ureter
    Primary obstructed megaureter with or without reflux
    Primary nonobstructed megaureter with or without reflux
    Ectopic ureter
        With duplicated renal moiety with or without ureterocele
        Single renal moiety
    Secondary hydronephrosis
        Posterior urethral valves
        Neurovesical dysfunction
        Prune belly syndrome
        Extrinsic bladder compression

Hydronephrotic Renal Involvement with Megaureter

In all children discovered to have a dilated ureter, the specific etiology of this abnormality is established by a combination of ultrasonography, VCUG, and renal scintigraphy, as previously described for children with hydronephrosis (Fig. 10). Primary nonrefluxing obstructed megaureter may be the result of a distal ureteral narrowing, an adynamic distal ureteral segment, or an ectopically inserted ureter. In the usual circumstance, the terminal 3 to 4 cm of the ureter is abnormal, but the muscular fibers proximal to the obstructive segment are normal. This entity occurs more commonly on the left side, is bilateral in 20% of cases, and is associated with a 10% incidence of contralateral renal agenesis. Excretory urography is not routine but occasionally helps to define the anatomy (Fig. 11).

Nonobstructive ureteral dilatation occurs more frequently than previously appreciated, and in all likelihood, this high incidence is a direct result of the almost routine use of prenatal ultrasound. Many of these dilated ureters normalize or improve with time and cause no symptoms. When the diuretic renal scan demonstrates prompt drainage of the dilated collecting system, no surgery is performed, and the children are followed with a combination of ultrasound examinations and renal scintigraphy. Surgery is performed when there is documented evidence of obstruction on the diuretic renal scan, increasing hydronephrosis, or decreasing renal function.

Ectopic insertion of a ureter occurs most commonly in association with a duplex collecting system with or without a ureterocele, and, as with the majority of renal malformations today, is most commonly identified during a prenatal sonogram. The postnatal sonogram (Fig. 12) is the preferred initial imaging study for defining the anatomy of a duplicated collecting system associated with hydronephrosis, the presence of the ureterocele, and the segments involved. A VCUG and a functional renal scan are performed routinely to identify reflux and evaluate the function in both the abnormal and the normal renal segments. Typically, it is the upper-pole moiety that is ectopically positioned, obstructed, or associated with the ureterocele. The lower-pole moiety of the duplex system is usually the one demonstrating reflux (Fig. 13), although hydronephrosis in the lower pole of the duplex kidney without reflux suggests a UPJ obstruction involving the lower-pole segment.

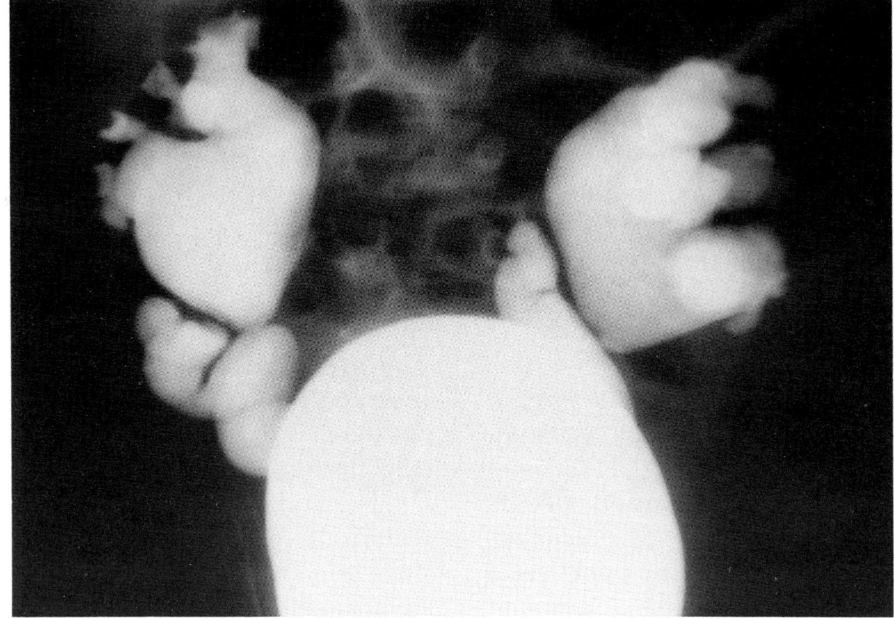

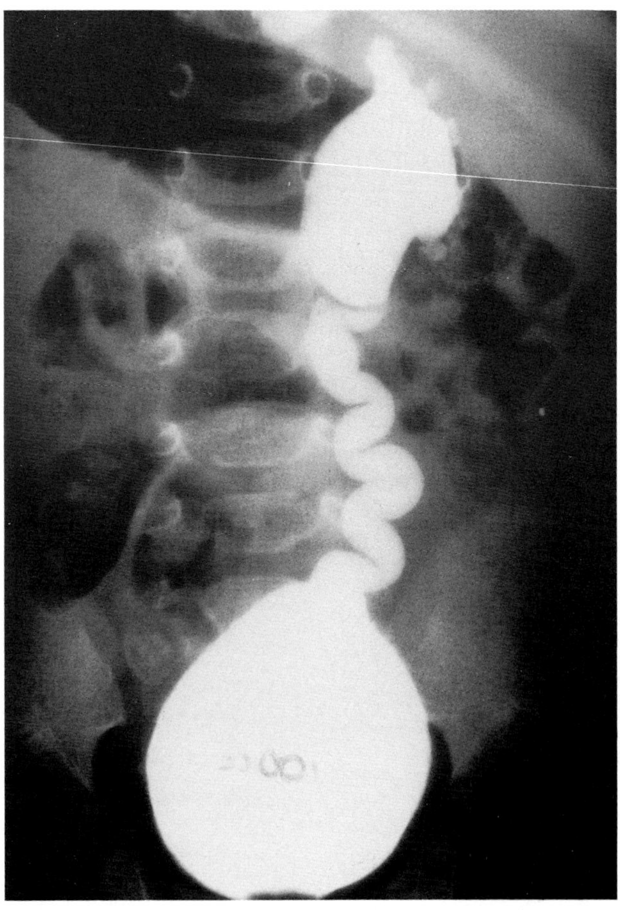

Figure 7. Each of these children had hydronephrosis detected prenatally. Postnatal ultrasound scans confirmed the presence of bilateral (A, top) or unilateral (B, bottom) hydronephrosis. The VCUGs in both children demonstrate that hydronephrosis is secondary to vesicoureteral reflux.

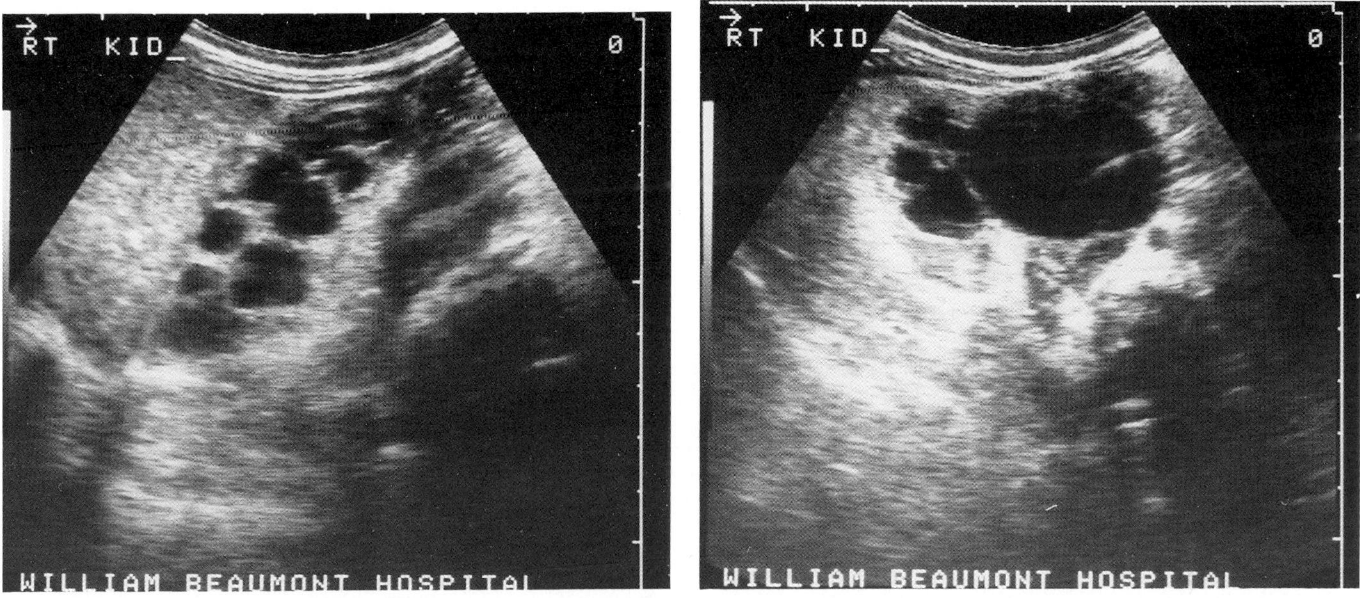

Figure 8A.   This newborn male had a possible right UPJ obstruction identified prenatally. His postnatal ultrasound scan confirmed findings, and his diuretic renal scan demonstrated UPJ obstruction.

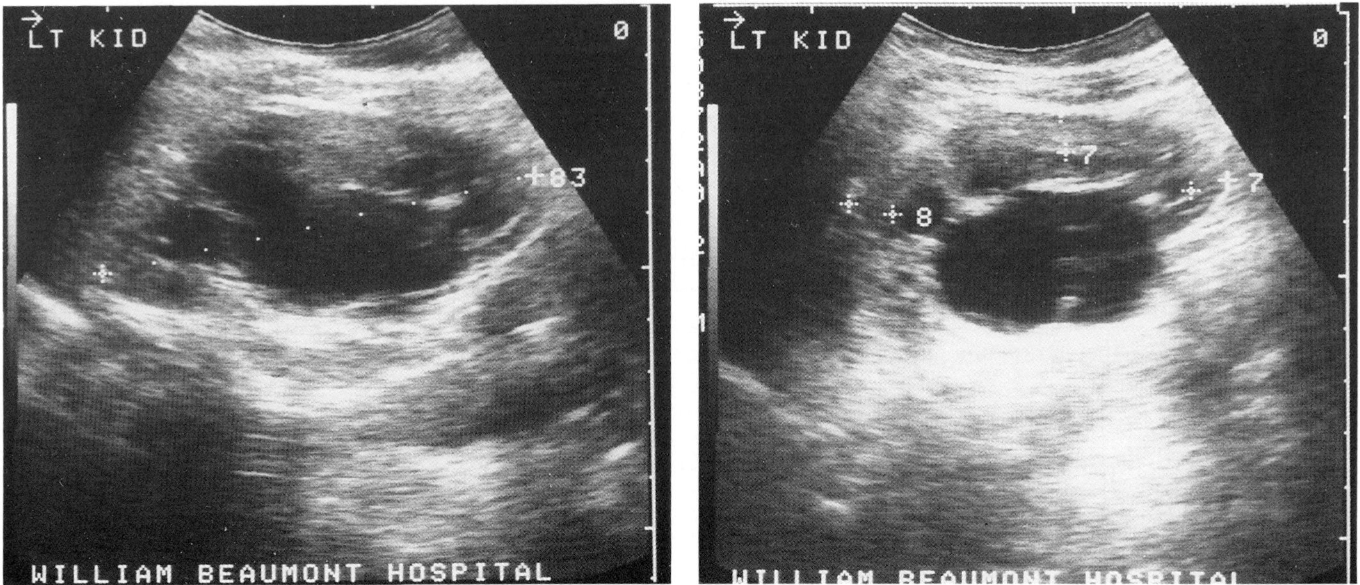

Figure 8B.   This child had a similar degree of hydronephrosis, yet diuretic renal scan does not demonstrate obstruction. She is being followed nonoperatively and remains asymptomatic with normal function in the hydronephrotic kidney.

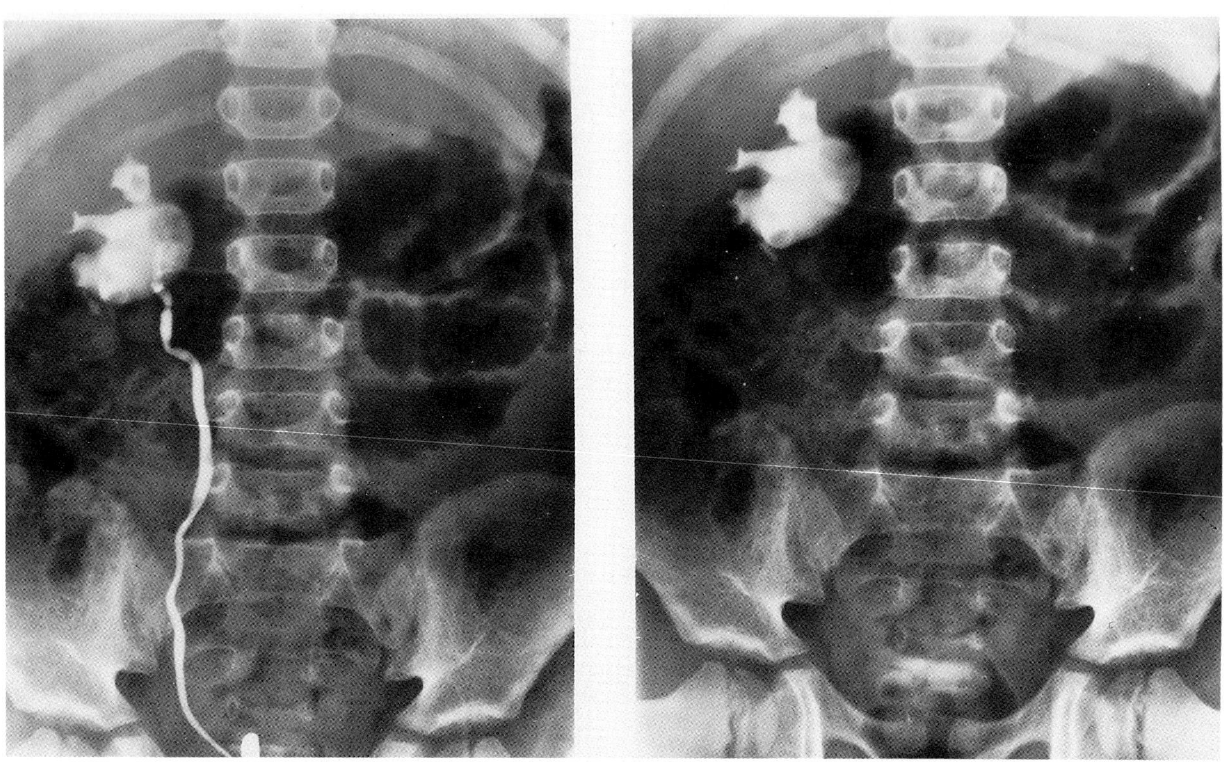

Figure 9.   This female infant had possible UPJ obstruction detected prenatally. Postnatal ultrasound scan confirmed the findings but did not demonstrate a dilated ureter. The VCUG was normal, and diuresis renogram confirmed UPJ obstruction. This retrograde pyelogram, performed just prior to surgery under the same anesthesia, demonstrates normal-caliber ureter. In this setting, retrograde study will rarely provide significant information.

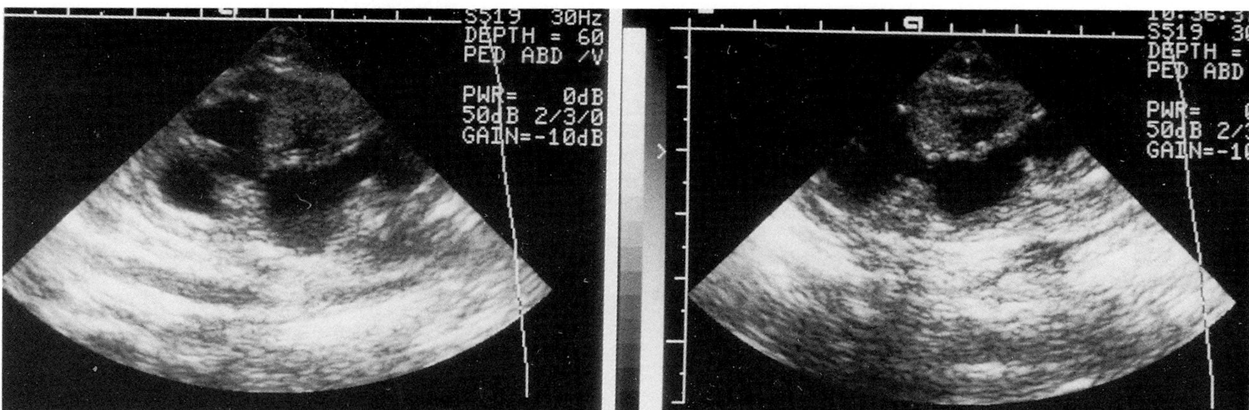

Figure 10A.   Evaluation of megaureter. This postnatal ultrasound scan demonstrates moderate bilateral hydronephrosis with good rim of overlying renal parenchyma.

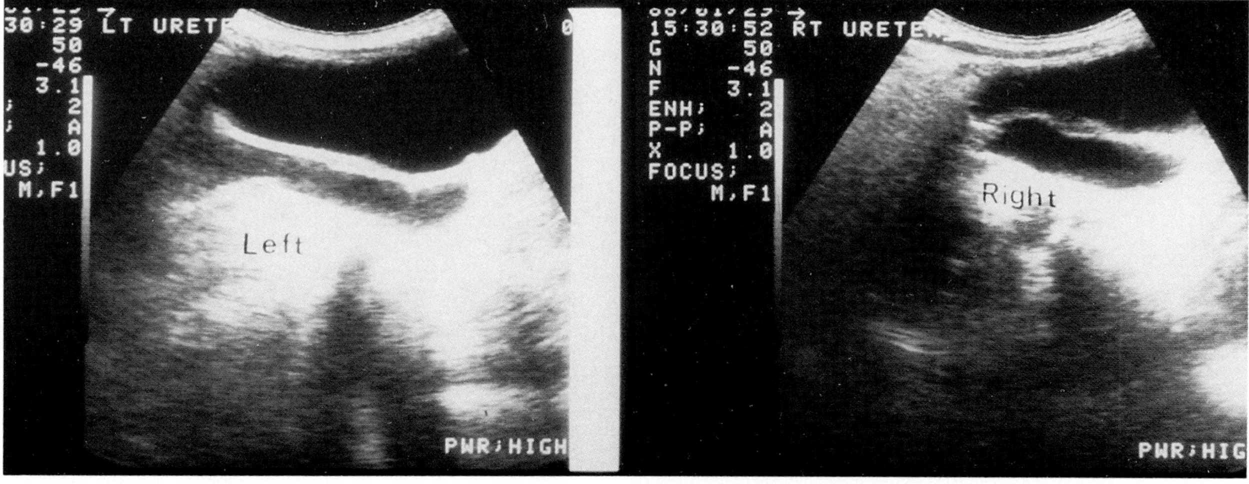

Figure 10B.   Dilated ureters are seen posterior to the bladder suggesting bilateral ureterovesical junction (UVJ) obstruction. The VCUG did not demonstrate vesicoureteral reflux or a urethral valve.

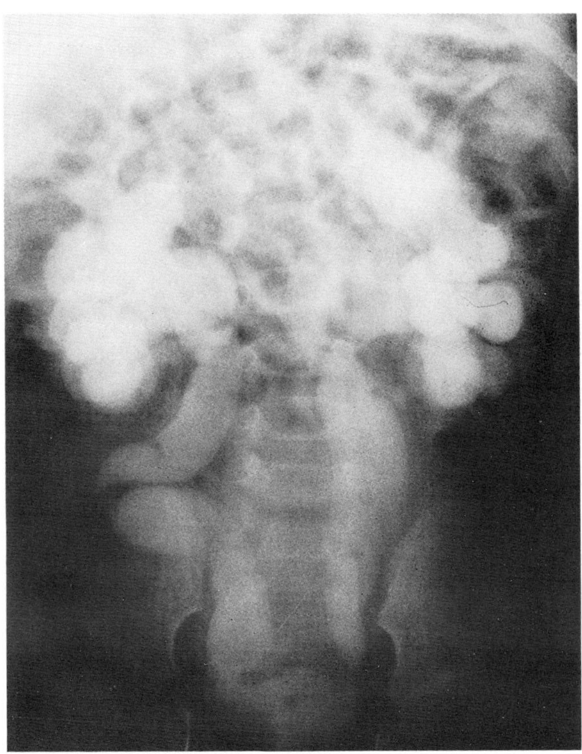

Figure 11.   Patient described in Figure 10 had this IVU. It again suggests bilateral UVJ obstructions, but whether it provides significant additional information that was not obvious on ultrasound scan is questionable.

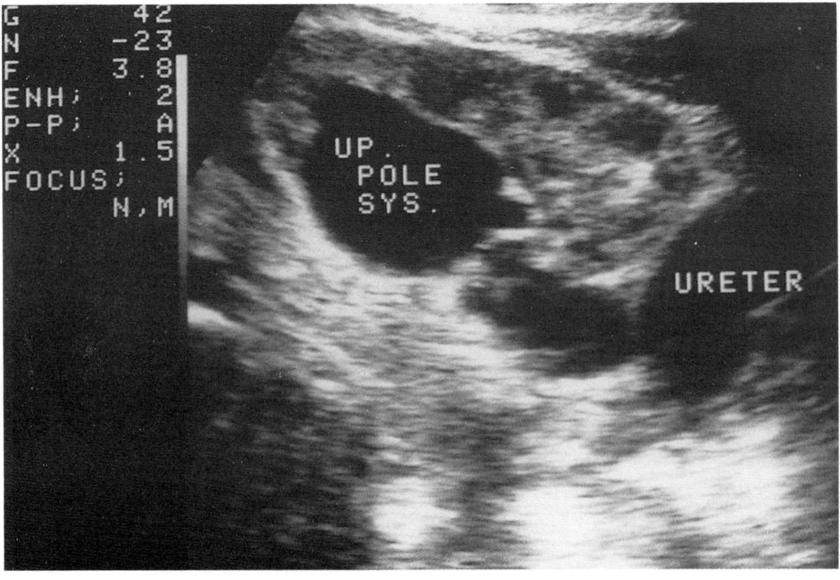

Figure 12.   This newborn had hydronephrosis detected prenatally. Postnatal ultrasound scan clearly demonstrates duplex kidney with hydronephrotic upper-pole segment and normal lower-pole segment. There is a markedly dilated ureter associated with upper-pole segment. No ureterocele was identified. The VCUG was normal. A Tc-99m DMSA scan showed no significant function in the upper-pole segment, and upper-pole nephroureterectomy was performed.

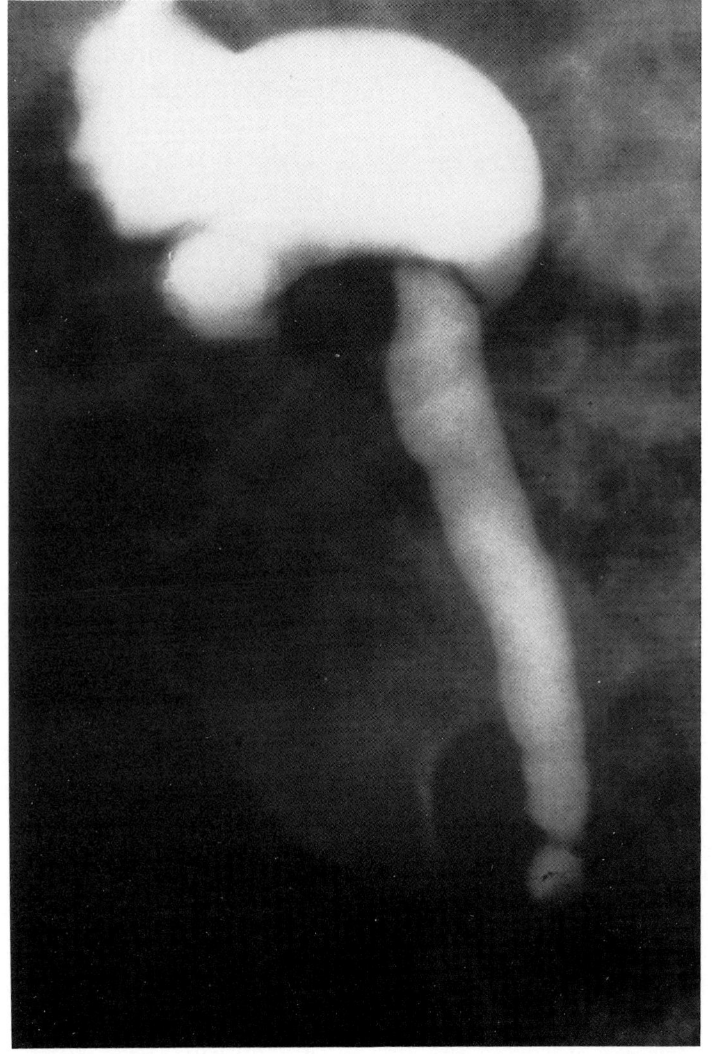

Figure 13. This child had hydronephrosis detected prenatally and confirmed postnatally. The VCUG demonstrates reflux into the lower pole of the duplex collecting system as etiology of hydronephrosis.

Secondary Hydronephrosis

Urethral Valves

The most common form of congenital urethral obstruction in the male is the posterior urethral valve. Three types of valves have been described.

Type 1 (most common) consists of thickened folds extending distally from the verumontanum and fusing anteriorly.

Type 2 (rare) consists of folds extending cranially from the verumontanum to the bladder neck.

Type 3 valves are diaphragms or membranes located below the verumontanum.

Seventy-five percent of children with posterior urethral valves present within the first year of life, and 50% present in the first 3 months. An increasing number of these cases are being diagnosed prenatally and present as an apparently healthy male neonate with bilateral hydroureteronephrosis. Occasionally, the increased pressure from the obstruction produces a rupture of a caliceal fornix (point of least resistance), with resulting extravasation of urine into the perirenal space, peritoneal cavity (Fig. 14), or even the pleural space (urothorax). The most common presenting symptom in the neonate or infant is urinary tract infection or failure to thrive. Only rarely is there evidence of impaired voiding. The physical examination may demonstrate an abdominal mass (hydronephrosis or distended bladder) or, rarely, ascites. In the more severe cases, renal failure may be present.

Imaging of these infants begins with ultrasound examination, which usually demonstrates bilateral hydroureteronephrosis and a thick-walled bladder. Occasionally, a dilated posterior urethra is seen. However, the VCUG is the study that establishes the diagnosis (Fig. 15). The most important findings are a dilated posterior urethra, marked discrepancy in size between the normal anterior and the dilated posterior urethra, and visualization of the valve. One should also note the presence or absence of reflux, and the size and configuration of the bladder.

Anterior urethral valves are discovered in a similar fashion but are much rarer. Again, it is the VCUG that establishes the diagnosis (Fig. 16).

The evaluation of global renal function is based on the creatinine level (which reflects the mother's renal function for the first few days after birth). Differential renal function is monitored by renal scintigraphy.

Neurovesical Dysfunction

The majority of children with congenital neurovesical dysfunction resulting from one of the variants of spinal dysraphism have normal upper urinary tracts at birth. It is only with the passage of time that hydronephrosis, vesicoureteral reflux, and incomplete bladder emptying develop. Neonatal hydronephrosis is rarely the result of neurovesical dysfunction but must be considered as part of the differential diagnosis, particularly when deformities of the lumbosacral spinal cord are present. A VCUG should be part of the routine evaluation.

Prune-belly Syndrome

The prune-belly syndrome is characterized by the congenital absence or deficiency of the abdominal wall musculature, bilateral hydroureteronephrosis with some degree of renal dysplasia (Fig. 17), a large bladder, various degrees of vesicoureteral reflux (Fig. 18), a dilated prostatic urethra (Fig. 19), and bilateral cryptorchidism. The degree of abdominal muscular deficiency and the level of renal impairment are highly variable and are not correlated. Ultimately, it is the degree of renal dysplasia and the level of renal function that determine the long-term prognosis for these children. Despite the apparent magnitude of the upper tract dilatation, obstruction does not play a major role here; one should be very cautious when attempting to diagnose obstruction in these children.

Extrinsic Bladder Compression

Extrinsic compression of the bladder can result in bilateral hydronephrosis and may be the result of a pelvic tumor, such as neuroblastoma, teratoma, or other neoplasm. However, most commonly, it is the result of hydrometrocolpos.

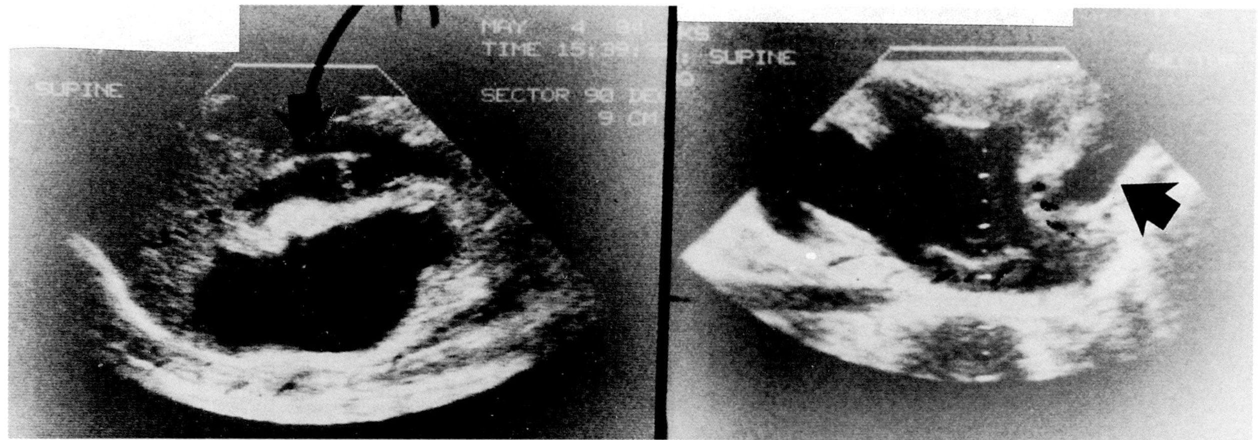

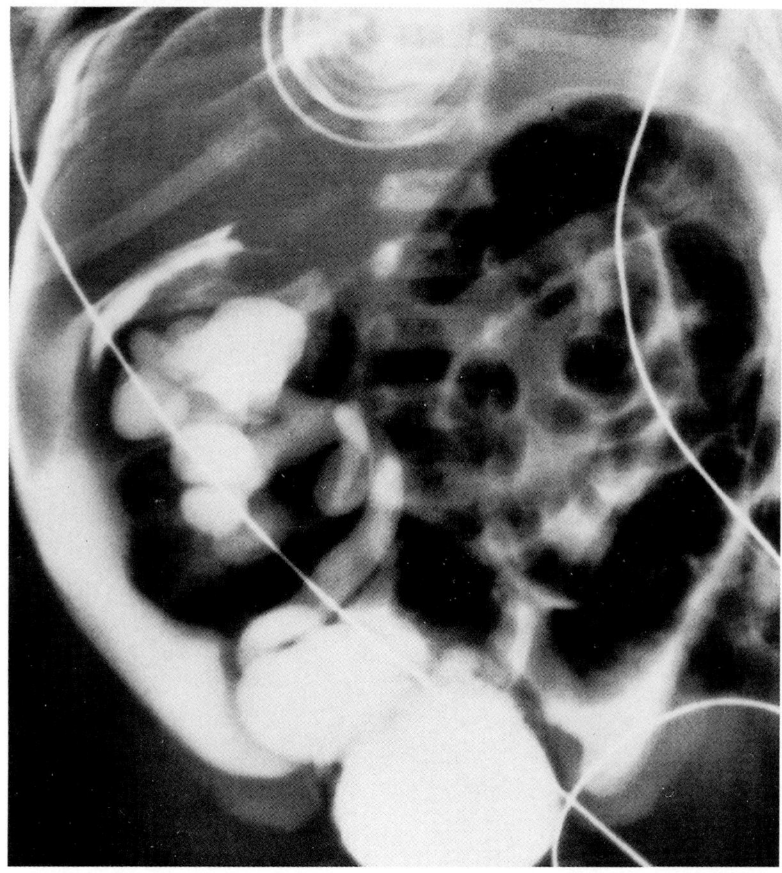

Figure 14.   This male newborn presented with ascites. (A, top) Renal ultrasound scan demonstrates bilateral hydronephrosis. One can see accumulation of urine outside the urinary collecting system (arrow) consistent with diagnosis of urinary ascites. (B, bottom) The VCUG demonstrates right-sided vesicoureteral reflux with urinary extravasation. Child had posterior urethral valve.

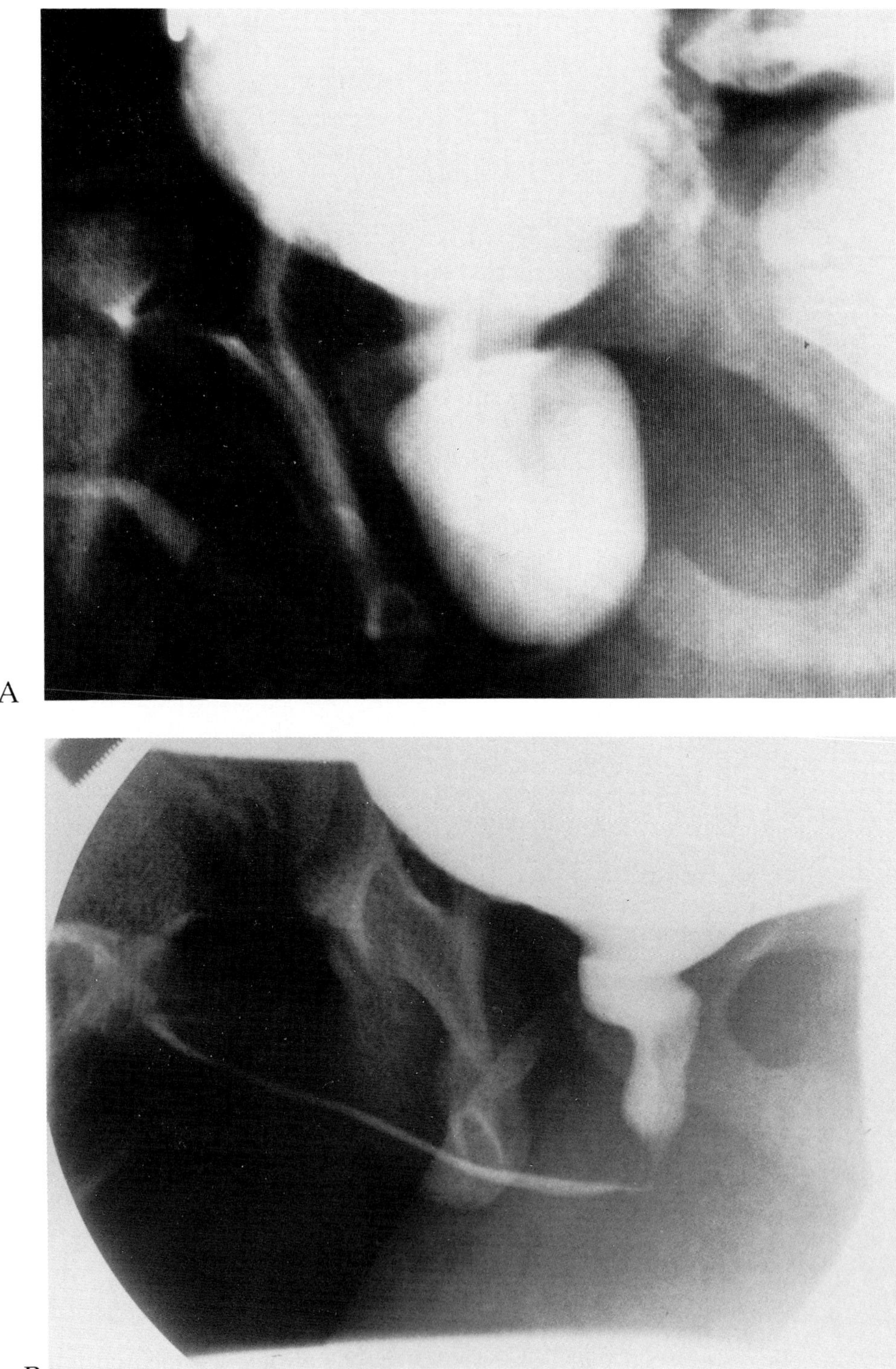

Figure 15. Voiding cystourethrograms in two infants with posterior urethral valves demonstrate enlargement of prostatic urethra and relative narrowing of the bladder neck (A, top) and (B, bottom). Note that the caliber of urethra distal to valve is markedly diminished.

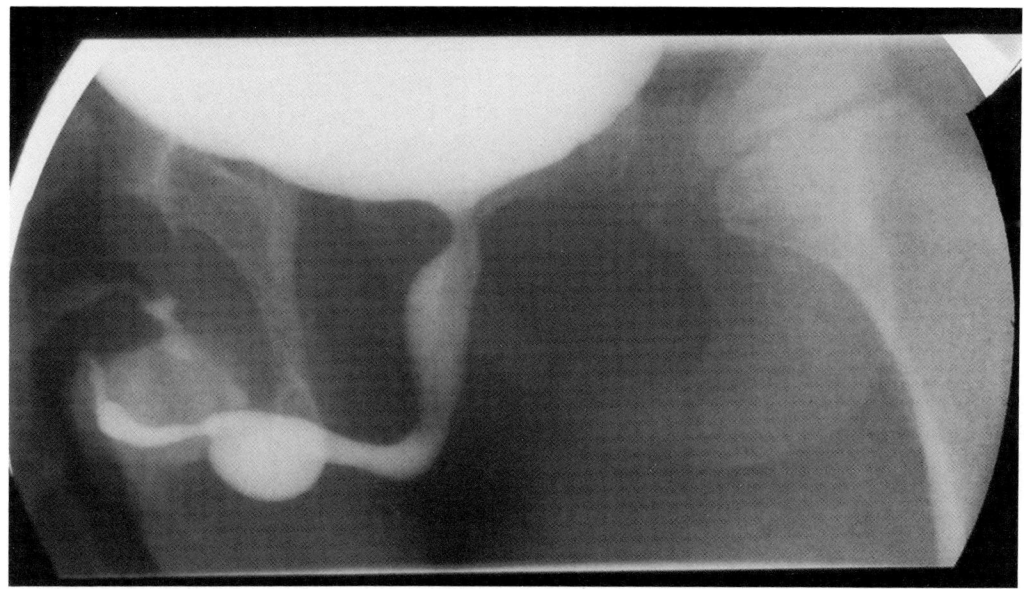

Figure 16.   Voiding cystourethrogram demonstrates anterior urethral valve, which was discovered during evaluation for prenatally detected hydronephrosis. The child was clinically well.

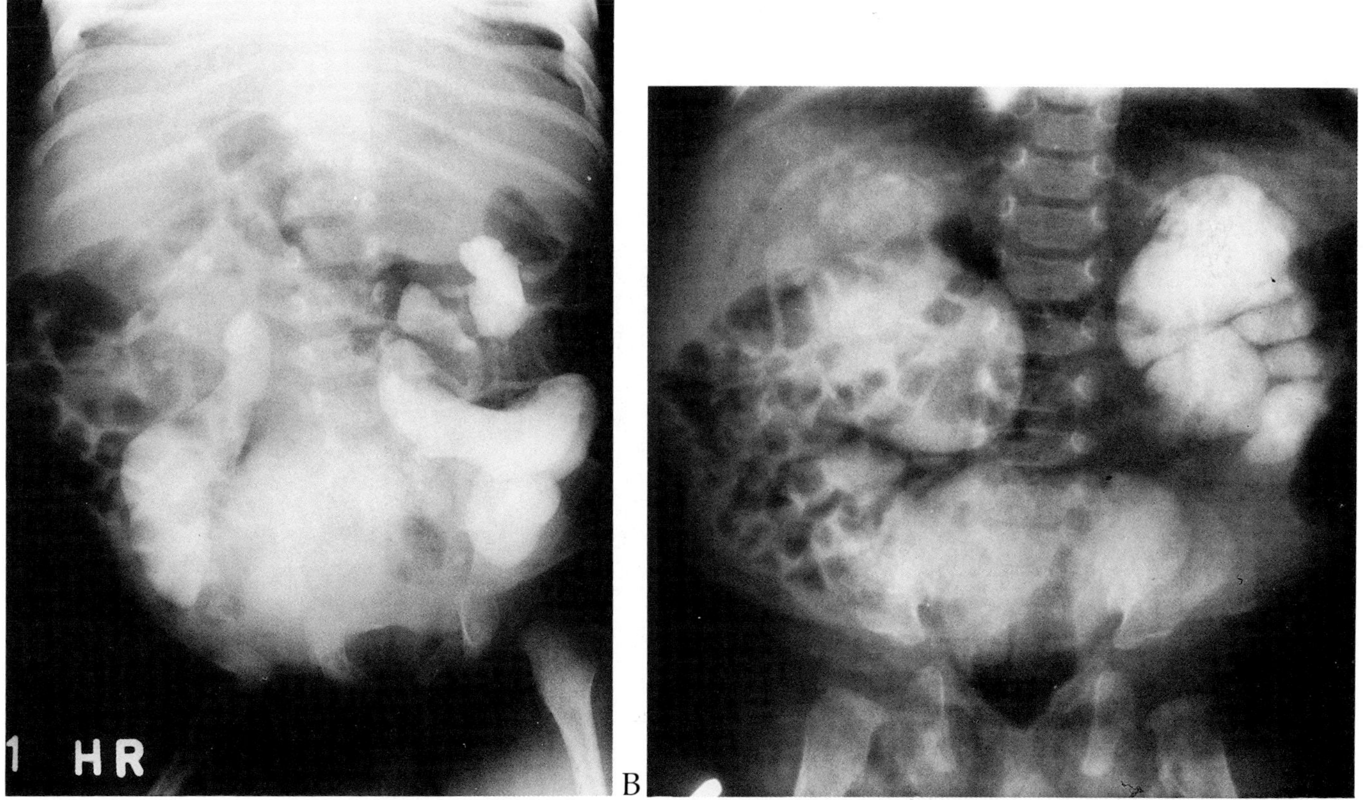

Figure 17.   These IVUs (A, left and B, right) demonstrate bilateral hydroureteronephrosis and ureteral tortuosity often observed in children with prune-belly syndrome.

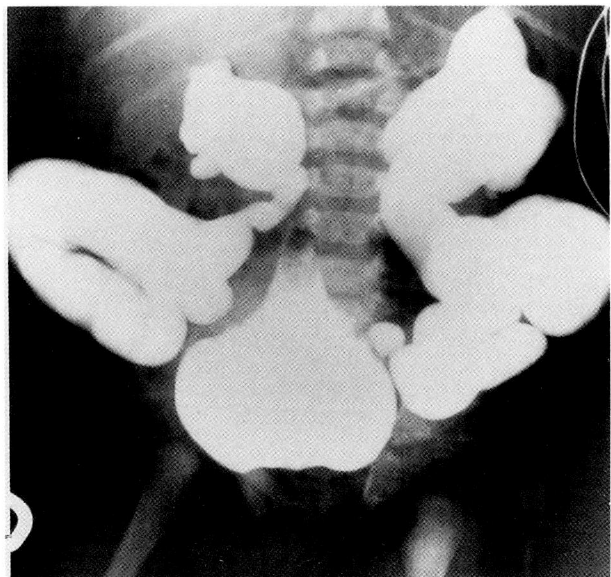

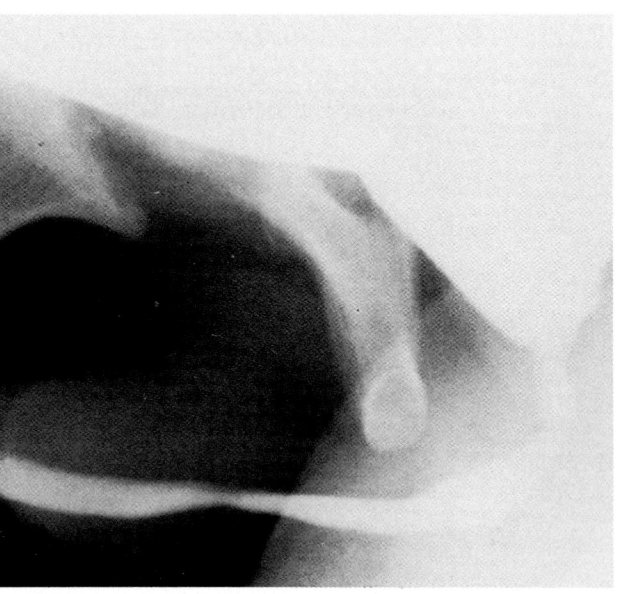

Figure 18. This newborn has bilateral hydronephrosis that was identified prenatally and confirmed postnatally. Physical examination demonstrated typical wrinkled abdomen of prune-belly syndrome. This VCUG demonstrates massive bilateral vesicoureteral reflux with tortuous ureters that is quite characteristic of the syndrome.

Figure 19. Dilated prostatic urethra often is demonstrated on VCUG in children with prune-belly syndrome. This dilatation should not be confused with that seen in children with a posterior urethral valve.

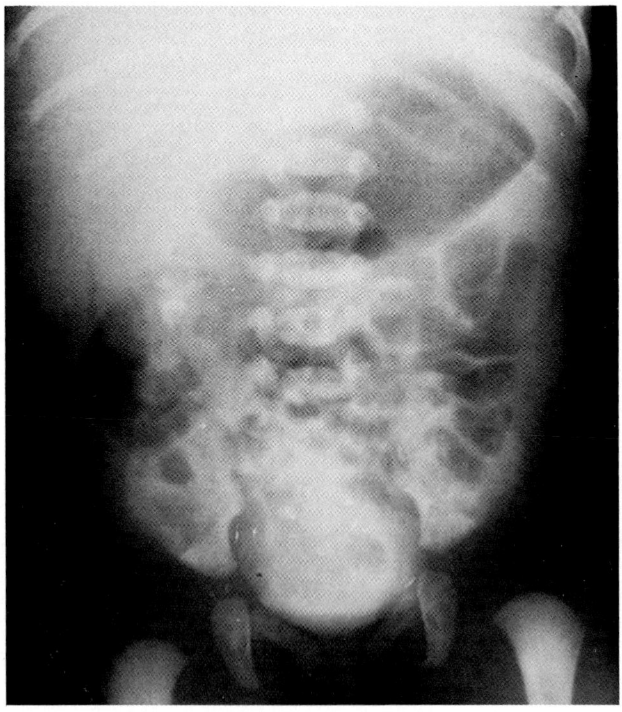

Figure 20. This newborn infant had gross hematuria. The IVU demonstrated a normal right kidney and nonvisualization of the left kidney. Ultrasound scanning demonstrated a left kidney, but there was no function on the renal scan. These findings are diagnostic of renal vein thrombosis.

Maternal hormonal stimulation produces secretions from the genital tract, which, if prevented from draining by an imperforate hymen (most commonly), vaginal stenosis or atresia, or a cloacal anomaly, may cause distention of the vagina (hydrocolpos) and the uterus (hydrometrocolpos).

Nonhydronephrotic Nephromegaly

Enlargement of the kidneys without hydronephrosis may be the result of renal vein thrombosis, tumor (fetal renal hamartoma, Wilms' tumor), cystic kidney disease (recessive, dominant, MCDK, simple renal cysts), or adrenal hemorrhage.

Renal vein thrombosis may be caused by dehydration, decreased renal perfusion and oxygenation, and the high hematocrit of the newborn. This entity is more prevalent in infants of diabetic mothers. The infant typically presents with gross hematuria and a palpable flank mass. If the problem is unilateral, renal function may not be abnormal. A variable degree of proteinuria is present. The diagnosis is suggested in this clinical setting when the ultrasound examination demonstrates an enlarged kidney(s) with various areas of increased and decreased echogenicity. Recently, color Doppler ultrasound has proved useful in evaluating perfusion of the kidney and blood flow within the renal vein and artery. The IVU typically demonstrates unilateral nonvisualization (Fig. 20). A renal scan will demonstrate diminished function. Nonfunction suggests total vascular occlusion.

Solid tumors in the neonate are rare lesions. The most frequent are fetal renal hamartomas. The child presents with a unilateral solid renal mass; rarely, there may be hematuria or hypertension. The imaging studies reveal a solid tumor with various degrees of renal displacement and distortion. In the great majority, there is no calcification. The differential diagnosis should include clear-cell sarcoma, rhabdoid tumor, Wilms' tumor, neuroblastoma, and lymphangioma (Fig. 21).

Renal cystic disease can be of several types. Autosomal recessive (infantile) polycystic kidney disease is a congenital abnormality affecting both kidneys. Liver pathology of some degree also is present in all cases. The newborn typically has bilateral flank masses or is discovered to have bilaterally enlarged kidneys prenatally. The level of renal function as well as the amount of amniotic fluid is extremely variable. The ultrasound examination demonstrates large, homogeneously hyperechoic kidneys (Fig. 22). The renal cysts typically are too small to be seen with any imaging modality, and the kidneys retain their reniform shape. Intravenous urography demonstrates the accumulation of contrast in dilated collecting tubules, producing a characteristic radial striation (Fig. 23). Ultrasound screening of the parents usually does not demonstrate any renal abnormalities, but sibling screening will occasionally detect renal or liver abnormalities.

Autosomal dominant (adult) polycystic kidney disease usually is first diagnosed in teenage children or adults. However, with the increased use of ultrasound as a prenatal or postnatal screening device, the identification of asymptomatic infants with this disease is increasingly more common. Occasionally, these enlarged kidneys present as a unilateral or bilateral abdominal mass. The ultrasound study may demonstrate an enlarged kidney(s) without a distinct corticomedullary junction and with macroscopic cysts (Fig. 24); however, in some individuals, the ultrasound scan is normal in childhood, and the characteristic cystic changes do not appear until they are 20 years of age. When the diagnosis is not clear from the family history or the child's ultrasound findings, a screening ultrasound scan of the parents can be used to demonstrate cystic changes in the kidneys of either the mother or the father.

Prior to the advent of prenatal ultrasound, the most common presentation for MCDK in the neonatal period was a palpable renal mass. Today, the majority of these children are identified prenatally. Sonography usually is diagnostic and demonstrates a clustering of various-sized macrocysts that do not interconnect (Fig. 25A), whereas in a UPJ obstruction, the "cysts" connect with the infundibulum and a dilated renal pelvis. In a few instances, a definite distinction between hydronephrosis and MCDK cannot be made by ultrasound. In this circumstance, renal scintigraphy is helpful in that nonfunction is consistent with MCDK (Fig. 25B). However, occasionally in MCDK, there is minimal function present, and either percutaneous cyst puncture with contrast injection or surgical exploration may be required to establish the diagnosis.

Simple renal cysts are rare in the newborn. They usually are discovered prenatally (Fig. 26) or incidentally as they do not typically produce any symptoms. The differential diagnosis includes a duplex collecting system, dominant polycystic renal disease, caliceal diverticulum, and cystic neuroblastoma or Wilms' tumor. The long-term significance of these cysts is unknown, and it is reasonable to follow these patients with annual ultrasound examinations.

Urinary Tract Changes Secondary to Other Anomalies

Genital Abnormalities

In females, there is a significant correlation between genital and urinary abnormalities. In the Mayer-Rokitansky-Kuster-Hauser syndrome, duplication, atresia, or agenesis of the uterus and vagina frequently are associated with unilateral renal agenesis. All girls with renal agenesis, therefore, should be screened for these anomalies.

Exstrophy of the Bladder

The pubic bones are widespread, and the bladder and urethral mucosa are exposed in exstrophy of the bladder, but the upper urinary tracts are typically normal. Vesicoureteral reflux is identified typically after bladder closure.

Urachal Anomalies: Patent Urachus, Urachal Cyst or Sinus

When the urachus remains patent, urine may leak from the umbilicus. Typically, these children present with a clear fluid accumulating within the umbilicus. If part of the urachus closes, the remaining portion may become encysted and form a urachal cyst. In this circum-

stance, the children present with an asymptomatic subumbilical mass. Ultrasonography will demonstrate an elongated hypoechoic structure at the anterior superior surface of the urinary bladder. A VCUG should be performed to determine if there is a communication with the dome of the bladder (Fig. 27).

Imperforate Anus

A fistulous tract between the terminal intestinal segment and the genitourinary tract is characteristic of imperforate anus. All children with a high imperforate anus have a urinary fistula: the termination in males is most commonly in the prostatic urethra (Fig. 28), whereas in females, the fistula connects to the vagina. Because of the high incidence of other genitourinary anomalies, a renal ultrasound scan and VCUG should be part of the routine evaluation of all of these children. The most common associated urologic anomalies are renal agenesis and vesicoureteral reflux. There is also an increased potential for deformities of the lumbosacral spine and if such are present, neurovesical dysfunction must be considered (Fig. 29).

Adrenal Hemorrhage

Adrenal hemorrhage is the most common neonatal adrenal lesion. In clinically apparent cases, the hemorrhage is right-sided in 70% and bilateral in 5% to 10%. Bilateral hemorrhage is found more frequently in males. The etiology of adrenal hemorrhage is uncertain, but it is known that the normal fetal adrenal gland is one-third the size of the kidney at the tenth gestational week and even at birth remains relatively enlarged (Fig. 30). It is apparent that trauma, bleeding or clotting abnormalities, or abrupt venous pressure changes may cause this vascular organ to hemorrhage. The neonatal adrenal can almost always be imaged sonographically, and occasionally, the adrenal hemorrhage is identified on a prenatal ultrasound scan (Fig. 31).

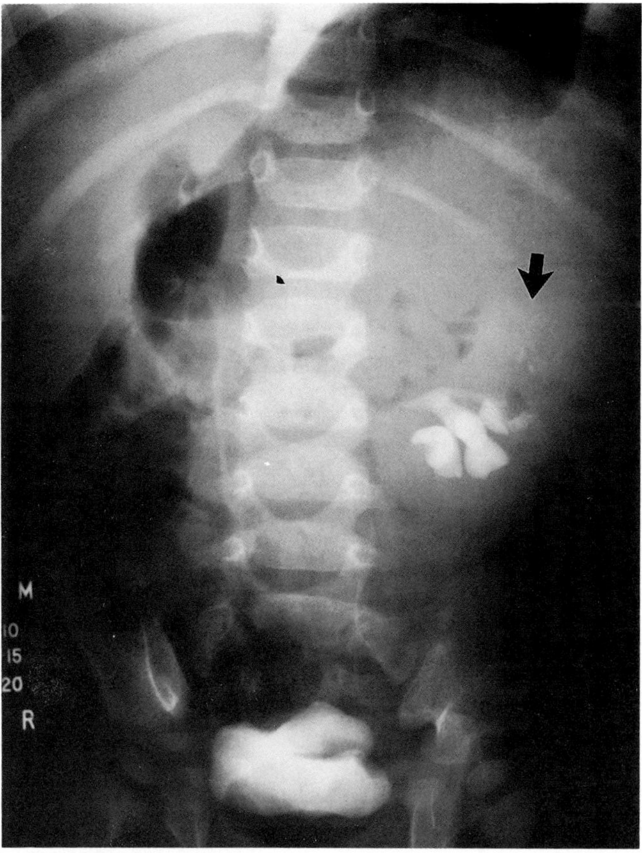

Figure 21A.   Tumors in infants presenting with asymptomatic abdominal mass. The IVU demonstrates inferior displacement of the left kidney by suprarenal mass with calcification (arrow). Ultrasound scan demonstrated that the mass was solid, thereby excluding duplication. Neuroblastoma was diagnosed.

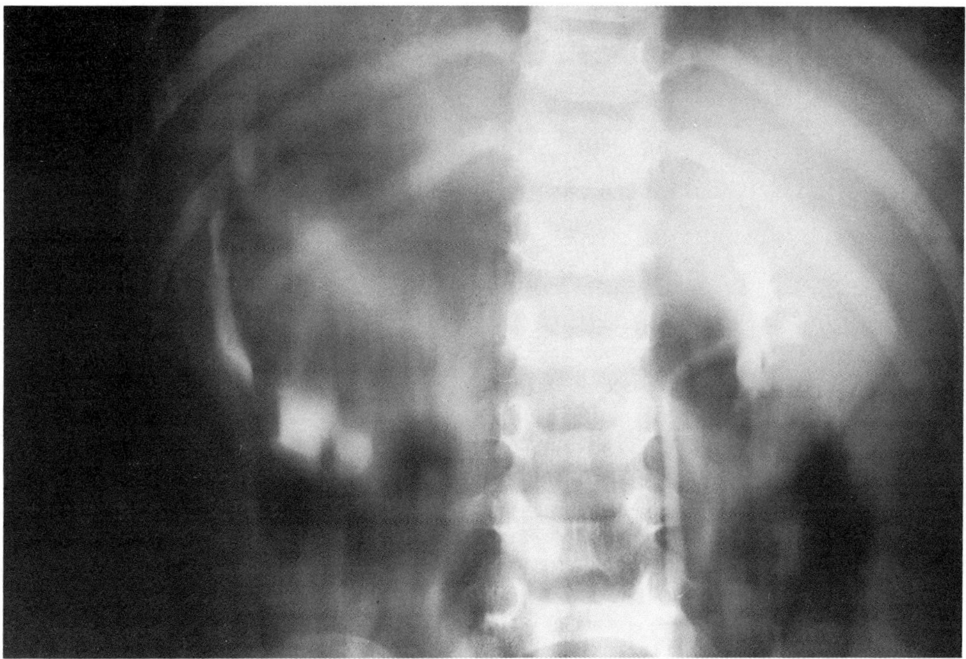

Figure 21B.   The IVU in another infant demonstrates distortion of the intrarenal collecting system by a solid mass (as seen on ultrasound). Wilms' tumor was diagnosed.

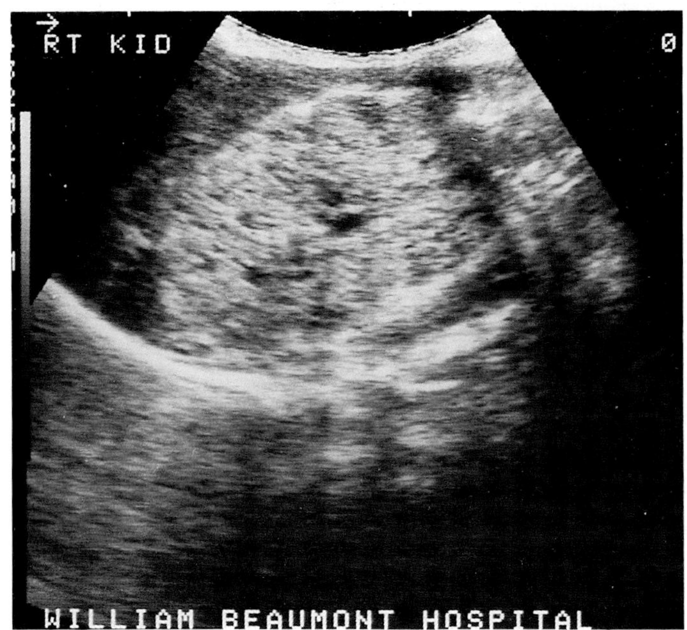

Figure 22.   Sagittal sonogram demonstrates enlargement of the right kidney, which is also diffusely hyperechoic, suggestive of infantile (recessive) polycystic kidney disease.

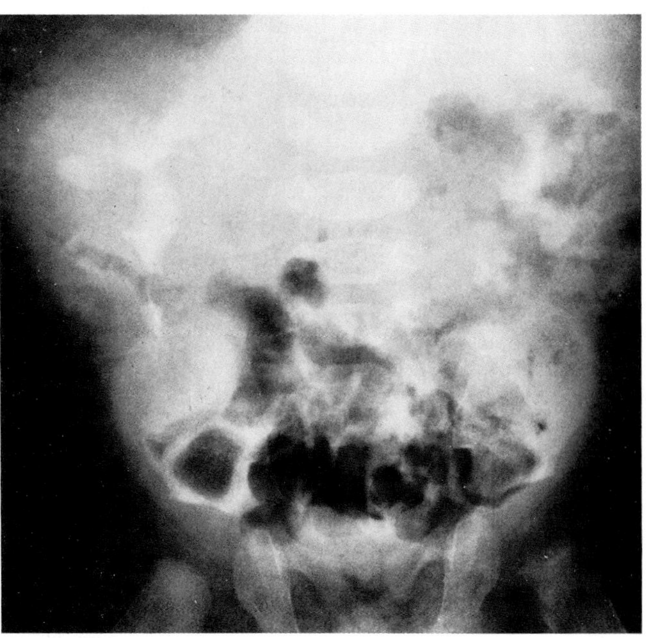

Figure 23.   The IVU of the same patient seen in Figure 22 shows bilaterally enlarged kidneys with splaying of calices and small bilateral parenchymal collections of contrast secondary to collecting tubule ectasia. These findings are characteristic of recessive polycystic kidney disease.

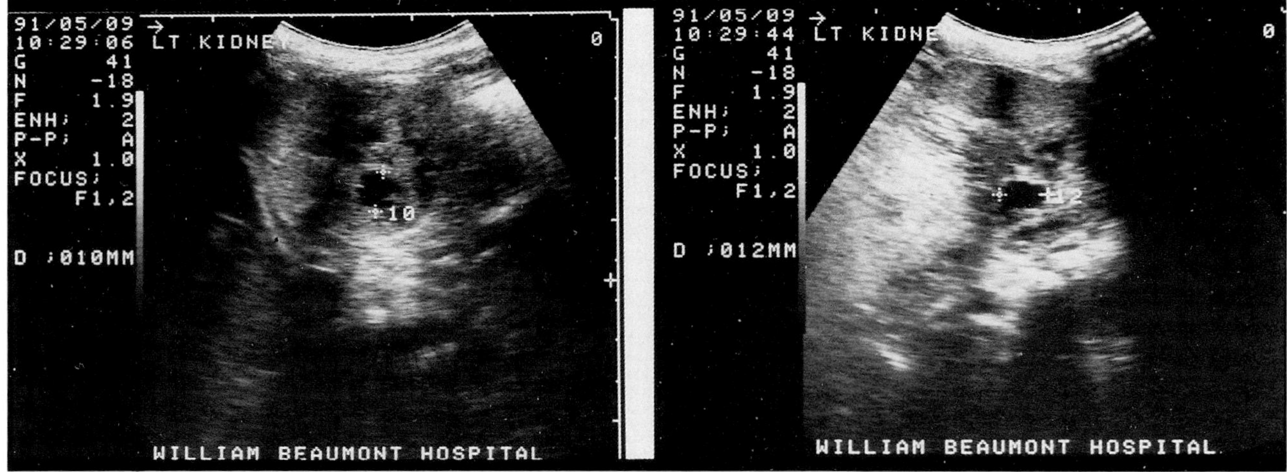

Figure 24.   This child had several renal cysts identified prenatally in each kidney. Postnatal ultrasound scan confirms the presence of two or three cysts in each kidney. Family history was consistent with diagnosis of dominant renal polycystic kidney disease. Physical examination, urinalysis, blood pressure, and serum creatinine were all within normal limits.

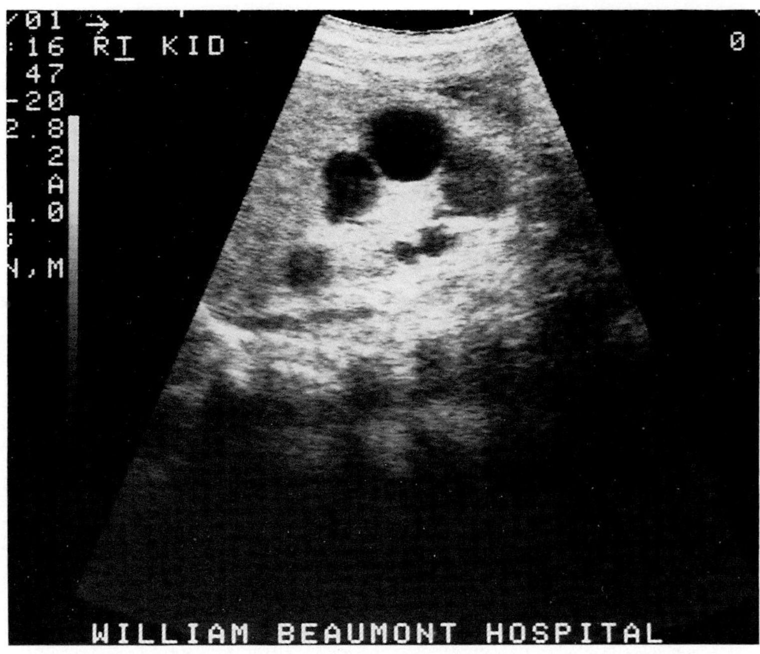

Figure 25A. A child had a right hydronephrotic kidney identified prenatally. Postnatal ultrasound scan demonstrates several cysts of various sizes that do not connect with each other. Dilated ureter was not seen, and VCUG was normal.

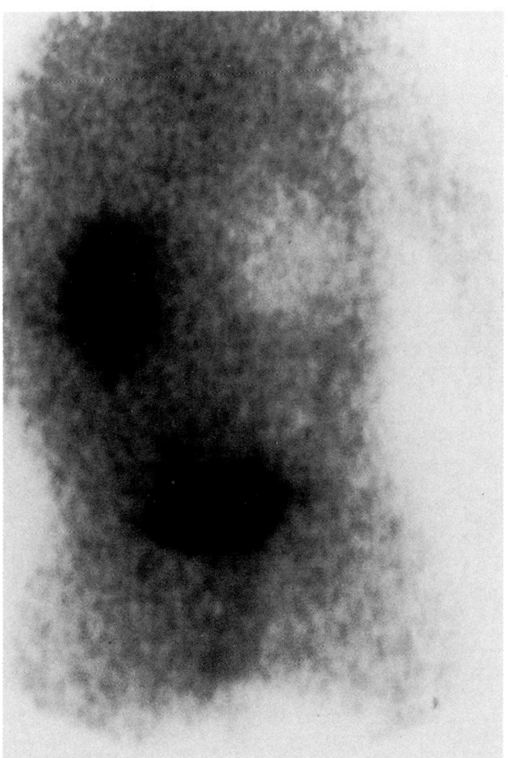

Figure 25B.   Renal scan in this child demonstrates a normally functioning left kidney. However, on the right side, there is a photon-deficient region consistent with diagnosis of MCDK. Diagnosis was confirmed at surgery.

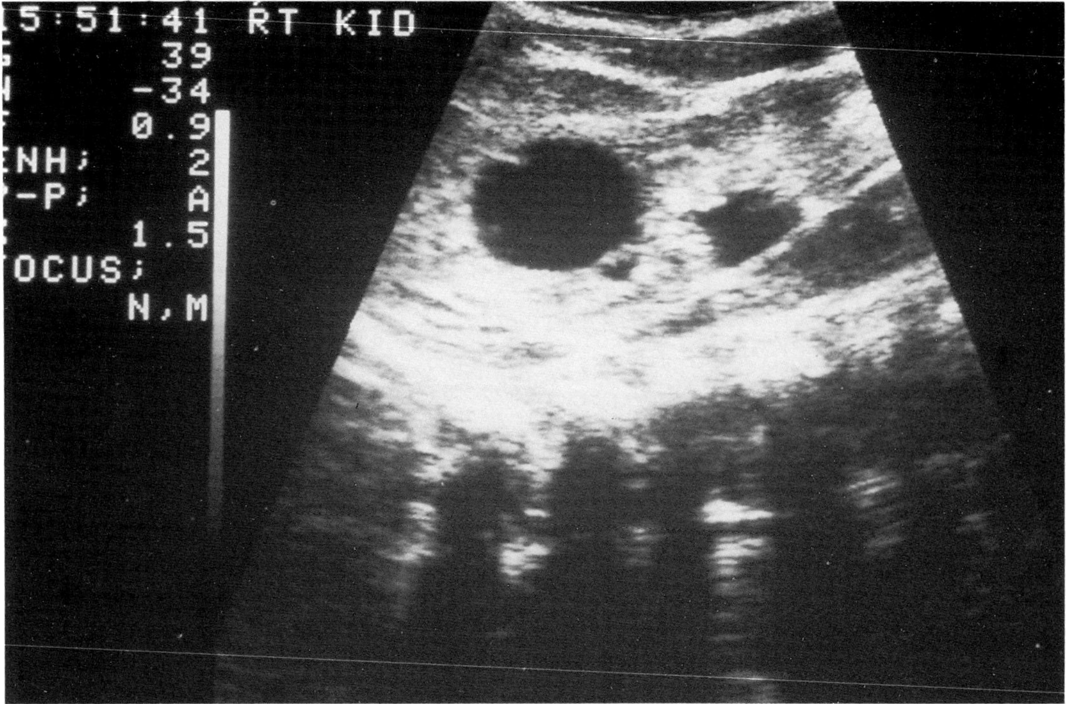

Figure 26.   This male infant was discovered to have hydronephrosis prenatally. Ultrasound scan demonstrates single simple renal cyst at upper-pole of the right kidney. There was no family history of cystic renal disease. No dilated ureter was identified. The VCUG was normal, as was Tc-99m DMSA scan. Child has been followed for 3 years, and cyst has not changed in size.

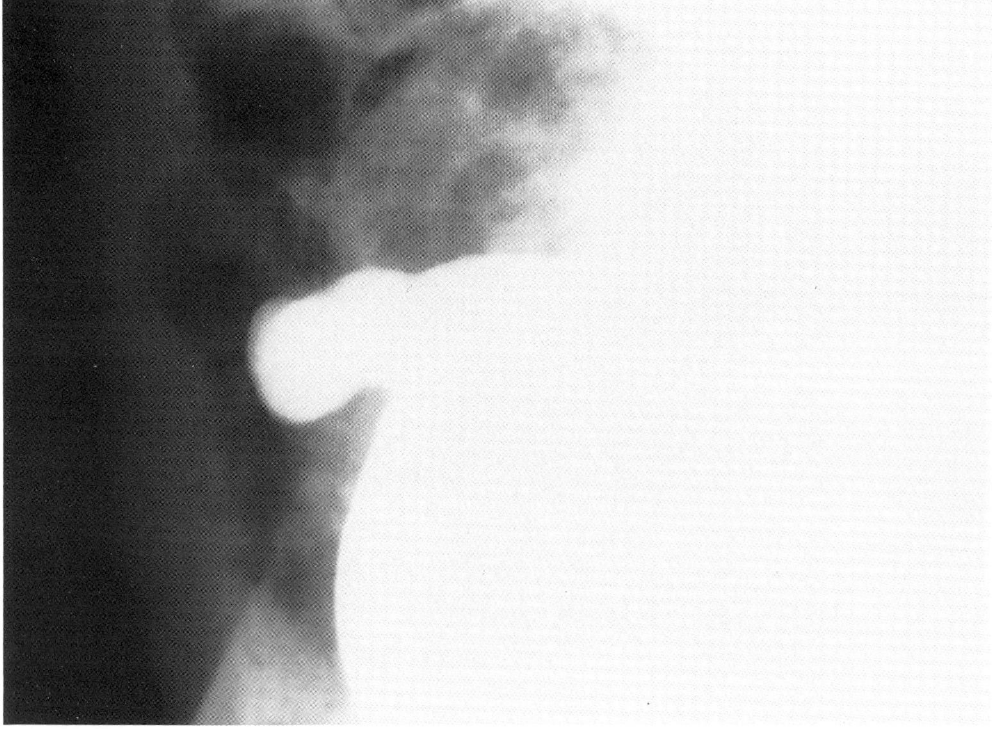

Figure 27.   The VCUG demonstrates urachal remnant at the dome of the bladder.

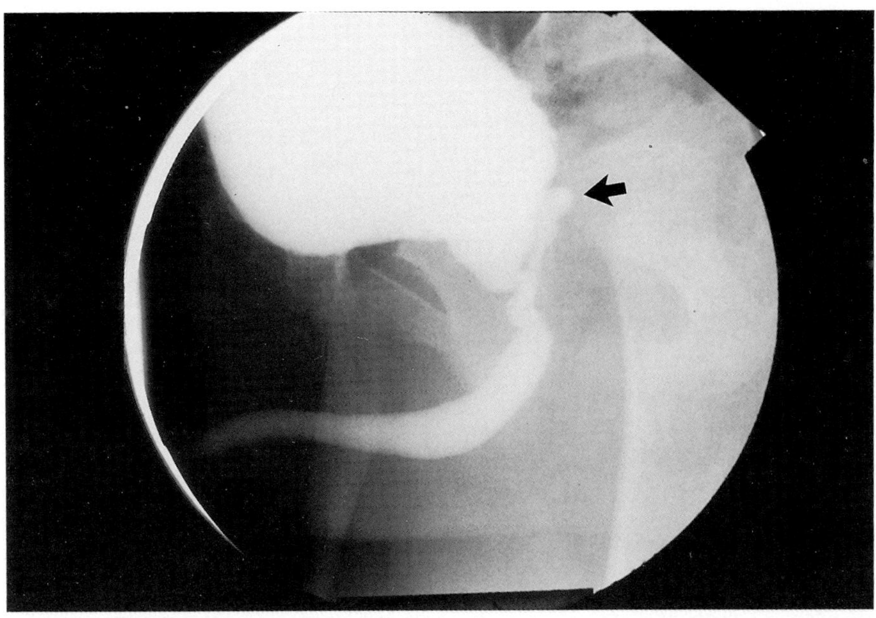

Figure 28.   This VCUG demonstrates fistula connecting terminal colonic segment to prostatic urethra (arrow).

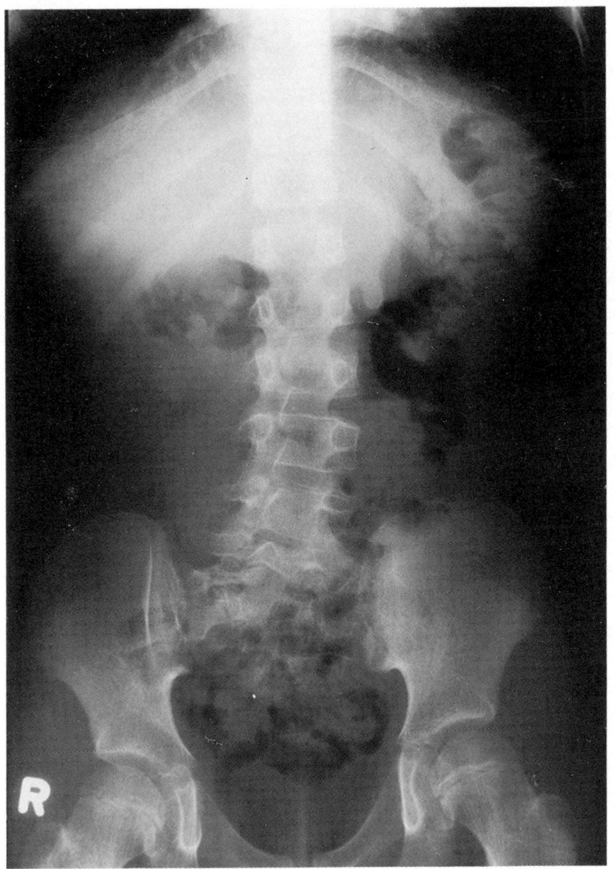

Figure 29.   Note sacral abnormalities in this child with imperforate anus. Despite absence of neurologic abnormalities, one must be concerned about potential neurovesical dysfunction.

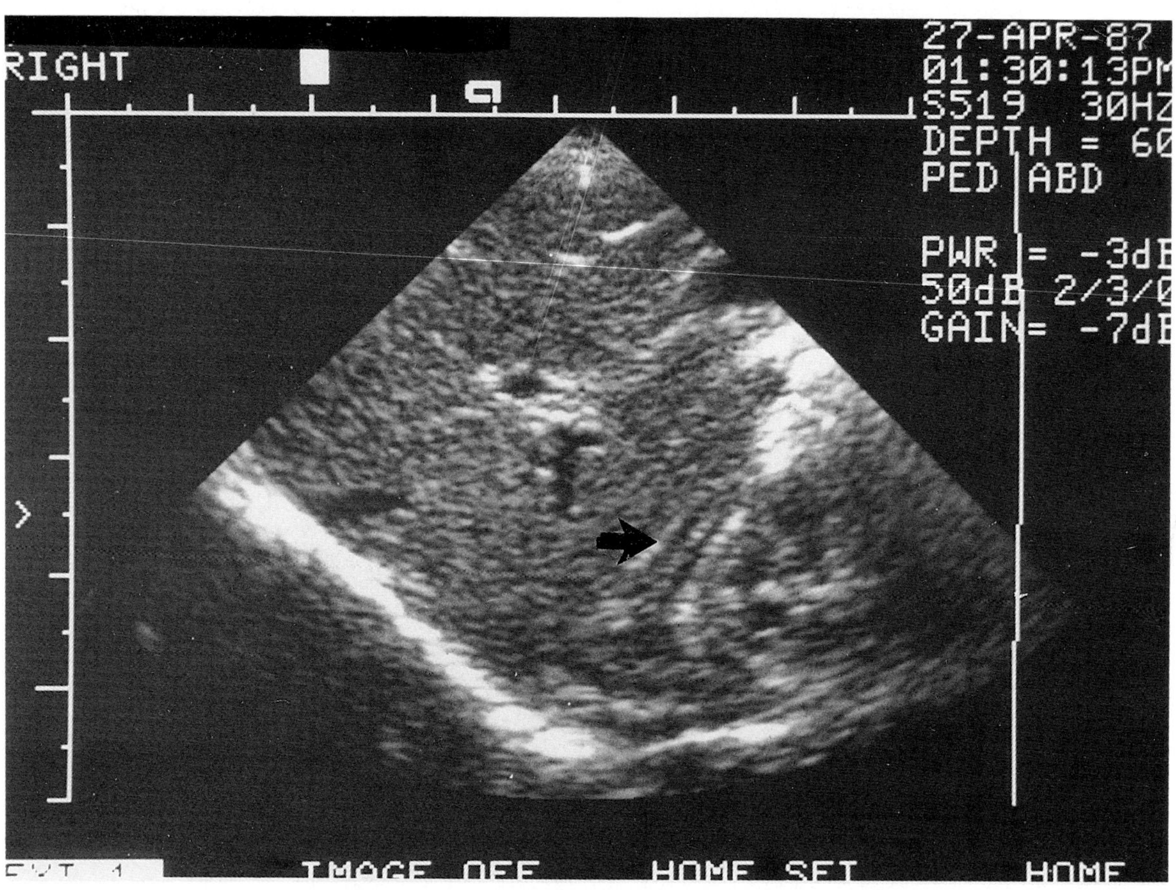

Figure 30.   Normal ultrasonographic appearance of the adrenal gland (arrow) in newborn.

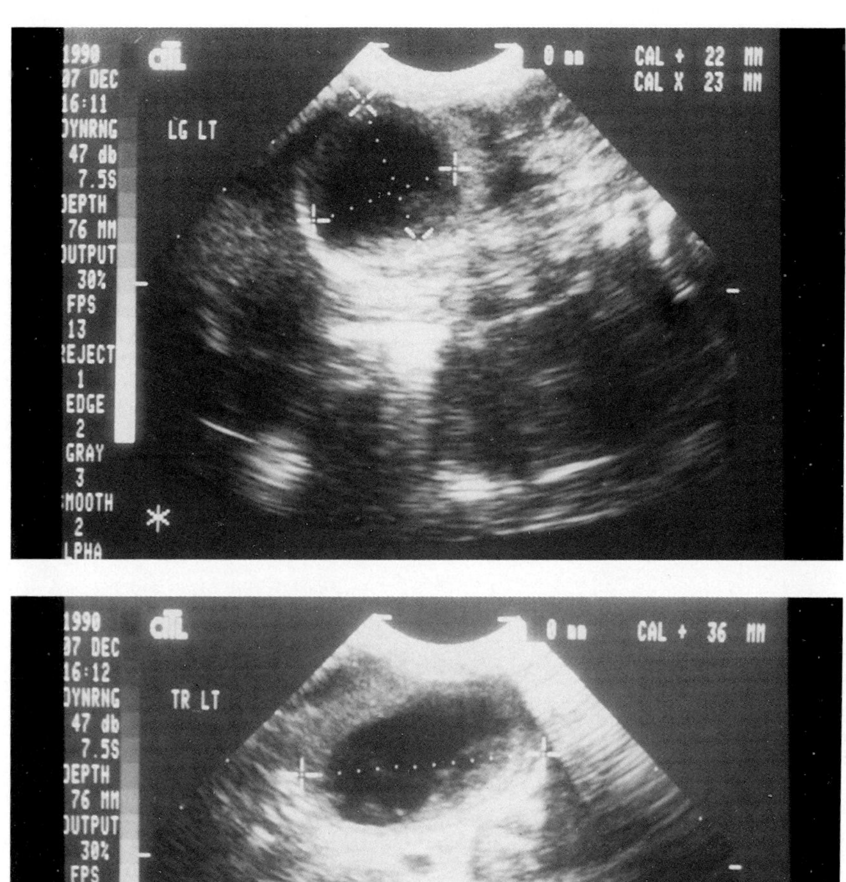

Figure 31. This child had a suprarenal cystic mass detected prenatally. Postnatal ultrasound consistent with adrenal hemorrhage. During the first few months of life the mass resolved completely and the patient remained asymptomatic.

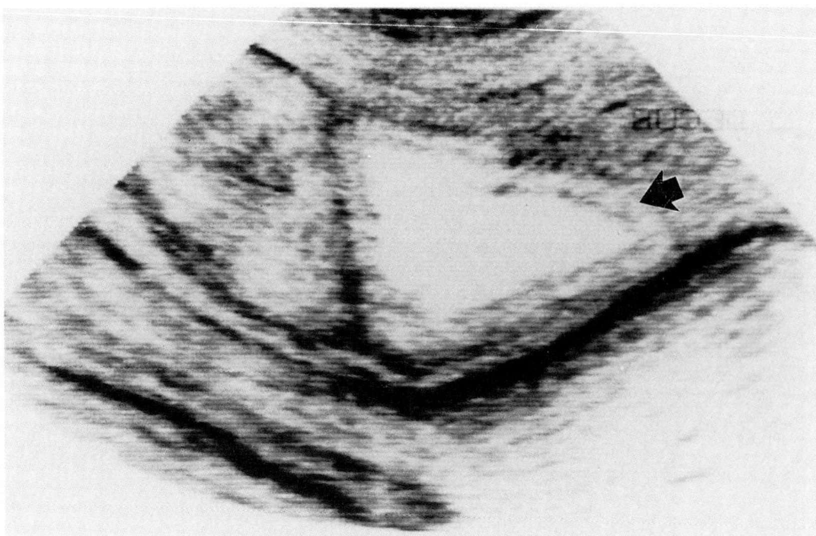

Figure 32A.   Sonogram demonstrating hyperechoic mass representing adrenal hemorrhage (arrow).

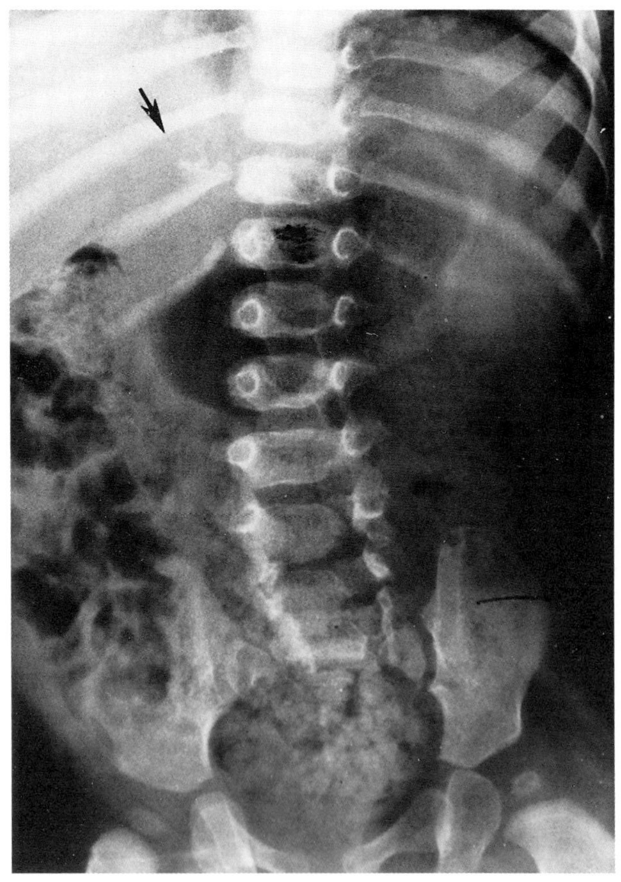

Figure 32B.   Follow-up scout film at 6 months demonstrating calcification in suprarenal area. Ultrasound scan showed that mass had resolved.

The newborn with adrenal hemorrhage may be identified because a mass is palpated, there is prolonged jaundice, or an abnormality is detected during an ultrasound study performed for some other purpose. It is rare for these patients to present with anemia or shock from bleeding. This entity rarely, if ever, leads to adrenal insufficiency. Initially, the hemorrhage appears hyperechoic (Fig. 32A) but rapidly (within days) becomes hypoechoic as the clot lyses; frequently, calcification in the suprarenal areas is all that remains (Fig. 32B). The principal differential diagnoses are neuroblastoma; duplex collecting system with a cystic, dysplastic, or hydronephrotic upper-pole moiety; adrenal cyst; retroperitoneal teratoma; and lymphangioma.

References

1. Hellstrom WJG, Kogan BA, Jeffrey RB Jr, et al: The natural history of prenatal hydronephrosis with normal amounts of amniotic fluid. J Urol 1984; 132:947.
2. Diamond DA, Sanders R, Jeffs RD: Fetal hydrone-phrosis: considerations regarding urological intervention. J Urol 1984; 131:1155.
3. Duckett JW, Harrison MR, Lorimier AA, et al: Fetal intervention for obstructive uropathy. Dialogues Pediatr Urol 1982; 5:2.
4. Kass EJ, Fink-Bennett D: Contemporary techniques for the radioisotopic evaluation of the dilated urinary tract. Urol Clinics North Am 1990; 17:273.

Chapter 2

Infections of the Urinary Tract

Joaquim Vieira, M.D.

Infections of the Kidney

Infectious interstitial nephritis is generally known as "pyelonephritis," which implies an inflammatory reaction to pathogenic organisms. The term "pyelonephritis" includes many variants such as acute, chronic, and tuberculous pyelonephritis and pyonephrosis (obstructive lesion with superimposed infection). Renal inflammatory disease also includes entities such as infected cyst, and intrarenal and perirenal abscess.

Acute Pyelonephritis

Acute pyelonephritis is the most frequent renal disease and is most common in the female patient 15 to 35 years old. The clinical features (sudden onset of fever, flank pain, and costovertebral tenderness) together with pyuria and bacteria constitute strong evidence for a correct diagnosis of simple, uncomplicated, acute pyelonephritis. Imaging tests are usually not necessary.

Infection ascending along the lymphatics adjacent to the mucosa of the collecting system, facilitated by reflux, obstruction, or congenital renal anomaly, has been postulated to be the most common route of infection; occasionally, infection is hematogenous. The most common organism is *Escherichia coli*. The presence of other gram-negative organisms or fungi suggests chronic infection, and culture of *Staphylococcus aureus* suggests hematogenous origins.

If the response to therapy is not prompt, the possibility of complicating factors such as congenital urinary anomalies (duplication), obstructive lesions (calculi), and ureteral reflux must be considered. Urographic abnormalities are only found in 25% to 28% of patients with uncomplicated acute pyelonephritis. The radiologic studies usually are done chiefly to look for the changes of chronic pyelonephritis, and to investigate those cases in which complicating factors are the reason for a poor response to the proper antibiotic treatment (Fig. 1). Urography is also indicated in male patients who develop acute pyelonephritis for the first time, even when the response to therapy is rapid since complicating factors usually are present in these cases.

The most common urographic abnormalities are: (1) renal enlargement; (2) unilateral functional impairment (decrease and delay in contrast excretion) general or segmental; (3) "spidering" (spasticity) of the pelvicaliceal system; (4) hypotonic (nonobstructive) dilatation of the calices, pelvis, and ureter with marked vascular impressions; and (5) ridging (striation) of the mucosa of the pelvicaliceal system and upper ureter.

Acute localized pyelonephritis without liquefaction of the renal parenchyma is known as

From *Imaging of Urologic Disorders* edited by Alexander S. Cass, MBBS, © 1992, Futura Publishing Inc., Mount Kisco, NY.

"acute focal bacterial nephritis" and usually involves only one portion of the kidney. The focal lesions appear radiologically as renal masses on urography, ultrasound (US), or computed tomography (CT). Computed tomography usually demonstrates a wedge-shaped mass of decreased attenuation with no enhancement or with a mottled, macrostriated appearance which is secondary to the ischemia of the affected area.

Emphysematous pyelonephritis may result from acute pyelonephritis developing in the presence of urinary tract obstruction or in patients receiving immunosuppressive therapy. It occurs in patients with diabetes with or without obstruction. The patient is usually septic, and the mortality rate is high (greater than 50%). In this serious condition, gas is present in the renal pelvis, caliceal system, interstitial tissue, and perirenal space (Fig. 2). The parenchymal gas often forms a peculiar lacework pattern. Ultrasound may be the first imaging modality used in such cases because of the patient's impaired renal function and will demonstrate multiple high-amplitude echoes in the renal fossa accompanied by acoustic shadows. Computed tomography or plain films can confirm the finding. The former should be used only in the confusing cases not as a routine modality to assess renal infection.

Aspiration needle biopsy may be necessary in the confusing clinical situation to determine the etiology of the infection or to rule out tumor.

Chronic Pyelonephritis

The clinical varieties of chronic pyelonephritis are: (1) chronic pyelonephritis with its onset in childhood known as atrophic pyelonephritis, or better known as reflux nephropathy; (2) chronic pyelonephritis with its onset in adulthood usually with urinary tract obstruction such as prostatic hyperplasia, calculi, or pregnancy ("obstructive chronic pyelonephritis"); and (3) chronic pyelonephritis the final result of severe acute bacterial pyelonephritis, which is rare and is seen chiefly in patients with septicemia and diabetes.

The primary atrophic type (reflux neuropathy) and the adult obstructive type are the most common forms of chronic pyelonephritis. The ascending route (via the ureter) generally is thought to be responsible for the large majority of renal infections, both acute and chronic.

Scarring in primary atrophic pyelonephritis occurs primarily in kidneys with moderate to severe (grades 3 or 4) vesicoureteral reflux that is associated with intrarenal reflux of sterile or infected urine, although it occurs faster and more severely with infected urine.

The majority of patients is young females because of the preponderance of vesicoureteral reflux in this group. In young males, outlet obstruction (posterior urethral valves) is the most common cause. Although the roentgenographic findings may be seen first in the adult, it is assumed that almost all cases of renal damage began in infancy or childhood. Therefore, it is important to diagnose urinary tract infections in infants as early as possible and to study patients properly by a urinary diary, urine cultures, and radiographic examination. Chronic pyelonephritis may involve both kidneys or only one. If the disease is unilateral, the contralateral kidney may be hypertrophied. Because of its focal nature, the disease usually progresses at different rates into two kidneys if it is bilateral which results in asymmetrically scarred kidneys. When one kidney is very small and coarsely scarred, the condition is referred to as "atrophic pyelonephritis" (Fig. 3).

The characteristic urographic findings in chronic pyelonephritis are as follows: (1) scattered, flat, or punctate focal scarring of the cortex, most often polar; (2) areas of normal or hypertrophied intervening cortex which occasionally mimic a mass (pseudotumor); (3) irregular, narrow, renal parenchyma; (4) blunting and clubbing of the calices, especially those in the area of cortical scarring (Fig. 4); and (5) dilatation of the pelvicaliceal system, especially in cases with advanced destruction of the renal parenchyma. This dilatation usually is secondary to an obstruction or to vesicoureteral reflux. Strictures in the infundibula or ureter do not usually occur in chronic pyelonephritis; however, they are common in renal tuberculosis.

Sonography in chronic pyelonephritis shows a small, irregularly outlined kidney with increased echogenicity of the parenchyma. However, it usually is not possible to distinguish chronic infection from other causes of renal atrophy. A small kidney with evidence of pelvicaliceal dilatation favors the diagnosis of long-standing reflux and pyelonephritis.

Cross-sectional imaging methods are now commonly employed early in the evaluation of patients with unexplained fever, atypical lumbar pain, or hematuria of obscure origin. Patients with renal inflammatory disease may present to their physicians with any of these complaints, and CT may thus be the first radiologic examination to suggest the diagnosis. Scanning may display a contour defect, reflecting an area of prior infection that has healed with cortical scarring, which produces a characteristic "wavy" irregular renal contour. Fat may also infiltrate the region of the renal pelvis in a kidney shrunken by chronic pyelonephritis. Angiography is nowadays seldom indicated. Hypertrophic compensation or intervening parenchyma (pseudotumor) may resemble a solid renal tumor on urography, nephrotomography, and angiography; in the latter study, the picture is similar to that of hypovascular tumors. In certain cases, a renal radionuclide scan may be helpful, demonstrating normal uptake in the pseudotumor.

Intrarenal Abscess

An abscess is a localized collection of pus cells, ranging from a microscopic lesion to a gross mass. The acute renal abscess may be the end product of tissue necrosis in an area of acute focal pyelonephritis. However, most often, it results from the coalescence of multiple small suppurative foci with formation of a large collection of pus with a poorly defined wall, also known as a renal carbuncle. The acute renal abscess may be of a diffuse type in which the entire kidney is involved by a single abscess or may take the form of multiple abscesses of the localized type in which the disease is limited to one region of the kidney. Renal abscess is usually unilateral; it occurs twice as often on the right side as on the left and is usually polar. Any condition that leads to infection or obstruction of the urinary tract, such as prostatism, diabetes, neurogenic bladder, or pregnancy may be a predisposing cause.

Symptoms and signs include chills, fever, flank pain, malaise, and marked leukocytosis. Systemic symptoms, if severe, may mask local signs. Pyuria and bacteriuria are not present in as many as 20% of cases. Scout films of the abdomen may be normal or may show diffuse renal enlargement or the localized enlargement of a renal mass with poor delineation of the psoas muscle and scoliosis concave to the side of the involvement. Urography usually shows decreased opacification of all or part of the parenchyma of the affected kidney seen as a nephrogram deficiency. The calices may be poorly opacified or amputated. The renal abscess may also appear as a space-occupying mass with a lump, blurred segmental contours, and deformity of the calices (Fig. 5A). If the abscess drains into the pelvicaliceal system, the cavity will opacify during urography or retrograde pyelography. A normal urogram does not exclude the presence of an acute renal abscess.

Ultrasonography can demonstrate an acute abscess, especially if the focal collection of pus has become 2 or 3 cm in diameter or larger. The abscess will appear as a sonolucent or hyperechoic area within the renal parenchyma with poorly distinct margins (Fig. 5B). On CT, acute abscesses are low-attenuation (20 to 30 HU (Houndsfield units), ill-defined masses. The centers of such masses do not change in attenuation with intravenous injection of contrast and may contain gas bubbles that are virtually diagnostic for an abscess. The walls of abscesses demonstrate enhancement in 35% to 50% of the cases.

If the acute abscess is not resolved by treatment or the immune response, a reparative process with the formation of a thick wall of granulation tissue will take place. The acute abscess then becomes the chronic renal abscess. The radiologic findings are now those of a well-localized intrarenal mass. Nephrotomography usually shows a radiolucent area with a thick wall. If the abscess breaks into the pelvicaliceal system, which is unusual, the urogram and retrograde pyelogram show opacification of an irregular cavity connecting with the renal pelvis. Sonography usually shows hypoechoic masses with increased transonicity and thick, irregular walls or capsule.

Computed tomography usually shows a spherical mass containing material with a relatively homogeneous low attenuation value. Quite often, a rim of variable thickness and higher attenuation will be seen. Avascular or hypovascular neoplasms, especially those with necrotic liquid centers, may have CT findings similar to those of an abscess. Extension into the perirenal space suggests an inflammatory process, but renal cell carcinoma can cause spontaneous hemorrhage in a subcapsular or perirenal distribution. Inflammatory processes tend to follow fascial planes, whereas tumor is more likely to extend by bulk mass formation in violation of fascial planes. Whenever the diagnosis is in doubt, a fine-needle aspiration biopsy should be done.

Perirenal Abscess

Perirenal abscesses most often (approximately 70%) occur by direct extension from renal infections.

The most common sequence of pathological events is an acute pyelonephritis progressing to acute renal cortical abscess, which in turn breaks through the true renal capsule with subsequent extension to the perirenal space. If the process continues to break through Gerota's fascia, the abscess will extend to the pararenal spaces and possibly to the retrofascial spaces. Further extension to the anterior abdominal wall, subphrenic space, thoracic cavity, mediastinum, iliac fossa, and thigh may occur.

The onset is usually insidious, and the patient may not seek medical care until 1 to 3 weeks has elapsed. The classic symptoms and signs include fever, flank pain, dysuria, leukocytosis, and a flank mass with tenderness (70% of cases). However, more frequently, the picture is nonspecific with malaise, weight loss, low-grade fever, nausea and vomiting, and no localizing signs. The urinalysis and urine culture are unremarkable in 35% of patients.

A scout film may appear normal but in many instances (about 50%) shows loss of the renal or psoas outline, lumbar scoliosis with concavity toward the side of the abscess, loss of normal respiratory motion of the kidney, an upper abdominal mass (retroperitoneal in 25%), and urinary calculi (35%). On intravenous urography, 75% to 80% of patients have findings such as an absent or indistinct nephrogram, diminution in concentration of the contrast medium with poor filling of calices, caliceal displacement or compression by a mass, thickening of the

renal fascia, hydronephrosis, and displacement of the kidney. Sonography usually shows a complex mass with irregular borders within the perirenal and pararenal spaces.

The superior anatomic resolution of CT makes it the modality of choice for diagnosis and assessment of the extent of the infectious process in the retroperitoneum and surrounding tissues. The subcapsular, perirenal, or pararenal abscess appears as an ovoid, low-attenuation mass with a relatively radiolucent center and a thick, enhancing wall. This infectious mass usually presents a loculated appearance. The adjacent renal contours may be poorly defined with thickening of adjacent fascial planes. The presence of gas bubbles is virtually pathognomonic of gas-producing organisms. On occasion, the infectious fluid collection extends to other sites (psoas muscle, iliac fossa, thigh, subphrenic area, mediastinum, and thoracic cavity), which will be easily demonstrated on CT.

Percutaneous aspiration of an inflammatory mass (renal, perirenal, or pararenal) for diagnosis or therapy (drainage) should be guided by cross-sectional imaging, especially in acutely ill patients. Definitive surgery can then be performed when the patient's condition improves. The course of these inflammatory masses, which usually are found in already debilitated patients, is grave; mortality rates of 75% to 100% have been reported with medical therapy alone.

Pyonephrosis

Pyonephrosis is defined as the accumulation of pus in a dilated renal collecting system accompanied by advanced suppurative destruction of the renal parenchyma. It may be the end result of renal infection without obstruction; however, most often, obstructive hydronephrosis is a precursor of pyonephrosis. The etiology of the obstruction may be a calculus at the ureteropelvic junction, a staghorn calculus, a stricture, or a congenital anomaly.

Nonfunction or minimal function of the involved kidney is the usual finding on the urogram. The kidney usually is enlarged, although infrequently, it is small.

Retrograde pyelography reveals the point of obstruction usually a ureteral calculus at the ureteropelvic junction, and, when the obstruction is not complete, may demonstrate large, irregular calices at times containing multiple filling defects caused by the accumulation of necrotic tissue or pus. However, after the urogram, cross-sectional imaging (US or CT) now is the procedure of choice in a patient with suspected pyonephrosis.

Sonography readily demonstrates the presence of hydronephrosis. Pyonephrosis usually is not as transonic as uninfected hydronephrosis. Furthermore, low-amplitude echoes may be seen within the infected hydronephrotic collecting system. Another important finding consistent with pyonephrosis is the presence of a sludge-fluid interface in the dilated pelvicaliceal system.

The diagnosis of pyonephrosis may be highly suggested by the CT images, which will demonstrate a hydronephrotic system with an attenuating value higher than water. This study also is important in demonstrating the presence of fluid-fluid interfaces, gas, opaque or nonopaque stones, and the extent of the inflammatory process.

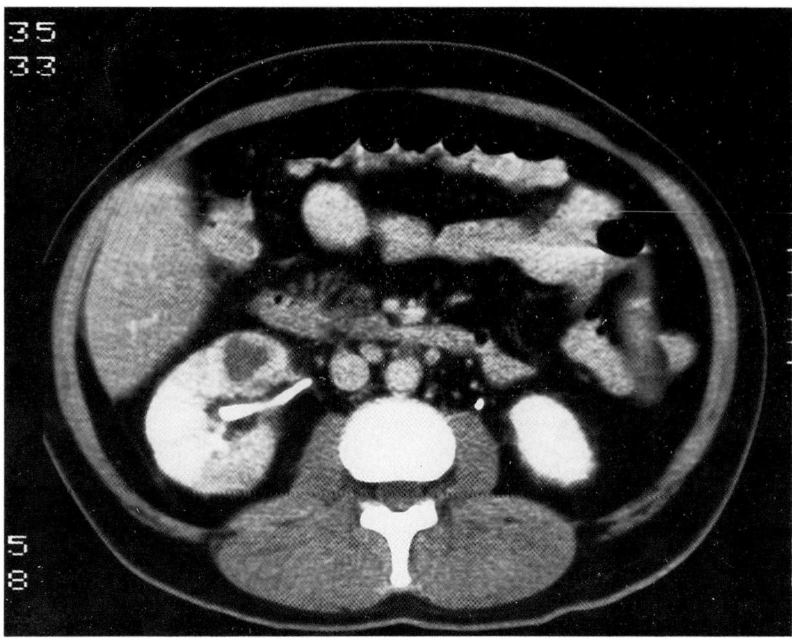

Figure 1A. Computed tomography scans of acute pyelonephritis of the right kidney with small abscess in a hemophilic patient with staphylococcal bacteremia who was admitted with right flank pain and fever. (A) Patchy areas of reduced attenuation involve the entire right kidney, with a small localized area at the anterior aspect of the middle third, consistent with pyelonephritis with a small abscess.

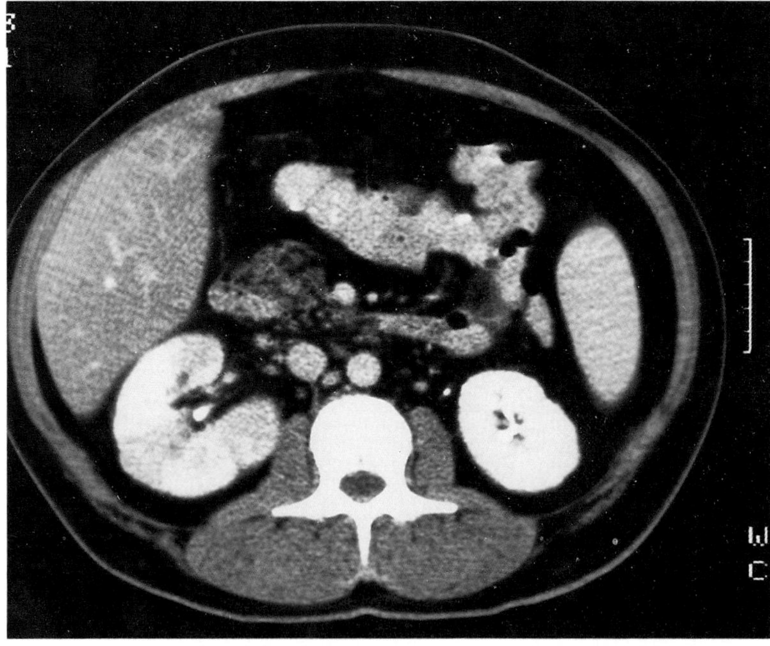

Figure 1B.   Enlargement of the right kidney secondary to diffuse edematous changes.

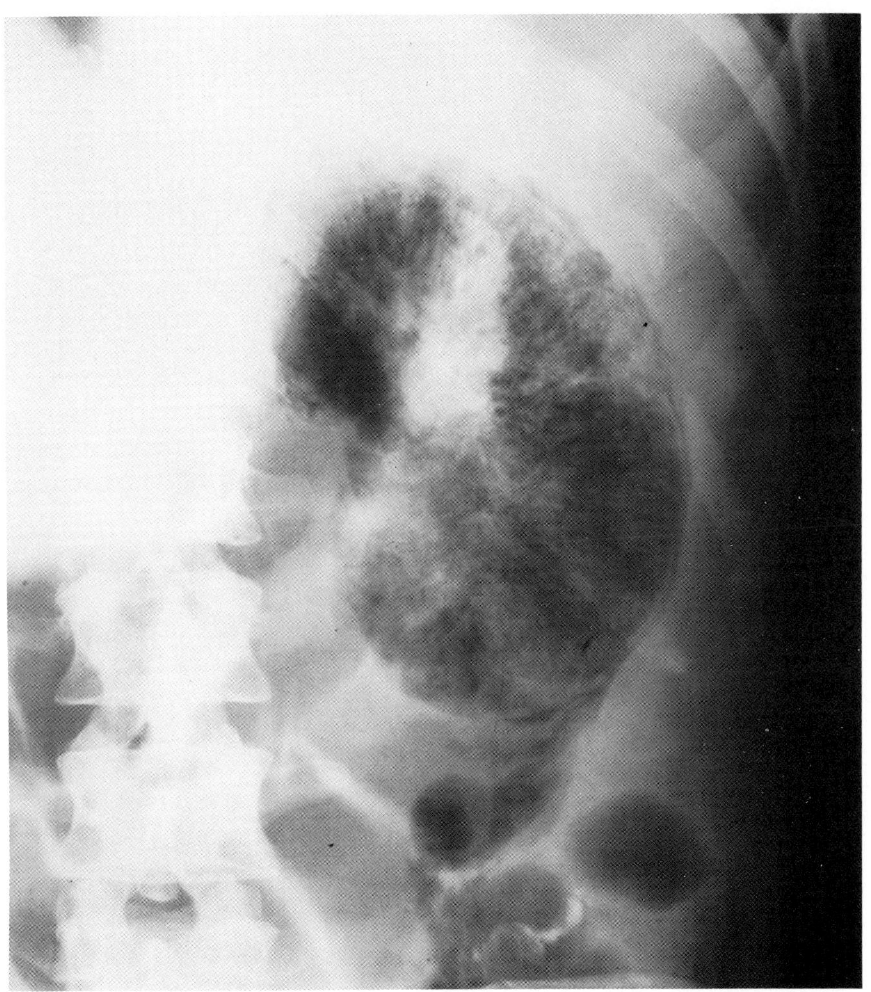

Figure 2.   Emphysematous pyelonephritis as seen on a flat plate; note the diffuse interstitial renal gas with perirenal extension.

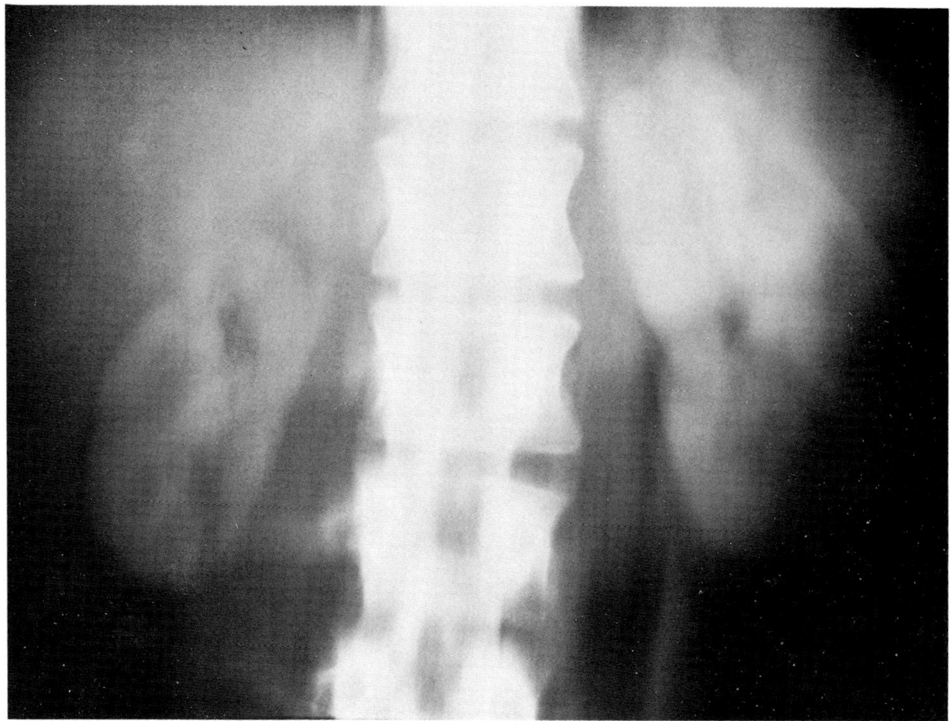

Figure 3A.   Atrophic pyelonephritis from reflux nephropathy. (A) Tomography shows an atrophic right kidney.

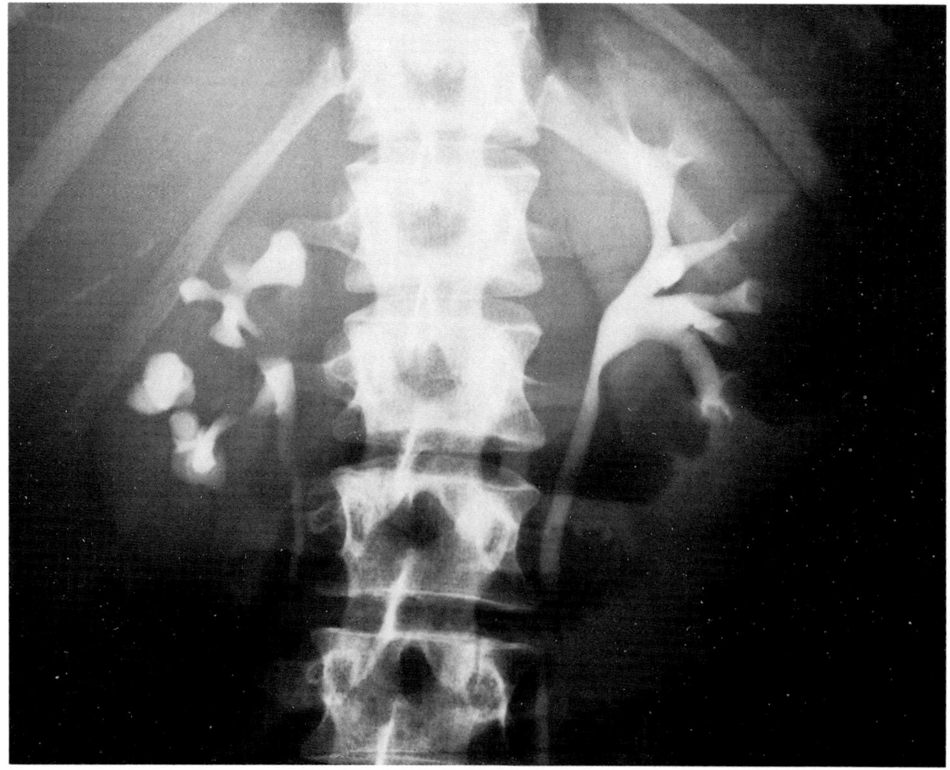

Figure 3B.   The 15-minute urogram reveals clubbing of several calices in the right kidney with associated cortical atrophy.

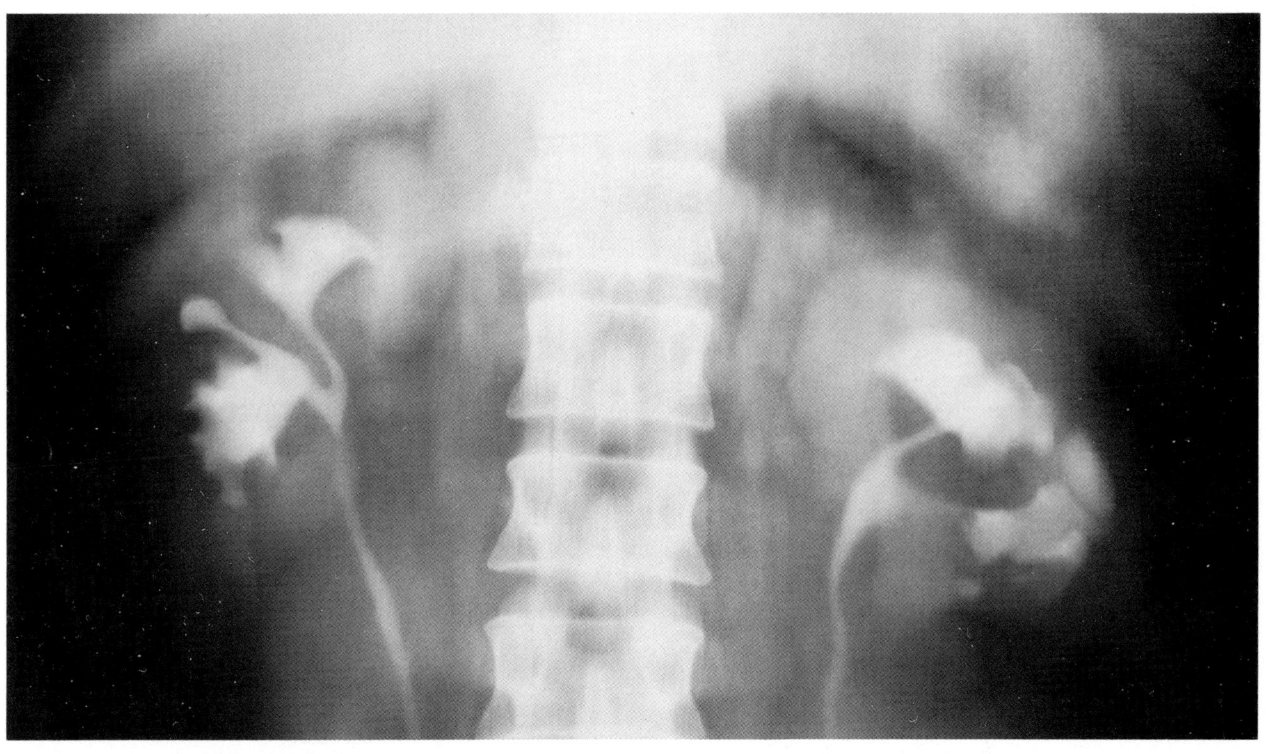

Figure 4.   Chronic pyelonephritis as seen by tomographic intravenous urogram. Clubbing (blunting) of several calices is apparent bilaterally with cortical atrophy of the left lower pole.

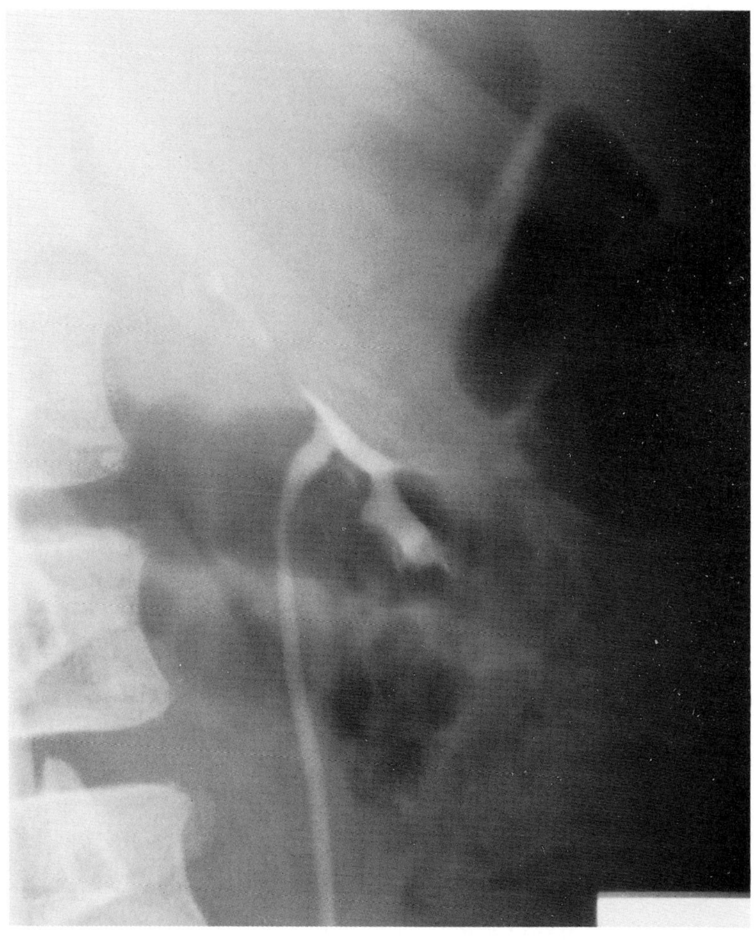

A

Figure 5. Abscess of the lateral aspect of the right upper-pole kidney in an 11-year-old admitted with right flank pain, fever, and leukocytosis. (A) On the intravenous urogram, a mass is apparent in the lateral aspect of the right upper pole, compressing and displacing the collecting structures medially.

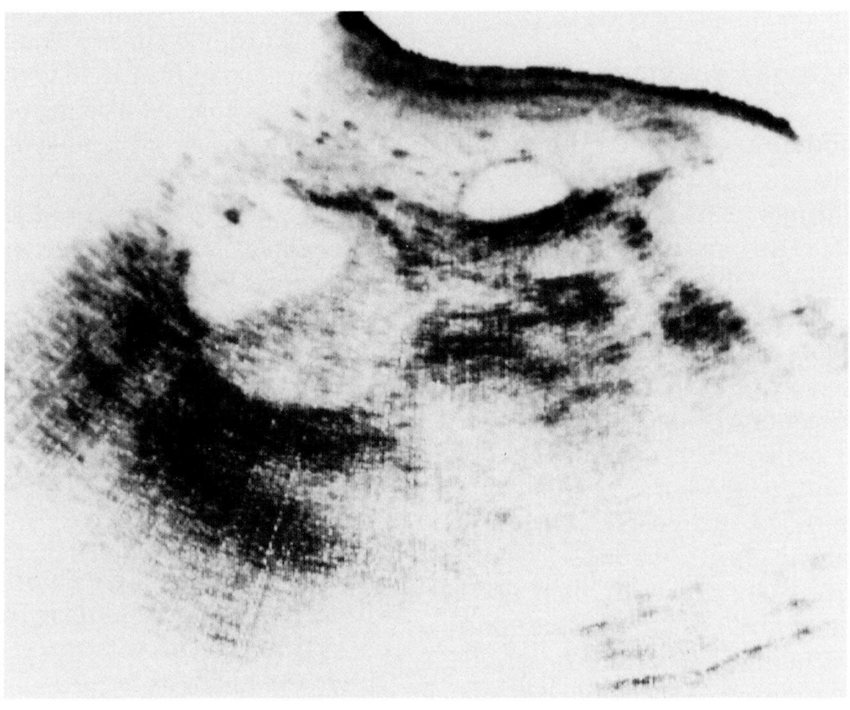

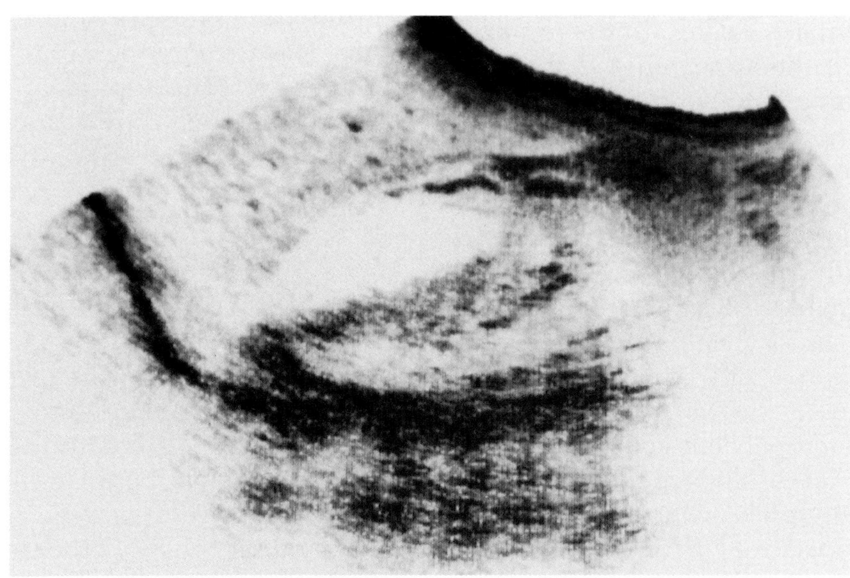

Figure 5B.   Ultrasound scans (top transverse, bottom longitudinal) show a cystic mass with few echogenic shadows consistent with a complex mass, most likely a renal abscess.

Inflammatory Renal Lesions with An Unusual Reaction Pattern

Xanthogranulomatous Pyelonephritis

Xanthogranulomatous pyelonephritis is an unusual chronic inflammatory disease with specific pathologic findings. The distinctive feature is the presence of xanthoma cells (large lipid-containing histiocytes), which usually are present in sheets, forming scattered yellow nodules a few millimeters to a few centimeters in size.

The condition occurs more often in female patients and is uncommon in children, usually being seen in the older age groups (sixth decade). The patient often gives a long history of renal infection (months to years). Urinalysis shows proteinuria and pyuria in most patients (about 85%) with positive cultures in the majority of cases (about 70% to 80%), the most frequently reported organisms being *Proteus* and *E. coli.*

Xanthogranulomatous pyelonephritis may present as either a diffuse or a localized (tumefactive) type. In the diffuse form, which is by far the more common (85% to 90%), the xanthoma cells are distributed in collections throughout the infected, nonfunctioning kidney, which is often obstructed and contains calculi. In the localized (tumefactive) form, the appearance is that of a mass in a functioning kidney, the mass consisting largely of xanthoma cells. The mechanism of production of xanthogranulomatous pyelonephritis is most probably related to both infection and obstruction. Probably, the obstructive process is primary, with secondary infection producing cell destruction and collections of lipids that are engulfed by histocytes, with subsequent formation of xanthoma cells. The obstruction is usually caused by a staghorn calculus or a calculus at the ureteropelvic junction; however, there are reported cases in which the obstruction was secondary to ureteral carcinoma or stricture. The infectious process may extend beyond the renal capsule with infiltration of the surrounding retroperitoneal tissues.

The diagnosis of xanthogranulomatous pyelonephritis should be suspected in a patient with an enlarged nonfunctioning kidney in the presence of renal calculi and evidence of urinary tract infection (Fig. 6).

Computed tomography can be highly suggestive of pyonephrosis by demonstrating some functioning of the renal cortex and maintenance of the kidney reniform shape. In xanthogranulomatous pyelonephritis, the affected kidney shows no cortical function and loses its reniform shape almost completely. Tumefactive xanthogranulomatous pyelonephritis is not easily distinguished from renal neoplasms. The presence of calculi together with a history of chronic infection should suggest the correct diagnosis.

Cystic Pyelonephritis or Pyeloureteritis Cystica

Cystic pyelonephritis is a benign process consisting of subepithelial cysts that elevate the urothelial mucosal layer of the pelvis, ureter, and, sometimes, the bladder and occurs in the presence of persistent or recurrent urinary tract infection. The cysts may range in size from microscopic to as large as 2 cm in diameter. They are usually multiple; however, a solitary cyst is seen occasionally. Grossly, the cysts are smooth and rounded and contain colorless or yellowish serous fluid with the consistency of mineral oil. The condition is seen mainly in the older age groups and is slightly more prevalent in women.

The roentgenographic findings are usually diagnostic. The typical appearance consists of multiple small, round, lucent filling defects in the opacified pelvicaliceal system and ureter at the time of urography or retrograde pyelography (Fig. 7).

Urogenital Tuberculosis

Tuberculosis of the urinary tract is the most frequent of all extrapulmonary manifestations of this infection. It continues to be an important clinical problem because the nonspecific clinical presentation and variable radiologic appearance often mimic those of other pathologic conditions.

Urinary tract tuberculosis is predominantly a disease of young and middle-aged adults, being recognized only rarely in children and older persons (>60 years of age). Frequently, there is a history of tuberculosis affecting other organ systems. Genitourinary tuberculosis usually arises from hematogenous spread of *Myco-*

bacterium tuberculosis from a distant source, most commonly from the lungs. However, the chest roentgenogram will be negative in 50% of patients. In the remaining 50%, evidence of healed or active tuberculosis will be seen. The absence of pulmonary pathology in a patient suspected of having genitourinary tuberculosis, therefore, should not discourage further workup for tuberculosis. A tuberculin skin test will be positive in almost all patients unless cutaneous anergy exists. Aseptic pyuria should always suggest the possibility of urinary tract tuberculosis.

The clinical diagnosis of genitourinary tract tuberculosis can be made only by demonstrating the presence of *M. tuberculosis* in the urine or in biopsy material. Urine cultures are positive in 80% to 90% of patients with active disease.

In the earliest stages of the disease, with tuberculous infection established in the renal cortex, the radiographic findings will be normal in spite of positive urine cultures. The most important radiologic findings in later genitourinary tract tuberculosis are: (1) absence or impaired imaging of the collecting structures either focally or generally; (2) fuzzy irregularity or "moth-eaten" calices; (3) blunting or clubbing of the calices (Fig. 8); (4) cicatricial deformity and obliteration of one or more calices; (5) papillary cavities that may or may not communicate with the collecting structures; (6) parenchymal scarring with abnormality of the underlying calices, similar to the changes of chronic pyelonephritis; (7) dilatation of segments of the pelvicaliceal system secondary to cavitations associated with parenchymal destruction or to obstruction secondary to strictures with subsequent formation of localized hydrocalycosis or generalized pyelocaliectasis, depending on the site of the stenotic lesion; (8) mass lesions associated with formation of tuberculomas, noncommunicating tuberculous abscess, or tuberculous pyelonephrosis, which may lead to a mistaken diagnosis of neoplasm; and (9) calcification of the renal parenchyma, which should always raise the suspicion of tuberculosis. However, the type of calcification usually is not specific for tuberculosis, and the pattern and density are highly variable. It rarely takes the form of renal calculi; more often, curvilinear or lacy calcification outlines all or part of a renal tuberculoma or a dilated obstructed calix in patients with au-

tonephrectomy. A reniform collection of amorphous calcification is produced that may outline both the renal parenchyma and the renal pelvis (Fig. 9). Calcified psoas abscesses are frequently associated with radiographic evidence of tuberculous spinal involvement (Pott's disease) and are quite specific for tuberculosis. Calcifications of the prostate, seminal vesicles, and vas deferens may be present in association with tuberculosis of the urogenital tract. However, these deposits usually cannot be distinguished from similar calcifications having other causes. Calcification of the vas deferens in a young nondiabetic patient is highly suggestive of tuberculosis. In far-advanced cases, calcification of the ureter (usually in the pelvic segment) or bladder may be seen.

Another radiologic finding is stricture of the ureter. Dilatation and a ragged, irregular appearance of the urothelium that extends from the renal pelvis to the bladder is the first sign of ureteral tuberculosis; and as healing occurs, ureteral strictures are formed. Strictures have a predilection for points of natural narrowing (infundibular, ureteropelvic and ureterovesical junctions, and distal ureter) but may occur anywhere in the ureter, and may progress to incomplete or complete obstruction. This complete obstruction may be associated with pyonephrosis with parenchymal destruction and calcified caseation, the "putty" kidney. Strictures are highly variable in length and may be single or multiple. Sometimes, areas of stricture and dilatation alternate, giving the characteristic image of a string of pearls (the beaded ureter). At times, the ureter presents with a tortuous course because of confluent strictures and ulcerations and then is known as the "corkscrew" ureter. In advanced cases, another variety of involvement is represented by a thick-walled, shortened ureter with a narrow lumen, which is known as the "pipestem" ureter. All of these patterns are strongly suggestive of ureteral tuberculosis. A final possible radiologic finding is significant bladder abnormalities, although these are infrequent in spite of cystoscopically apparent disease. The most common finding on the cystogram with an interstitial cystitis is a thickened, spastic bladder of small capacity. The wall is typically smooth at this stage; at times, however, one encounters asymmetric involvement of the bladder, which is secondary to localized deformity from cicatrization or to a hyperplastic inflammatory lesion simulating a neoplasm.

Infections of the Bladder

Cystitis cannot be diagnosed definitely by radiologic methods. The diagnostic role of radiology is mainly as a supplement to demonstrate predisposing factors such as a calculus, diverticulum, and vesical outlet obstruction or complications associated with cystitis.

The principal radiographic findings in cystitis are: (1) bladder edema characterized by thickening of the mucosal folds or a cobblestone appearance of the mucosa; (2) thickening of the bladder wall; (3) small bladder; (4) single or multiple mucosal or submucosal filling defects; (5) the presence of a ring-like calcium in the bladder wall, which is highly suggestive of tuberculosis or schistosomiasis; and (6) the presence of gas in the wall or lumen of the bladder, which is almost pathognomonic of emphysematous cystitis.

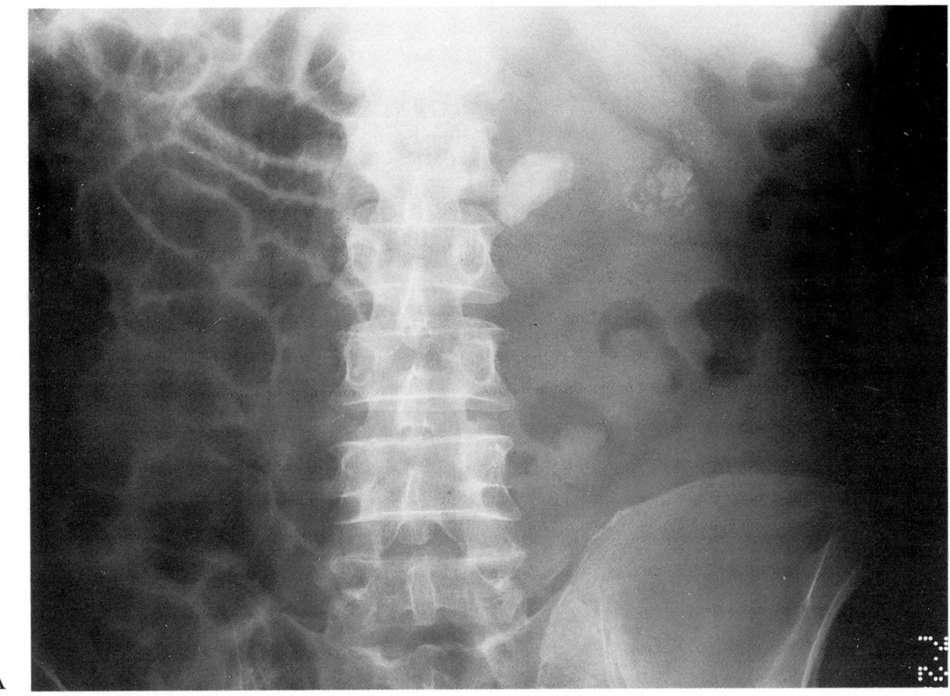

Figure 6.   Xanthogranulomatous pyelonephritis with invasion of the left psoas, left perirenal and postpararenal spaces, and soft tissues of the flank in a 77-year-old man admitted with left groin pain and a left lower-quadrant mass. (A) Flat plate shows multiple calcific masses in the left upper quadrant consistent with renal stones and a left-sided staghorn calculus, most likely causing obstruction.

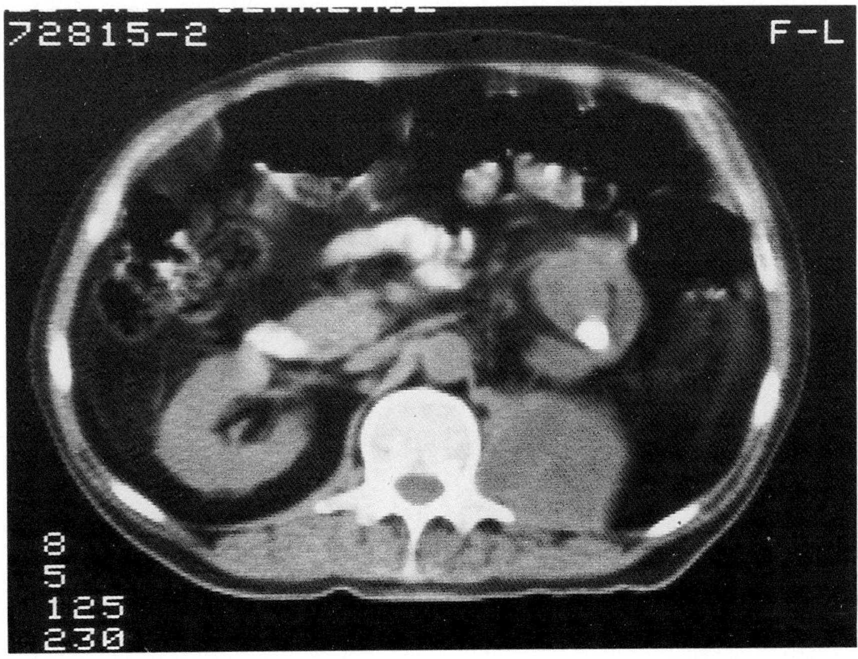

Figure 6B.   Xanthogranulomatous pyelonephritis on CT with left renal calculus, hydronephrosis, and invasion of the left psoas muscle.

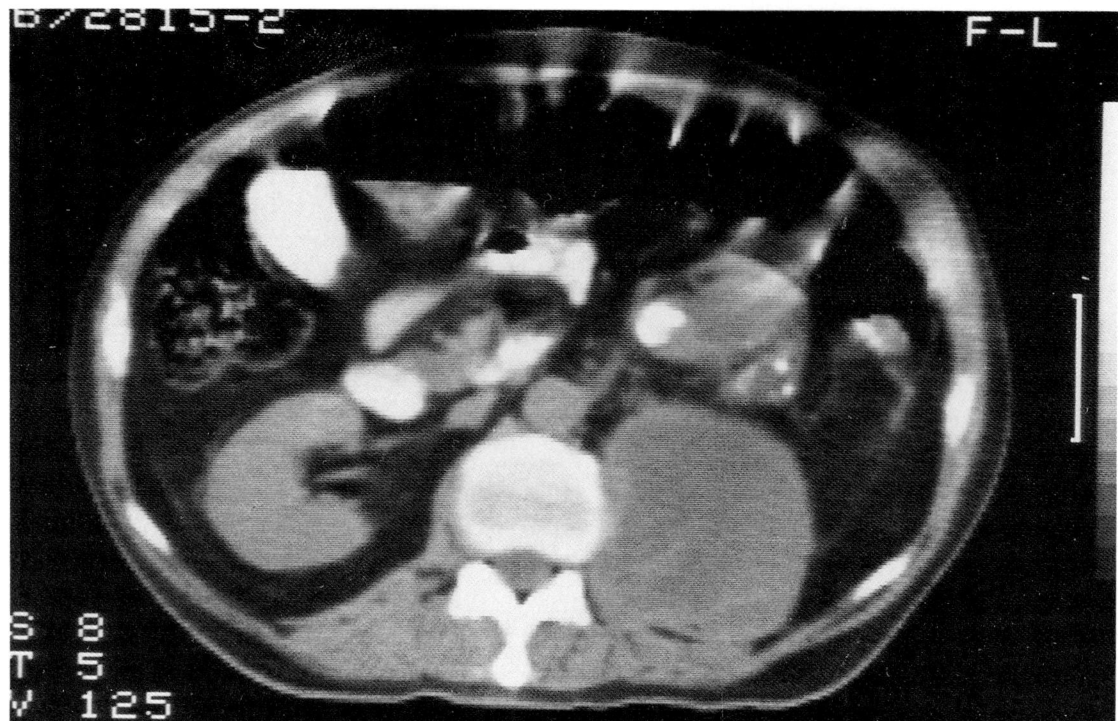

Figure 6C. CT showing calculus in left renal pelvis, multiple renal stones and xanthogranulomatous pyelonephritic invasion of the left psoas.

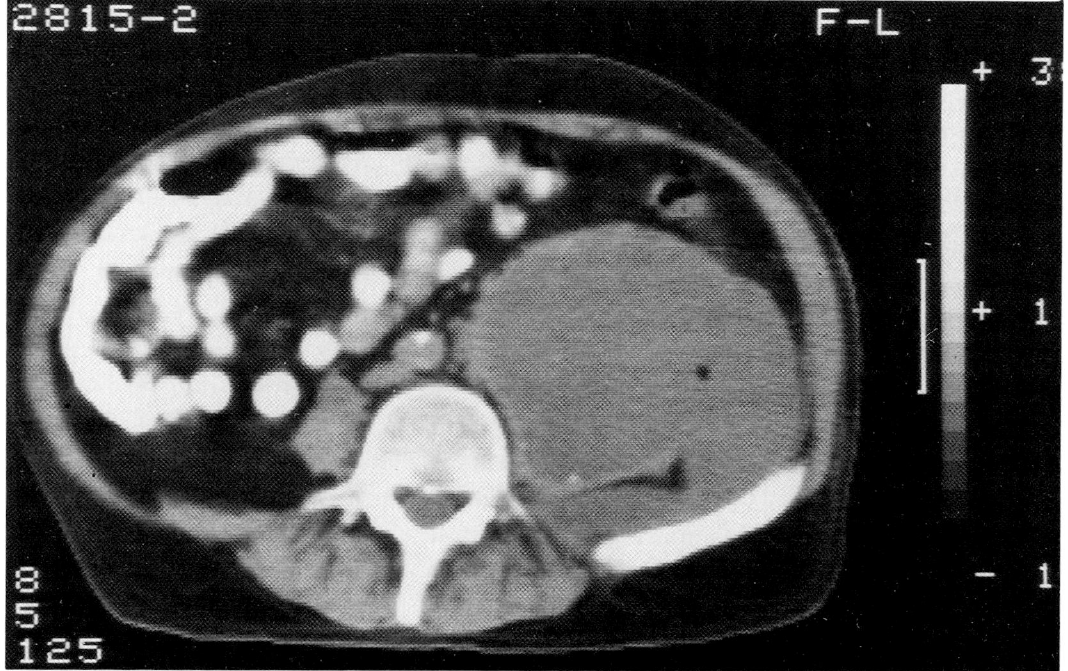

Figure 6D. Huge mass is seen on CT in the retroperitoneal space with an enhancing ring involving the psoas muscle, perirenal, and postrenal spaces, and soft tissues of the left flank.

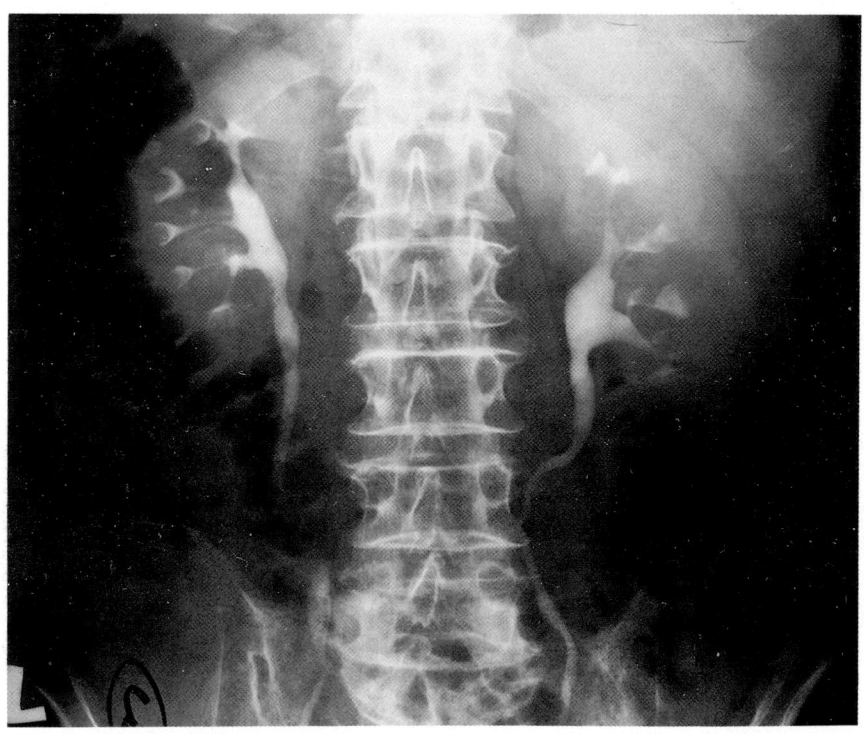

Figure 7.   Bilateral ureteritis cystica. An intravenous urogram demonstrates multiple small round filling defects in the upper ureters.

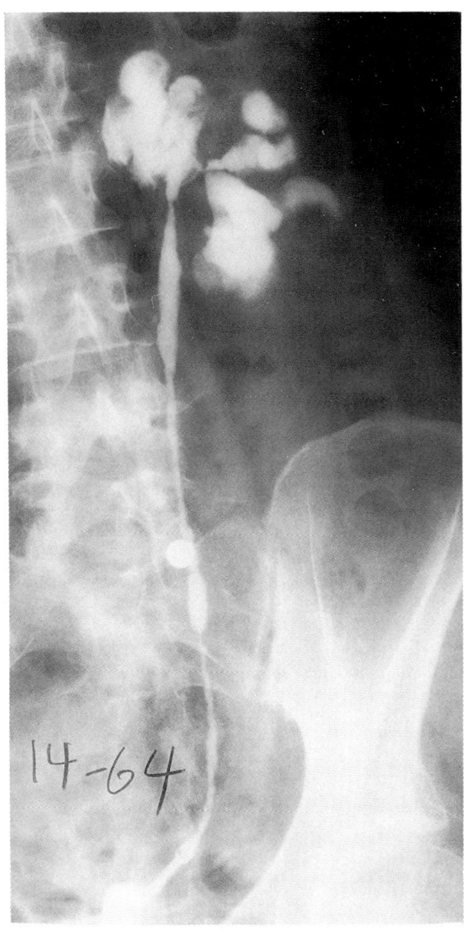

Figure 8.   Tuberculosis as seen on the retrograde pyelogram showing pipestem-type left ureter, marked stenosis of the left renal pelvis and a middle infundibulum and severe caliectasis with cavities.

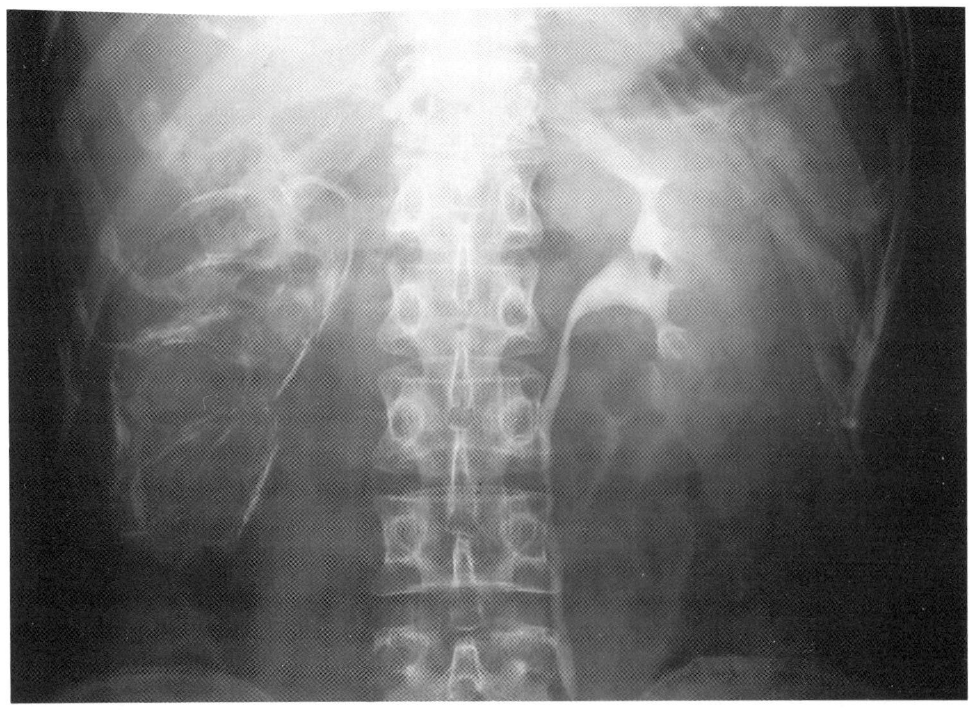

Figure 9.   Autonephrectomy caused by renal tuberculosis. Fifteen-minute urogram film shows nonfunctioning right kidney with reniform-like calcium deposits.

Chapter 3

Neoplasms of the Urinary Tract

Joaquim Vieira, M.D.

Tumors of the Kidney

Tumors of the kidney are usually carcinomas and together with tumors of the renal pelvis rank third in frequency among tumors of the urogenital system following carcinomas of the prostate and bladder. Most cases fall into one of four categories:

1. Adenocarcinoma of the renal parenchyma (hypernephroma) constitutes about 80% to 85% of all renal malignancies;
2. Carcinoma of the renal pelvis constitutes about 8% to 12% of all renal malignancies;
3. Nephroblastoma (Wilms' tumor) constitutes about 5% to 8% of all renal malignancies;
4. Sarcoma constitutes about 1.3% to 3.0% of all renal malignancies.

There also are benign renal tumors that are important primarily because it may be necessary to distinguish them from carcinomas.

Benign Tumors

Benign renal tumors, which are often found at autopsy, are generally smaller than 2 cm. Therefore, they rarely attain significant clinical importance. Larger benign tumors have symptomatology and radiographic findings similar to those of malignant neoplasms, and the benignity often is first recognized postoperatively. However, occasionally, adenoma, angioma, and angiomyolipoma may be suspected preoperatively.

Adenomas arise from the mature renal tubules and are divided histologically into three types: papillary, alveolar, and tubular. Because the majority of renal adenomas are less than 3 cm in diameter, they usually are asymptomatic, being discovered incidentally during surgical exploration or radiologic evaluation of other existing or suspected renal diseases. Almost half (55%) are associated with carcinomas. Adenomas are invariably cortical and may be cystic (cystadenoma). The different types are not distinguishable radiologically and show on the intravenous urogram (IVU) as a small mass with a thick wall, which differentiates them from simple cysts. Angiography usually shows a hypovascular mass with minimal neovascularization, and computerized tomography (CT) shows an isodense to hypodense nonenhancing mass.

In the last decade, attention has been given to the renal *oncocytoma*, which is a proximal tubular adenoma composed of oncocytes. These are considered altered epithelial cells and have eosinophilic, finely granular cytoplasm of large volume, filled with a great abundance of mitochondria under electron microscopy. Oncocytomas usually are asymptomatic, being discovered

---

From *Imaging of Urologic Disorders* edited by Alexander S. Cass, MBBS, © 1992, Futura Publishing Inc., Mount Kisco, NY.

as an incidental finding during physical examination, urography, or laparotomy for other complaints. They are slowly growing, benign, solid tumors without invasion of the perinephric fat, renal pelvis, or renal vein. They are characterized by long-term survival without evidence of metastatic involvement. Grossly, they are brown (similar to renal tissue), well encapsulated, and, usually, homogeneous in appearance except for an occasional central scar.

The angiography strongly suggests the features of an oncocytoma which are a spoke-wheel appearance of the vascular supply; a homogeneous capillary nephrographic phase (similar in density to the normal nephrogram); sharp, smooth margination with a lucent rim; and absence of arteriovenous shunting or puddling (Fig. 1). On CT examination, oncocytomas are round, well-marginated masses with homogeneous contrast enhancement. Some lesions, especially the bigger ones, show a stellate central scar that is highly suggestive of this type of tumor. It should be noted, however, that no radiologic finding is pathognomonic of oncocytoma, as all these characteristics can sometimes be found in renal carcinomas or angiomyolipomas. Even needle biopsy of a portion of the tumor is not definitive because well-differentiated renal cell carcinoma (RCC) may have portions with oncocytic features.

Hemangiomas are less than 2 cm in diameter in most cases, and in the greater majority (90%), they are located near the renal pelvis. Larger lesions have a tendency to be subcapsular and may result in a perirenal hematoma. On angiography, the majority of these lesions appear hypervascular, and on CT, a well-demarcated, round mass of low density without significant enhancement usually is seen. Clinical clues may be of help. For example, hemorrhage from a hemangioma frequently is intermittent and occurs over a long period of time. Also, the age of onset is between 20 and 40 years in approximately 70% of cases.

Angiomyolipoma is a hamartoma that, as the name implies, is composed of variable amounts of vascular, muscular, and lipoid tissue. This benign tumor occurs in the kidney in particular clinical settings including: (1) associated with tuberous sclerosis, in which case, the tumor is usually multiple and bilateral (about 80% of patients with complete or severe forms of tuberous sclerosis have renal angiomyolipomas) (Fig. 2); (2) associated with lymphangiomatosis; and (3) in a symptomatic form unassociated with any syndrome or disease (the most common type). In the last circumstance, the tumors are usually unilateral, solitary renal masses and appear especially in women during the third and fifth decades. The right kidney is more often involved than the left (80%). Bleeding and pain associated with that bleeding are the most common symptoms; and (4) an asymptomatic form, in which the tumor is found incidentally by CT or ultrasound or at autopsy (Fig. 3). The tumor might be tiny (less than 1 cm) or larger (up to 5 cm).

Hamartomas may recur locally and may invade the renal vein and metastasize to the regional lymph nodes, although distant metastases are unknown. Another characteristic that sets the hamartoma apart from other benign renal tumors is the tendency for spontaneous infarcts or hemorrhages to develop deep within the tumor and cause severe pain. Spontaneous rupture with profuse retroperitoneal hemorrhage is an uncommon feature of this tumor; however, perirenal hematomas occur in 25% of cases.

The majority of angiomyolipomas are hypervascular angiographically; the few (less than 5%) that are hypovascular usually are myolipomas. Angiographically, the lesions are very similar to RCC and because of this, in the past, they were often misinterpreted as malignant masses. There are several angiographic characteristics that are suggestive of angiomyolipoma: (1) the presence of aneurysms resembling a cluster of grapes; (2) the absence of arteriovenous shunts; and (3) the presence of a whorled onion-peel appearance of the pathologic vessels. However, these characteristics are not always present. Hence, in most instances, the angiographic findings are not distinctive enough to rule out the diagnosis of RCC, and the diagnosis is dependent on the detection of fatty constituents of the tumor by CT (see Fig. 3) except on the rare occasion when there is no mature fat in the tumor. Hemorrhage, a frequent early complication of this lesion, may be of sufficient volume to obscure the fatty elements within the tumor, in which case, the proper diagnosis cannot be made by CT. The differential diagnosis of liposarcoma and angiomyolipoma can be impossible by CT; in such cases, angiography will help. Liposarcomas usually are hypovascular, and angiographic diagnosis is characterized by tumorous vessel encasement.

Adenocarcinoma (Hypernephroma; Renal Cell Carcinoma)

Renal cell carcinomas constitute 3% of all malignant neoplasms. They arise from the proximal tubular epithelial cells, have their peak incidence in the fifth and seventh decades, and are more than three times more frequent in men than in women. The two kidneys are affected equally, and each pole is involved in 40% to 45% of cases. About 5% of renal adenocarcinomas have multiple cystic areas, but the occurrence of a small tumor in the wall of a cyst is rare.

The classic triad of hematuria, flank mass, and flank pain occurs in 10% to 15% of patients, and in almost half of these individuals, metastases will already be present. Calcification is noted radiographically in 10% of renal carcinomas: of all calcified renal masses, 58% are carcinomas; 90% of mottled calcified masses and 20% of those peripherally calcified are malignant.

Renal carcinomas metastasize most commonly (approximately 69%) and earliest to the lungs. Other frequent sites of spread are the liver (34%), bone (42%), para-aortic lymph nodes (35%), adrenal glands (20%), and brain (7%). In about 7% of patients, there is bilateral renal involvement, discovered either initially or at various times after treatment of the first lesion. It is not clear whether these contralateral lesions represent bilateral independent primary tumors or metastases from the first lesion.

Renal cell carcinomas are generally staged as follows:

Stage I: Confined to the kidney
Stage II: Perirenal fat involvement but not beyond Gerota's fascia
Stage IIIA: Renal vein invasion that may extend into the inferior vena cava
Stage IIIB: Involvement of regional lymph nodes
Stage IIIC: Both venous and lymph node involvement
Stage IVA: Spread to adjacent organs, excluding the ipsilateral adrenal gland
Stage IVB: Distant metastases

Staging of RCC can be accomplished by CT, but magnetic resonance imaging (MRI) has proved to be slightly more accurate, particularly for assessing the vascular extension of the tumor. Radiology with current techniques plays an important role in the detection, diagnosis, and staging of RCC. Small, low-stage carcinomas are now commonly identified during abdominal sonography or CT performed for nonrenal complaints. Indeed, almost as many new renal carcinomas are currently being detected incidentally as are being found by evaluation of the symptoms and signs usually associated with this tumor.

The roentgenographic diagnosis is made by different modalities. *Excretory urography* very often shows space-occupying masses; bulging or obliteration of the renal contours; enlargement and displacement of renal shadows; and displacement, compression, elongation, and amputation of the pelvicaliceal system. However, the nature of a renal mass usually cannot be determined by this method, although at times, there are urographic signs that suggest RRC: the presence of amorphous, patchy, central calcifications; a smooth or irregular filling defect in the renal pelvis and calices; or absence of renal function, which usually indicates renal vein occlusion by the neoplasm.

On *sonography*, RCC usually appears as a solid mass with poor transonicity. The mass may be hyperechoic, isoechoic, or hypoechoic compared with the normal renal cortex and often appears complex because of hemorrhage and necrosis. Sonography is inferior to CT as far as staging is concerned; however, very often, sonography is useful for showing proximal vena caval and right arterial tumor extension (Fig. 4).

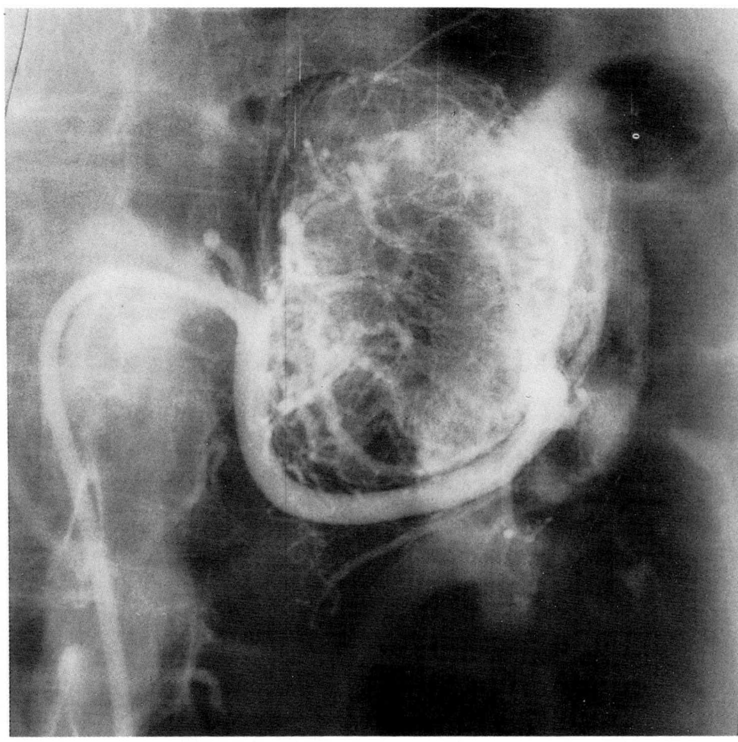

Figure 1A.   Oncocytoma. Arteriographic phase of the angiogram reveals a spoke-wheel appearance of the pathologic vessels.

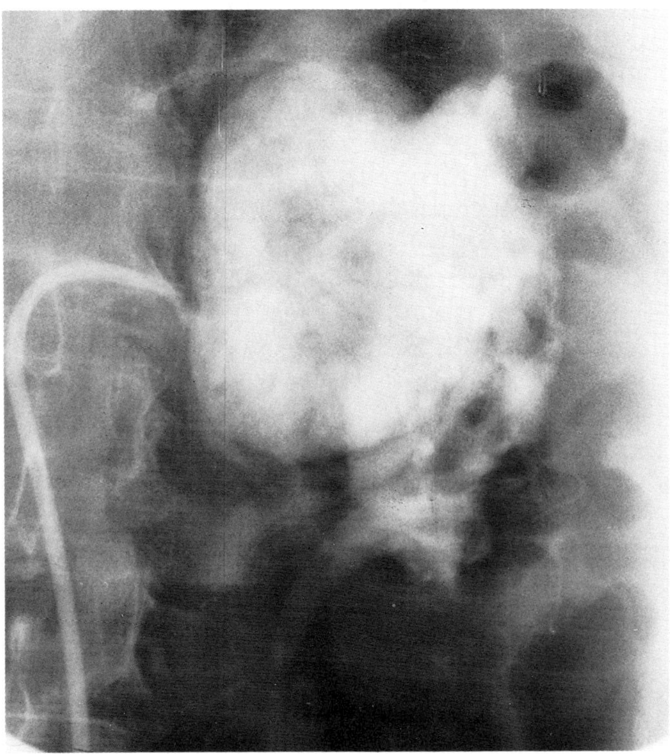

Figure 1B.   On nephrographic phase, homogeneous tumor staining is apparent except for its center, most likely because of central scarring.

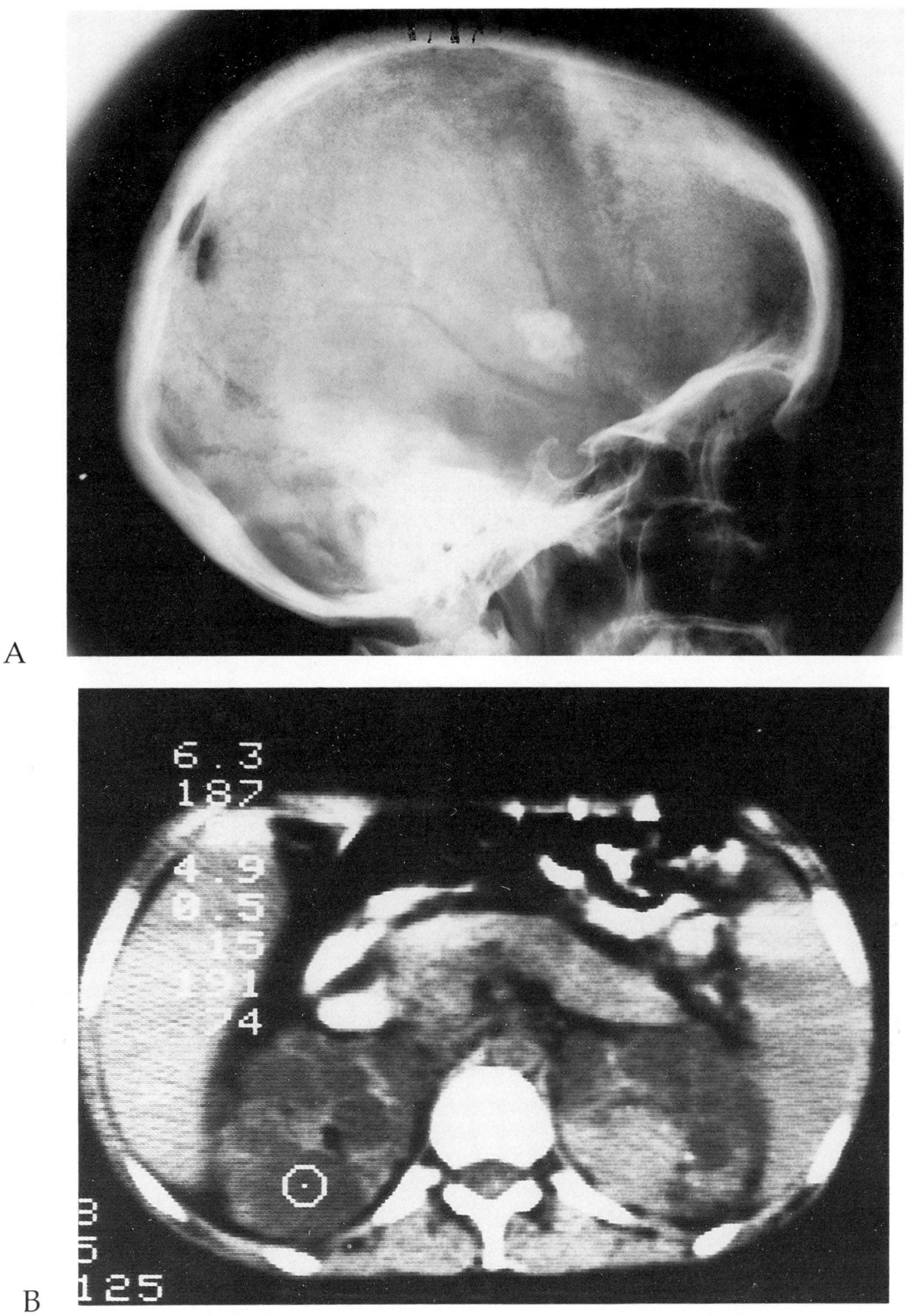

Figure 2. Multiple angiomyolipomas in a patient with tuberous sclerosis. (A,top) Skull films reveal periventricular calcium and thickening of the cranial vault. (B, bottom) CT shows multiple intrarenal fat masses consistent with angiomyolipomas.

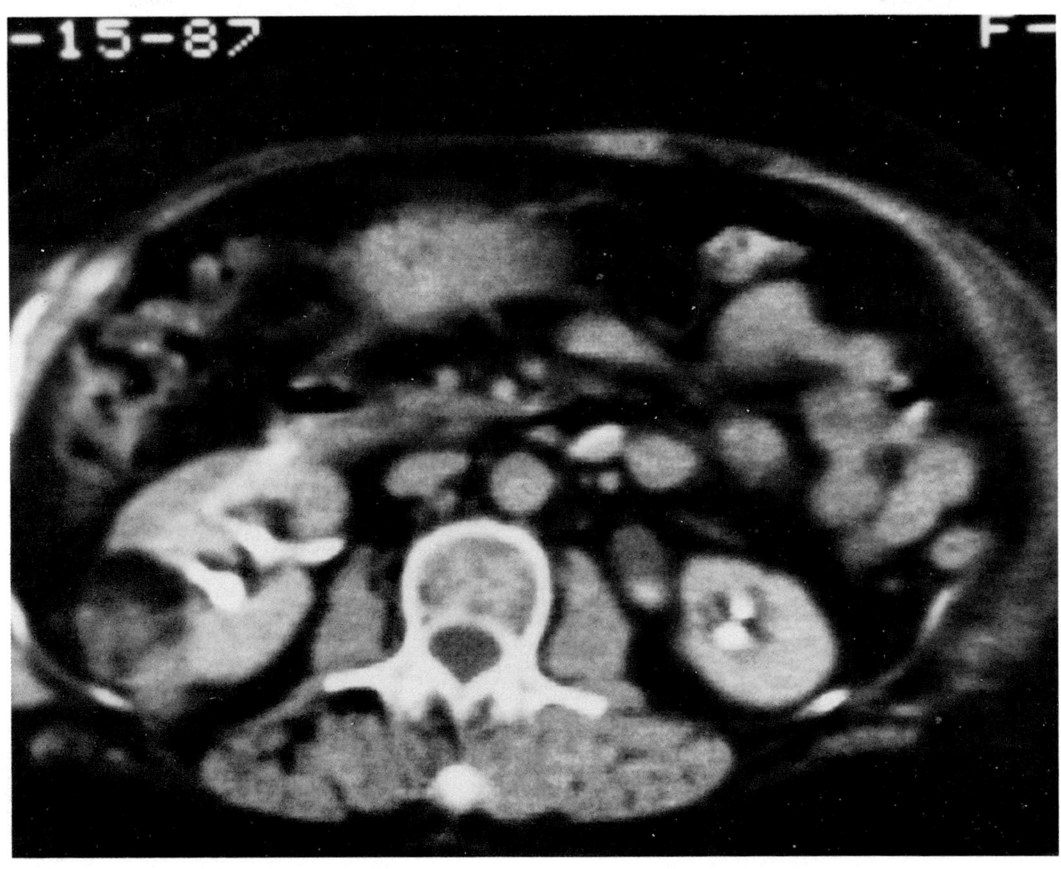

Figure 3.   Angiomyolipoma. CT shows mass in the middle third of the right kidney with fat component (129 HU [Hounsfield units]).

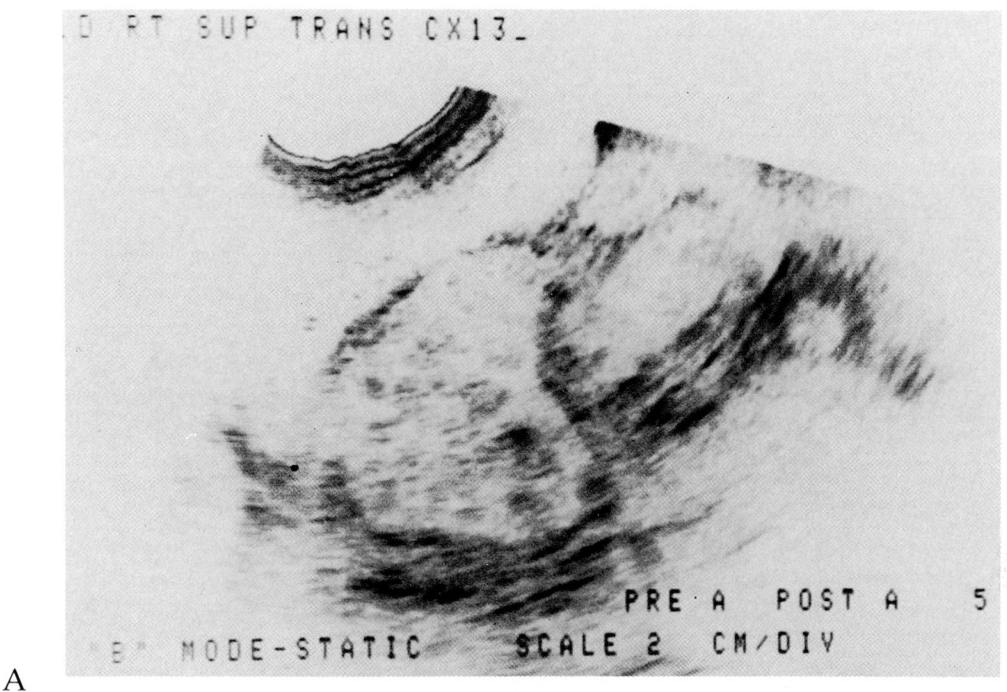

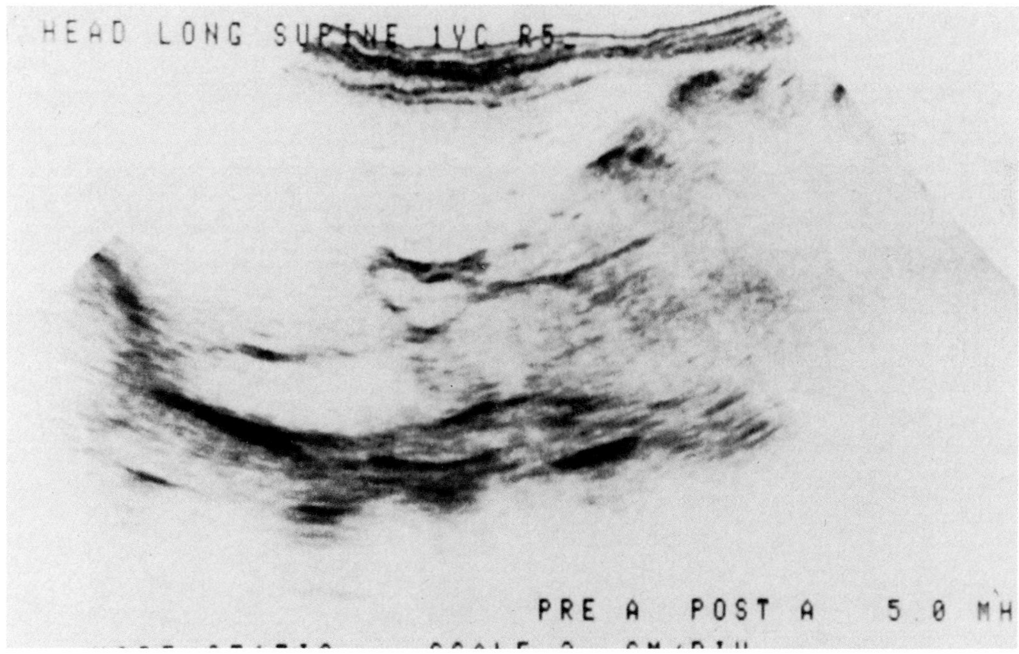

Figure 4.   Renal cell carcinoma with right renal vein and inferior vena cava thrombi. (A, top) Axial ultrasound shows an echogenic mass at the right upper pole with involvement of the right renal vein and inferior vena cava. (B, bottom) Longitudinal ultrasound shows echogenic shadows within the inferior vena cava consistent with malignant thrombi.

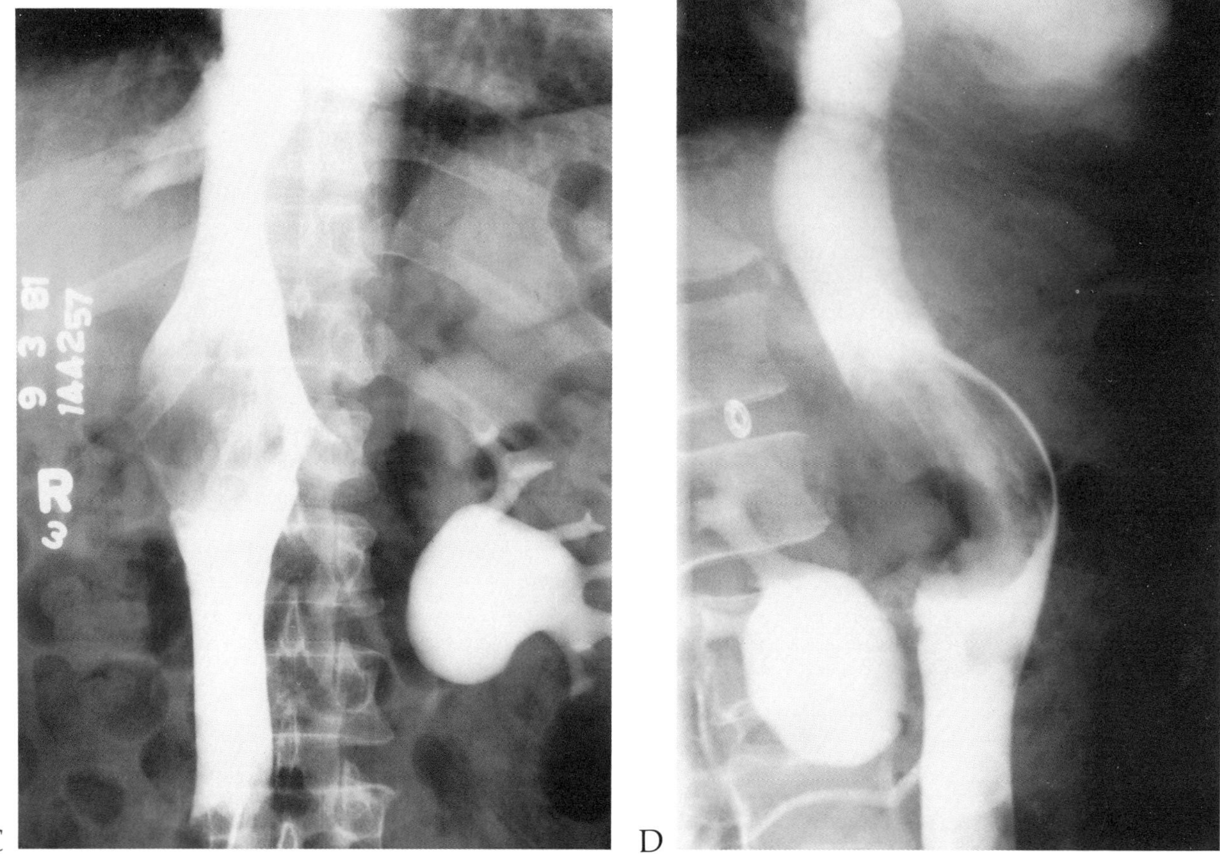

C

D

Figures 4C,D.   (C, left) Anteroposterior and (D, right) lateral inferior venacavographies show a huge filling defect consistent with malignant thrombus.

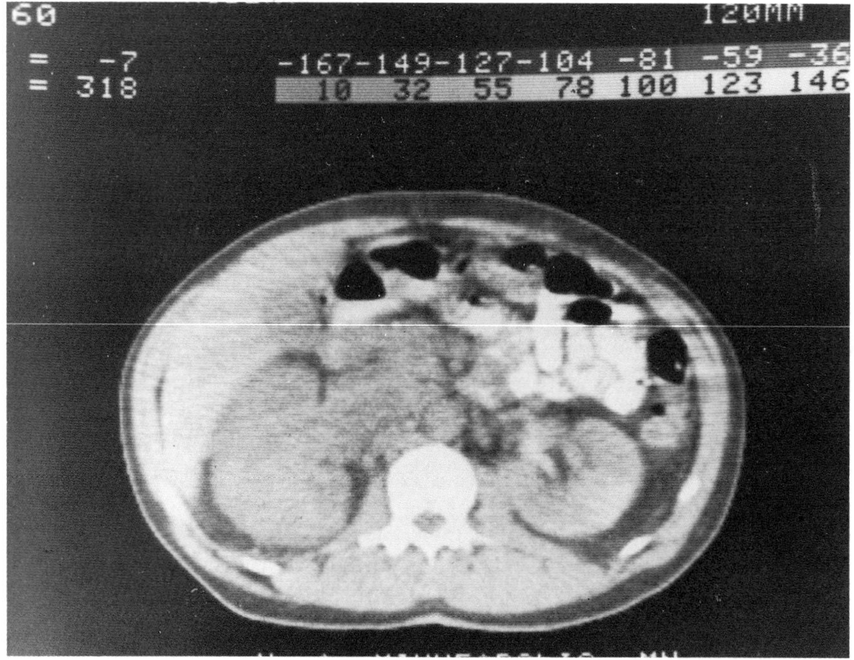

Figure 4E.   Computed tomography shows a mass at the right upper pole with involvement of the right renal vein and inferior vena cava.

Computed tomography can detect renal masses because they differ in density from the normal parenchyma or because they alter the contour of the kidney, projecting beyond the normal margin (Figs. 5 and 6). Because a tissue-specific diagnosis is not possible by CT, differentiation between RCC and other solid renal tumors cannot be accomplished in this way. However, CT has proved to be extremely accurate in distinguishing a benign cyst from a neoplasm. The features important for this differentiation are: (1) the attenuation value of the mass; (2) the presence or absence of enhancement; (3) the demarcation of the mass from normal renal parenchyma; and (4) the thickness of the wall of the mass. Computed tomography also is very useful in the differentiation of tumors and pseudotumors such as dromedary humps, fetal lobulation, lobar compensatory hypertrophy, and Bertin's column. All these pseudotumors contain functioning nephrons, and none produce a defect on the CT image. Also, unlike pathologic renal masses, they enhance after contrast injection to the same degree as functioning normal renal parenchyma. Some renal carcinomas are isodense with normal renal parenchyma on precontrast images. Therefore, a small tumor may not be visible, whereas large neoplasms usually produce a mass effect. On postcontrast scans, the RCC is enhanced but usually to a lesser degree than normal renal parenchyma, and enhancement is usually inhomogeneous because of tumor hemorrhage and necrosis. The malignant mass usually shows an indistinct interface with the surrounding parenchyma and often has lobulated or irregular outer margins. The CT scan shows amorphous central calcifications in 15% to 30%, but it is particularly helpful in evaluating a renal mass with a ring-like calcification. Demonstration of a soft-tissue mass extending beyond the calcification clearly indicates the neoplastic nature of the lesion. A diagnostic accuracy exceeding 95% can be reached by using strict CT criteria.

Magnetic resonance imaging is accurate in staging RCC (Fig. 7) and is especially useful in detecting venous tumor extension, particularly in evaluating the superior extent of the caval thrombus relative to the diaphragm, hepatic veins, and right atrium (Fig. 8). It will also be helpful in clarifying contiguous involvement of adjacent viscera.

Angiography should be reserved for renal masses that are indeterminate by nephrotomography, ultrasound, and CT. There are three patterns of abnormal vascularity of kidney tumors: (1) typical and usual hypervascular; (2) reticular neovascularity; (3) hypovascular (so-called "avascular"). Most RCCs show the typical hypervascular pattern characterized by "tumor" vessels, which are irregular in outline, tortuous with absence of normal tapering, variable in size, and unpredictable in branching (Fig. 9). Other angiographic possible characteristics are arteriovenous shunts; microaneurysms; pooling and puddling of contrast material; accentuated rim stain; diffuse tumor blush; parasitic vessels feeding the mass; nonopacification of the renal vein, thrombus in the renal vein, or streaking by neoplastic vessels in the confines of the vein; and early and rapid opacification of the main renal vein and inferior vena cava because of multiple large arteriovenous shunts.

Approximately 15% of RCCs are marked by a hypovascular or "avascular" appearance, and therefore, are confused with cystic lesions. Although they may appear "avascular", careful examination usually discloses abnormal vessels entering the mass from the periphery. The proper diagnosis in these cases can be made by paying proper attention to the marginal abnormal vessels, the thick rims of tumor, and an irregular interface of the tumor with the normal parenchyma. Ultrasound and CT are helpful in making the differential diagnosis.

The diagnostic accuracy of angiography can be enhanced by magnification, subtraction, liberal use of oblique views, and injection of epinephrine.

Tumorous involvement of the renal vein and inferior vena cava can be demonstrated by inferior *venocavography*, selective renal *venography*, and high-dose (30 ml) arteriography. Selective renal venography should not be attempted unless inferior venocavography has shown no extension of tumor into the vena cava to avoid dislodging fragments of the tumor thrombus to distant sites. Renal vein tumor extension, which happens in 25% to 45% of cases, may be suspected if the vein shows a filling defect, if it fails to opacify after high-dose arteriography, or vascularized tumor thrombus with streaking and a striated pattern is demonstrated (see Fig. 9). When the vena cava contains tumor, it is necessary to evaluate the upper extent of this thrombus, as resection of the renal tumor and its venous extension en bloc improves the survival rate.

Sarcoma of the Kidney

Sarcoma of the kidney is an uncommon neoplasm representing 1.3% to 3.0% of all primary malignant renal tumors. Most cases probably originate from the renal capsule. The most usual type has a tendency to produce large masses, often encapsulated or semiencapsulated, that compress and displace the kidney, metastasize early and widely, and usually grow rapidly.

Most renal sarcomas are radiologically indistinguishable, although there are a few exceptions. For instance, in small liposarcomas and osteosarcomas, fat and bone (starburst ossification) may easily be detected by either plain abdominal radiographs or CT. Absence of lymphadenopathy is to be expected. Angiographically, most renal sarcomas are hypovascular, the notable exception being the very vascular hemangiopericytoma. Arteriovenous shunts and tumor staining are seldom present. As expected, the primary blood supply to the mass is often through capsular vessels (Fig. 10). Magnetic resonance imaging offers promise in detecting fibrous neoplasms, since the signal intensity of these lesions will not increase with T2 weighting.

Renal Metastases

Metastases to the kidney are encountered twice as frequently as primary renal tumors. Most are small (<3 cm), multiple (80%), and bilateral (50%). Excluding renal infiltration by lymphoma and chronic leukemia, the neoplasms that most commonly metastasize to the kidneys are carcinomas of the lung (by far the most common), breast, and gastrointestinal tract (especially the stomach), and melanoma. However, almost any organ can be the site of the primary lesion, including, as noted above, the contra-

lateral kidney. There can be direct extension from a tumor of the pancreas, adrenal gland, or colon.

Renal metastases are of relatively minor clinical importance as they usually are a late finding in a patient with widespread cancer, and they rarely cause symptoms. Nonetheless, antemortem diagnosis is not uncommon owing to the frequent use of cross-sectional imaging (especially CT) for staging and follow-up studies in cancer (Fig. 11).

Differentiating a renal metastasis from a primary RCC or other condition that mimics metastases, such as diffuse renal lymphoma, infiltrating transitional cell carcinoma, and acute renal inflammation (pyelonephritis or renal phlegmon) may be difficult. In a few cases, aspiration biopsy may be necessary for the definite diagnosis, especially when there is no other evidence of metastatic disease.

Wilms' Tumor

Wilms' tumor is rarely suspected in adults, but even though it is uncommon beyond adolescence, physicians should always keep in mind that this lesion is not limited to the young. The microscopic features and imaging characteristics are similar to those of the tumors seen in infancy and childhood (Fig. 12).

Wilms' tumor is one of the most common intra-abdominal malignancies in children. The peak incidence of this tumor is between 2.5 and 3 years of age. The tumor is generally unilateral, but the bilateral variety has been reported in 5% of cases. The bilateral variety is very often associated with nodular blastema or nephroblastomatosis and also has a tendency to be associated with other congenital anomalies. Because of this, bilateral Wilms' tumors are considered by some authors to be familial.

A palpable abdominal mass is an important clue to the diagnosis, being present in 60% to 90% of patients. About 50% of the patients have low-grade fever and hypertension. Hematuria is uncommon (20%).

Approximately 15% of all children with Wilms' tumor have associated congenital abnormalities, which include congenital hemihypertrophy, sporadic nonfamilial aniridia, Beck-with-Wiedmann syndrome, cerebral gigantism, pseudohermaphroditism, neurofibromatosis, and several types of chromosomal abnormalities. All patients with these entities should be followed closely for the early diagnosis of Wilms' tumor.

Wilms' tumor is usually a triphasic embryonic neoplasm containing epithelial, blastemal, and stromal elements. It is usually solid with a pseudocapsule that separates it from the normal renal parenchyma. Frequently, it contains areas of hemorrhage and necrosis, and in many instances (30% to 40%), there is invasion of the renal vein. Spread to the lungs is frequent, with other less common sites of metastases being the liver, para-aortic and mediastinal lymph nodes, bones, and the brain.

Few studies are generally needed for the diagnosis of Wilms' tumor. A scout radiograph of the abdomen discloses a soft-tissue mass in the region of the kidney. Mottled or curvilinear calcifications occur infrequently (about 5% to 10%). Excretory urography very often shows an intrinsic lesion characterized by stretching and distortion of the pelvicaliceal system without renal displacement (Fig. 13). Nonfunction of the kidney is found in as many as 10% of the cases, usually secondary to a massive tumor with extension into the renal pelvis or renal vein involvement. Sonography demonstrates an echogenic complex mass. At the same time, the presence or absence of tumor thrombosis within the inferior vena cava and right atrium can be determined.

Computed tomography confirms the intra-renal location of the tumor, which presents as a mass of low attenuation with inhomogeneous contrast enhancement. Calcification is identified in 10% to 15% of cases. The study also allows evaluation of the renal arteries and veins, inferior vena cava, adjacent lymph nodes, liver, and contralateral kidney, which can be evaluated better by this method than by ultrasound. Chest CT should also be performed, because pulmonary metastases are present in more than 10% of patients at the time of initial diagnosis.

Magnetic resonance imaging may prove to be the favored primary imaging technique for Wilms' tumor. Its advantages include the absence of ionizing radiation, the large anatomic field of display, the capacity for multiple views, increased contrast sensitivity, and the ability to demonstrate blood vessels to look for venous thrombus and invasion and displacement of the aorta and inferior vena cava.

Angiography has practically lost its role in the radiologic diagnosis of Wilms' tumor.

Wilms' tumor must be differentiated from hydronephrosis, multicystic kidney, congenital mesoblastic nephroma, neuroblastoma, pheochromocytomic adrenal adenoma, carcinoma, and adrenal hemorrhage. When a neuroblastoma invades the kidney, it may be impossible to differentiate from Wilms' tumor. However, neuroblastomas are more likely to be calcified, and they tend to push the kidney inferiorly and laterally, causing displacement of calices but not intrarenal distortion. Also, they are more likely to cross the midline than is Wilms' tumor. Biochemical assays of the urine for the metabolites of the catecholamines (metanephrines and vanillylmandelic acid) are helpful in cases of suspected neuroblastoma.

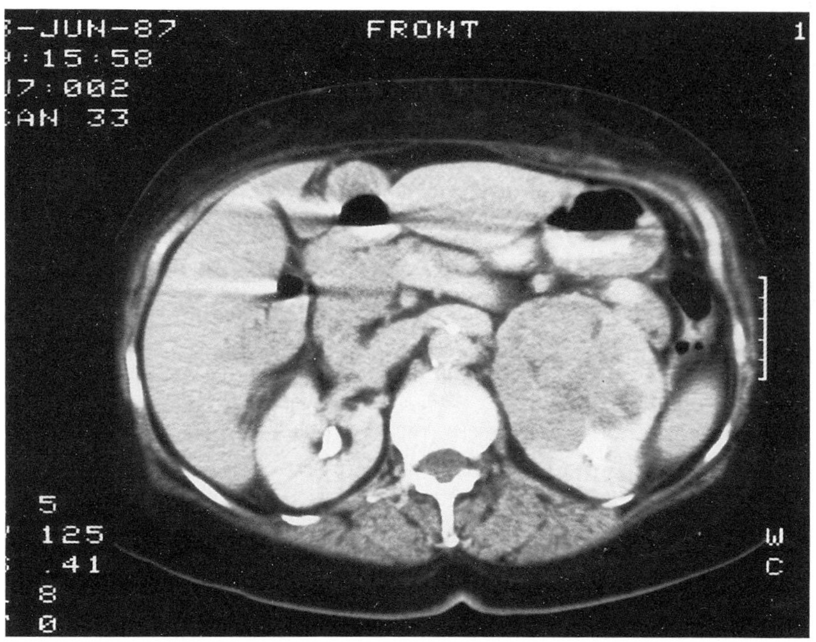

Figure 5A.   Computed tomography shows a necrotic mass at the left upper pole consistent with RCC. There is no evidence of enlarged regional lymph nodes, and the left renal vein is fairly well seen and normal.

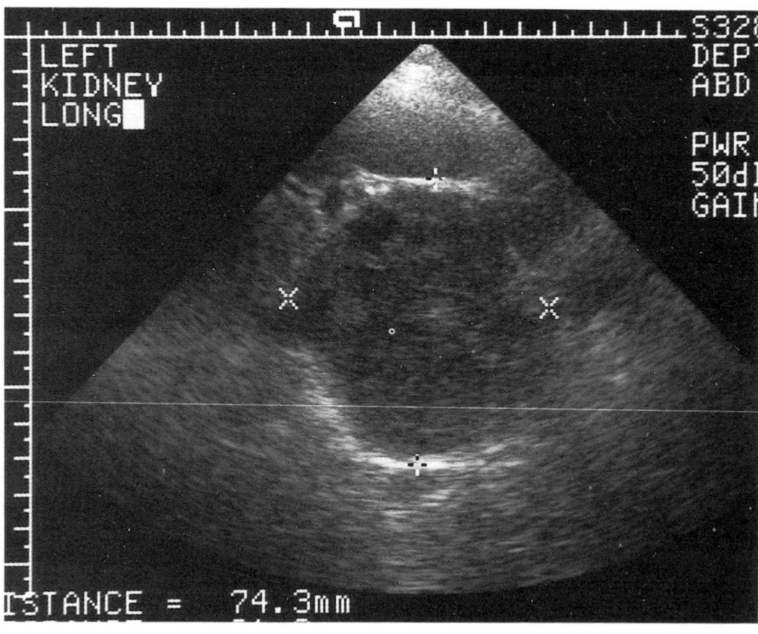

Figure 5B.   Ultrasound reveals an echogenic mass at the left upper pole measuring approximately 8 × 7.5 cm and consistent with a solid mass, most likely hypernephroma.

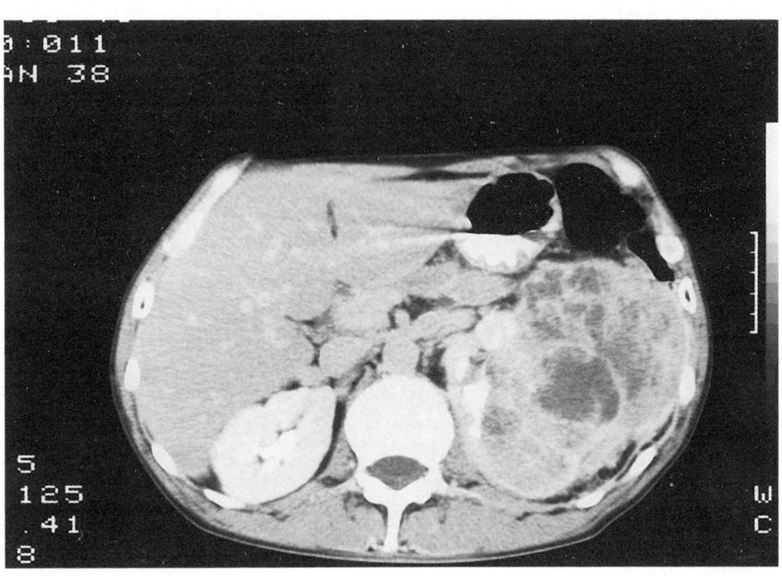

Figure 6.   Computed tomography shows a huge necrotic mass involving the left kidney consistent with RCC.

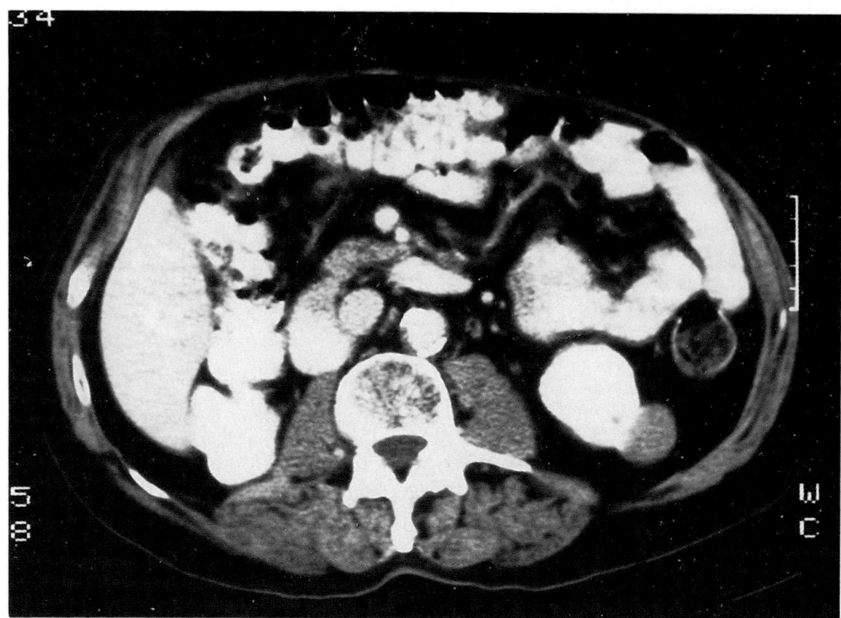

Figure 7A.   Contralateral renal metastasis after a right nephrectomy for renal cell carcinoma. Previous CT of this mass was interpreted as showing a cyst on the left kidney. CT scan with contrast revealed a mass on the lateral aspect of the lower pole.

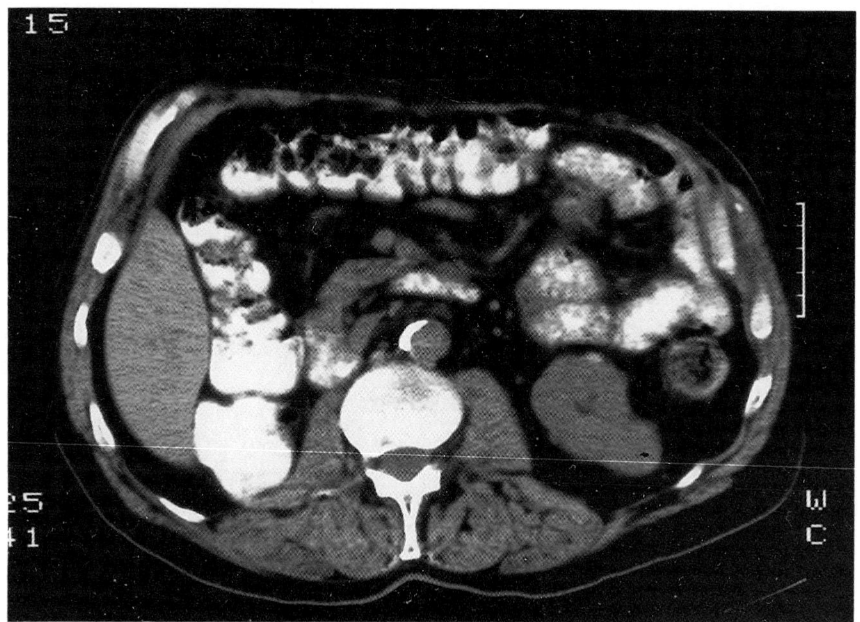

Figures 7B.   CT scan without contrast shows a mass on the lateral aspect of the left kidney. Density without contrast 22 HU; with contrast 67 HU, suggesting a solid mass.

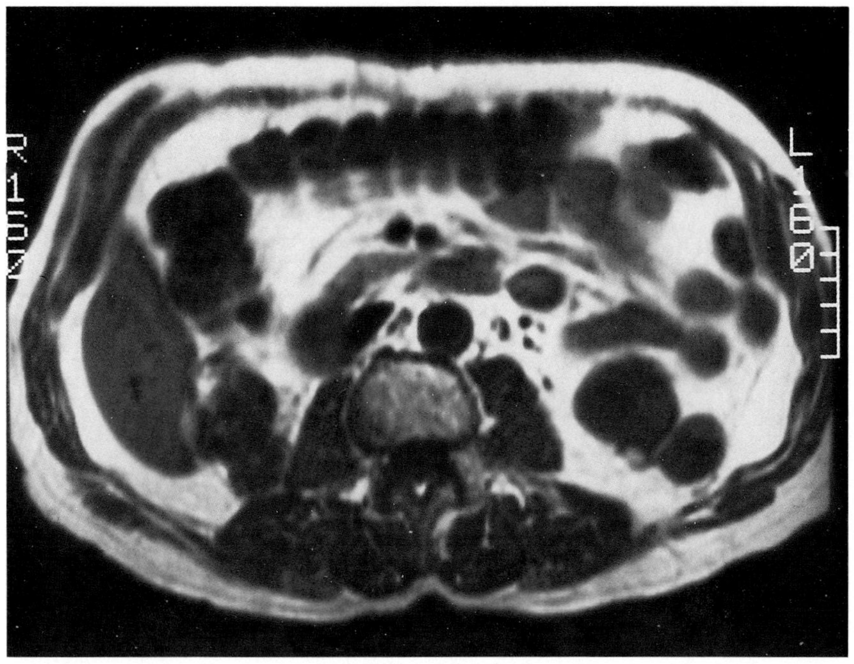

Figures 7C.   Axial MRI scan with T1 weighting reveals a mass of decreased signal at the lateral aspect of the left lower pole.

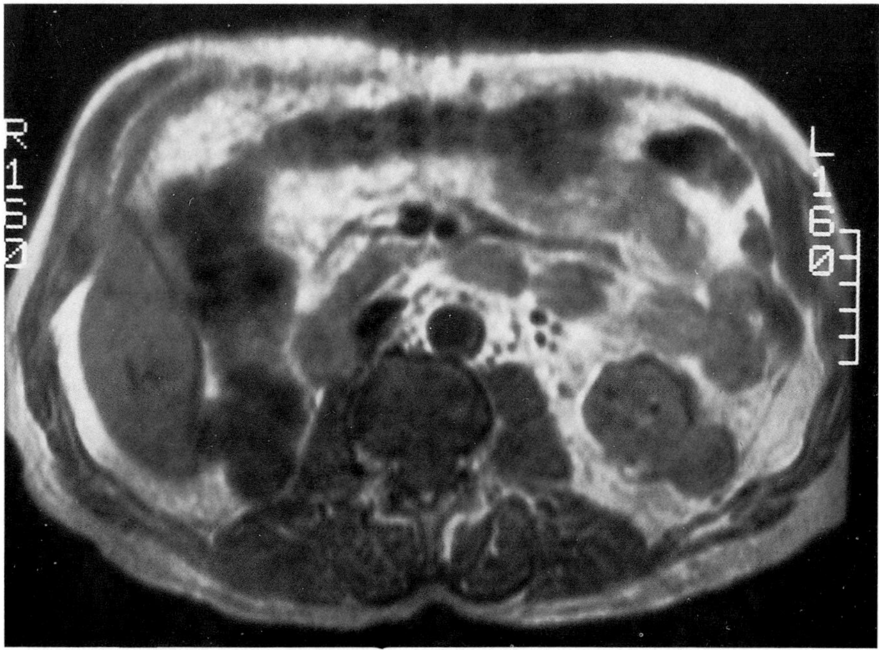

Figure 7D.   The U (proton) scan also shows a mass of decreased signal in same site.

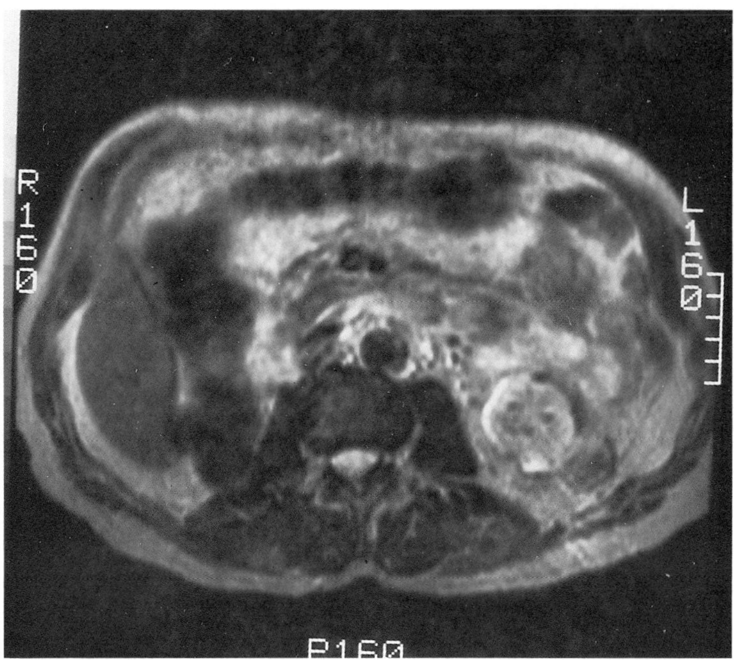

Figures 7E.   The mass is of intermediate signal intensity on T2-weighted scans.

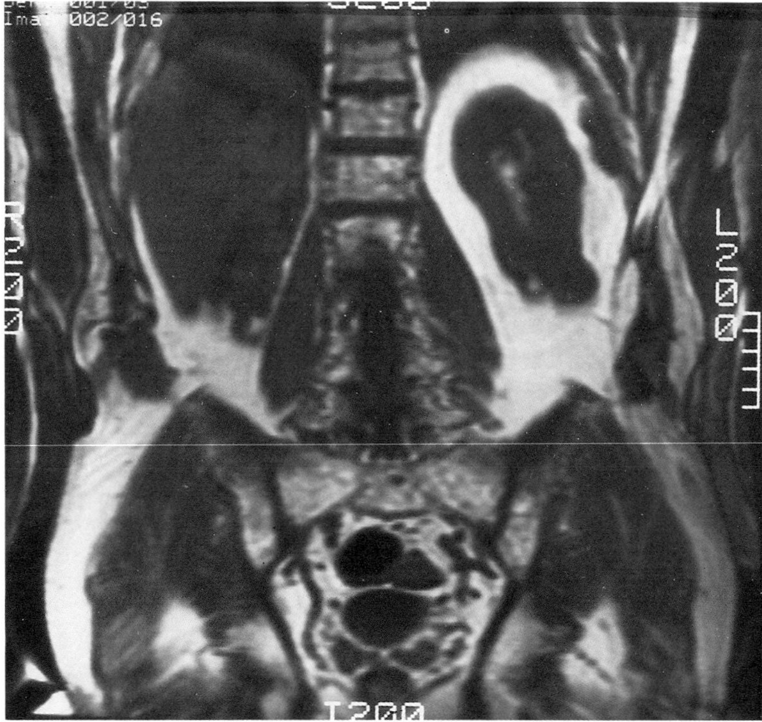

Figure 7F.   Coronal MRI scan with T1 weighting revealed a mass of decreased signal.

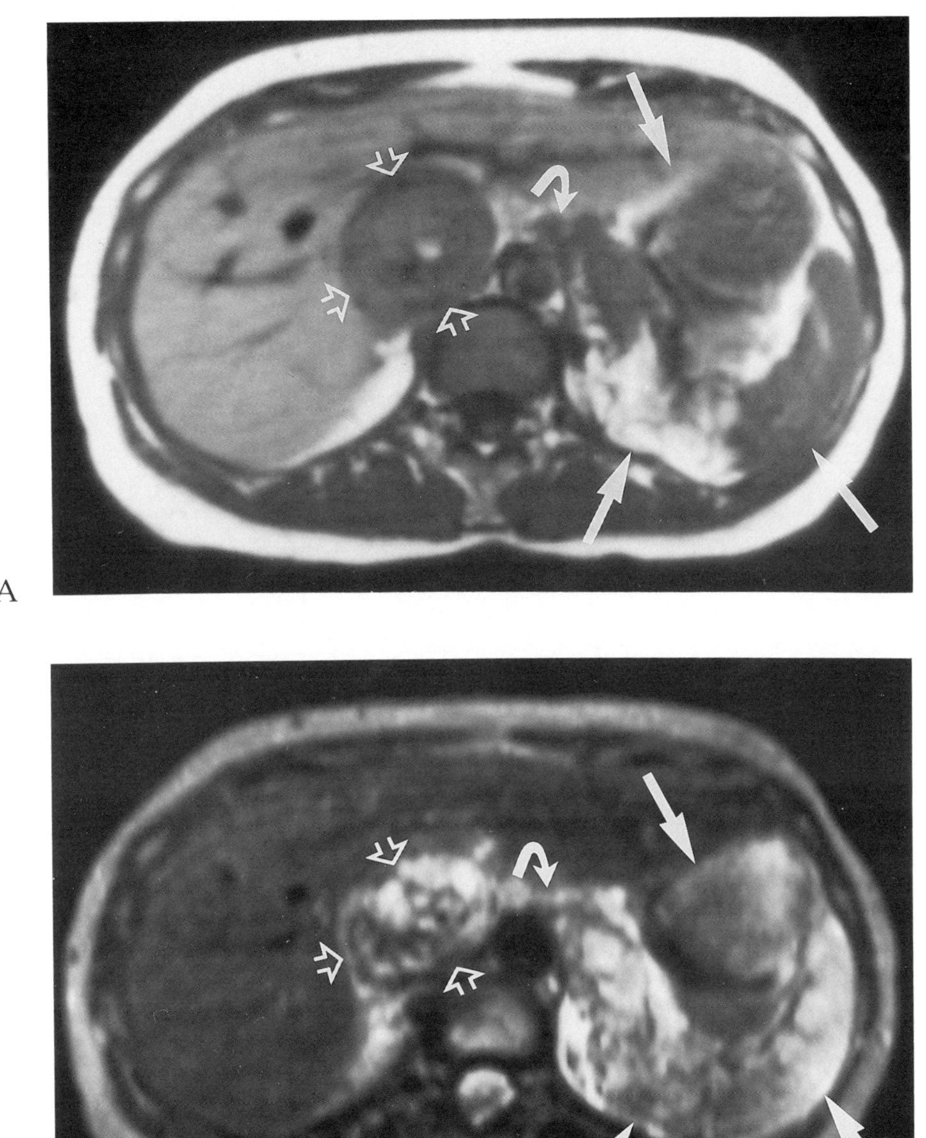

Figure 8. MRI examination of abdomen in a patient with an enormous left renal cell carcinoma, demonstrating left renal vein and inferior vena cava extension of tumor thrombus. In (A, top) axial T1-weighted image and (B, bottom) axial T2-weighted image, the primary tumor (arrows) renal vein (curved arrow) and inferior vena caval thrombus (open arrows) have a similar intensity on both T1-weighted and T2-weighted sequences. (Courtesy of John Cardella, M.D.)

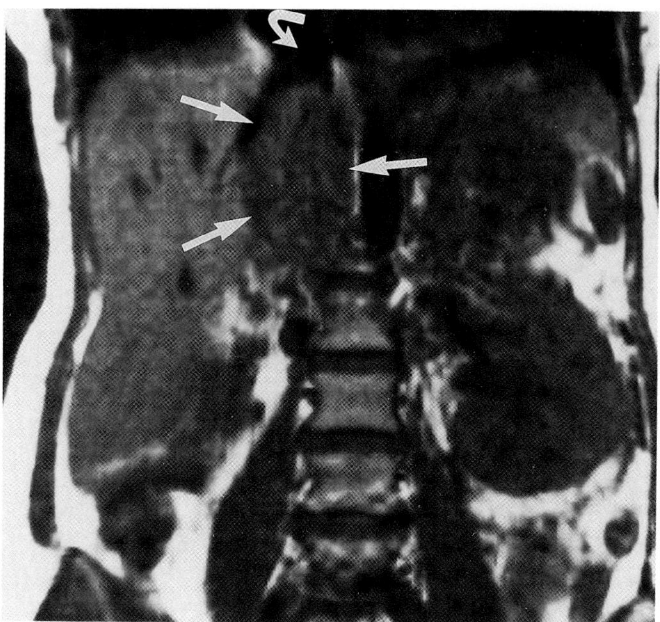

Figure 8C.   Coronal T1-weighted image shows the tumor thrombus (arrows) distending the inferior vena cava and extending superiorly to the right atrial junction (curved arrows).

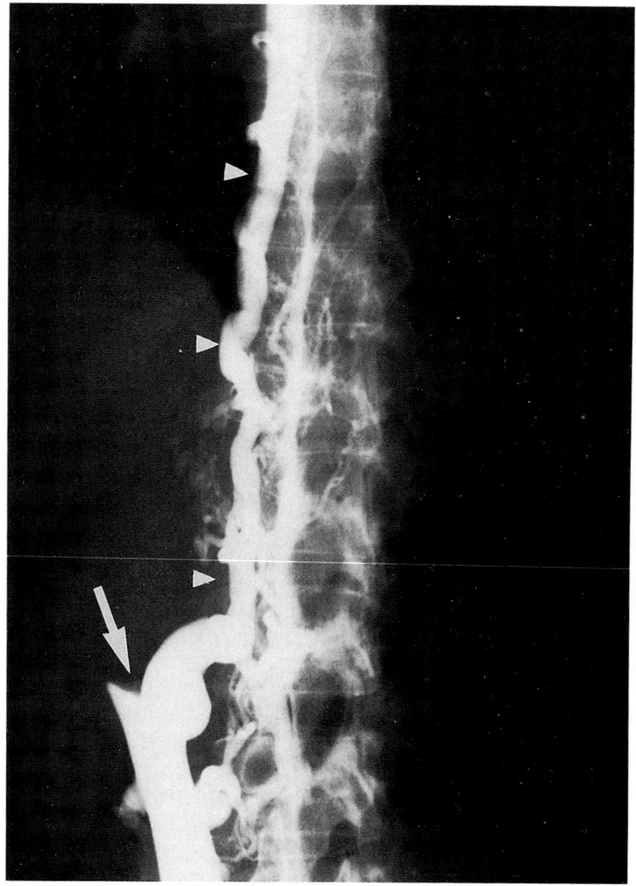

Figure 8D.   Inferior vena cavagram demonstrates total occlusion by tumor thrombus (arrow), and azygous vein continuation of flow (arrowheads).

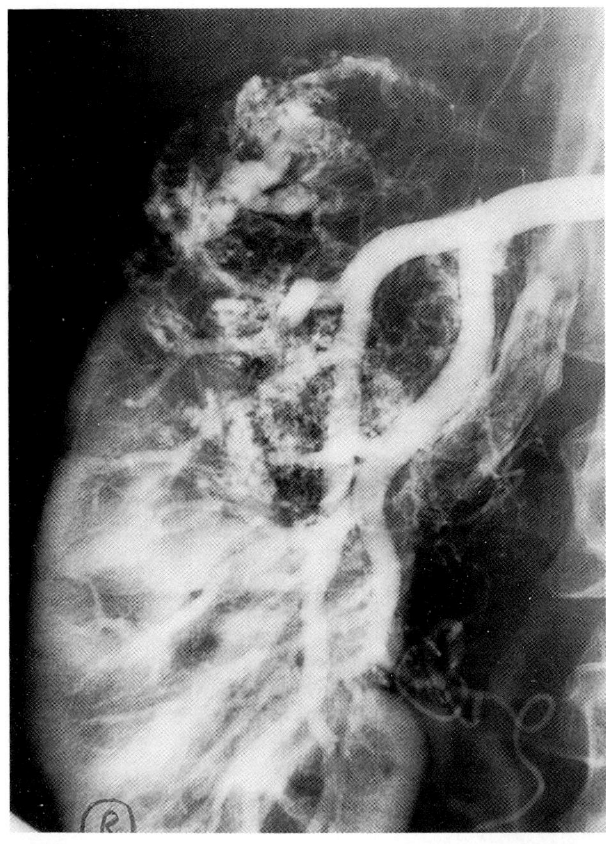

A

Figure 9. (A, left) Arteriogram showing hypervascular RCC with corkscrew vessels, AV malformations with early opacifications of the right renal vein with radiations, and striations within it consistent with malignant thrombus. (B, bottom) Intravenous urography showed a mass at the right upper pole.

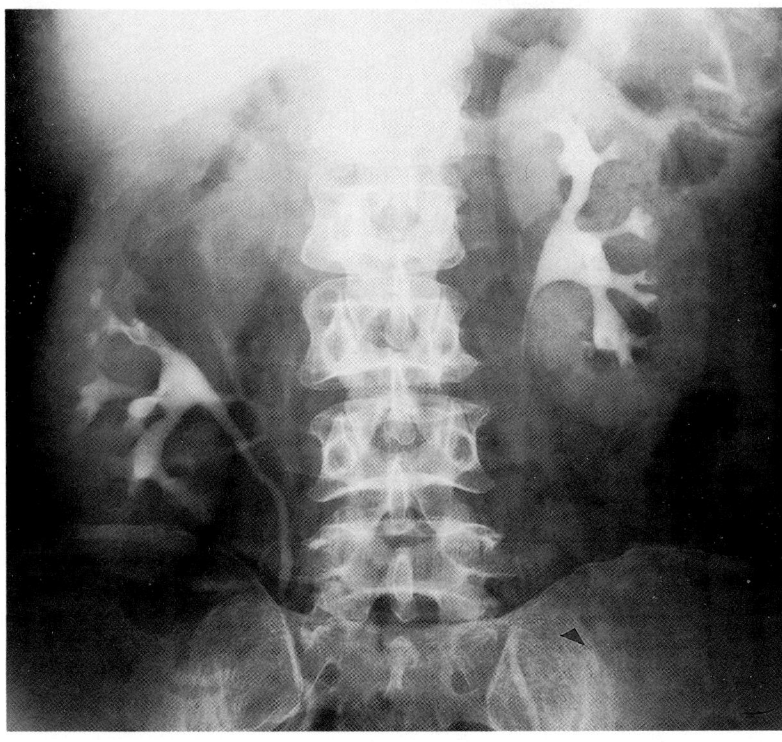

B

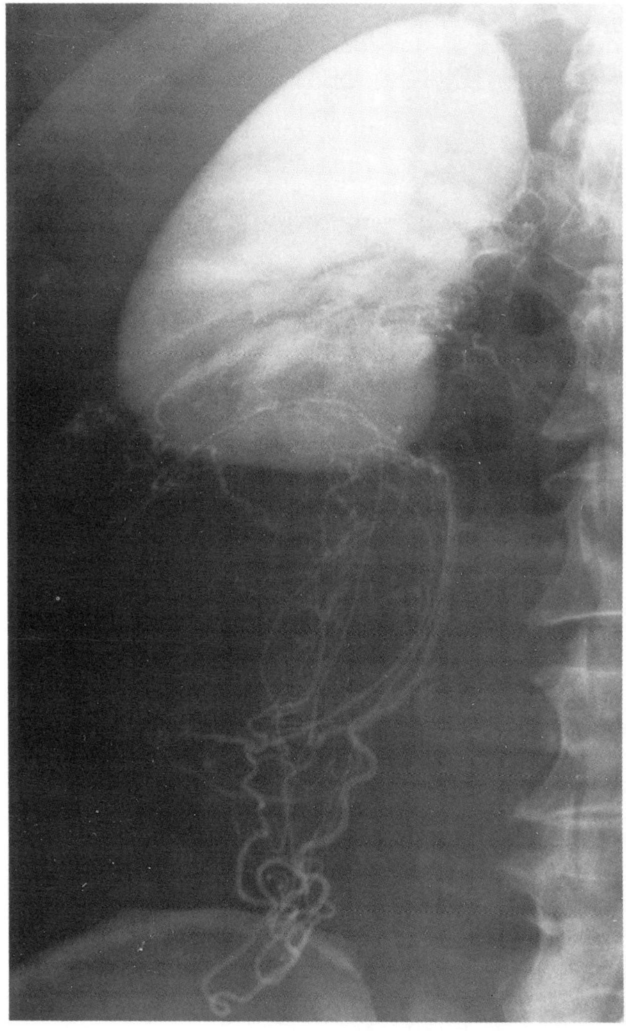

Figure 10.   Fibrosarcoma. Angiography reveals a mass at the right lower pole that displaces the kidney without intrinsic involvement and with prominent capsular pathologic vessels, almost pathognomonic of capsular sarcoma.

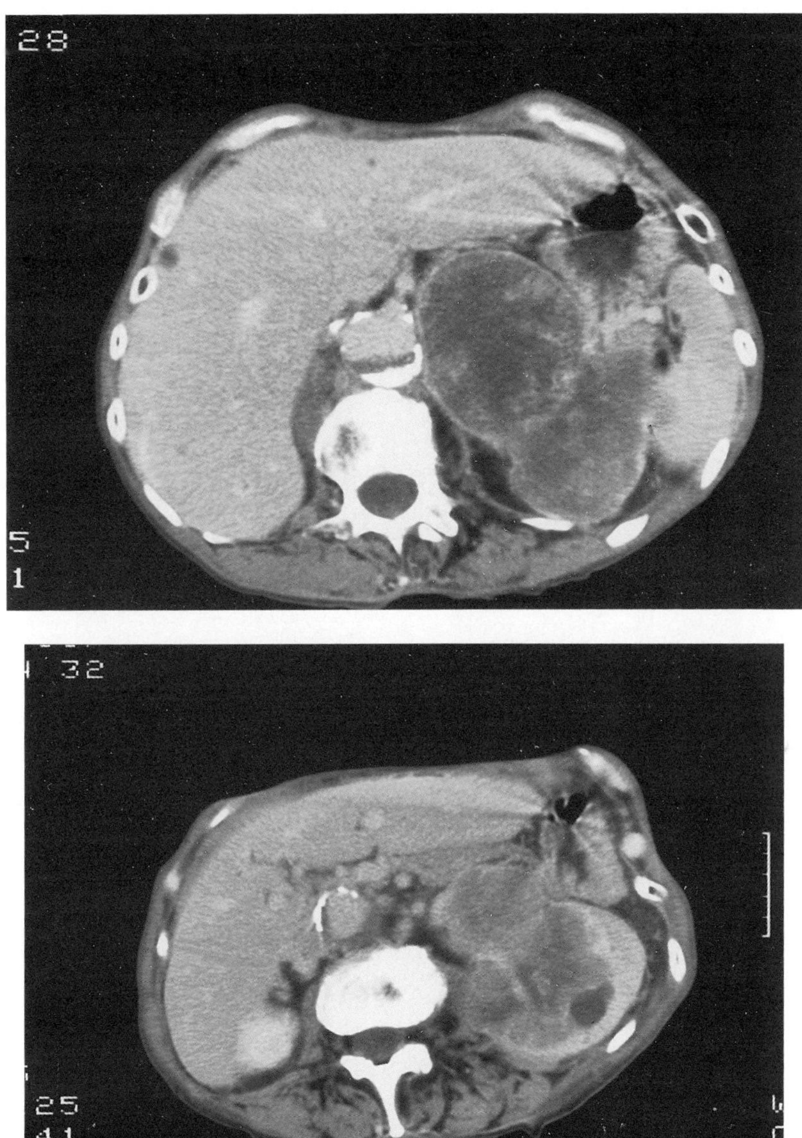

Figure 11.   (A, top) and (B, bottom) Computed tomography shows a huge necrotic mass occupying the upper half of the left kidney. Discharge diagnosis was oat-cell neuroendocrine tumor, metastatic to the left kidney.

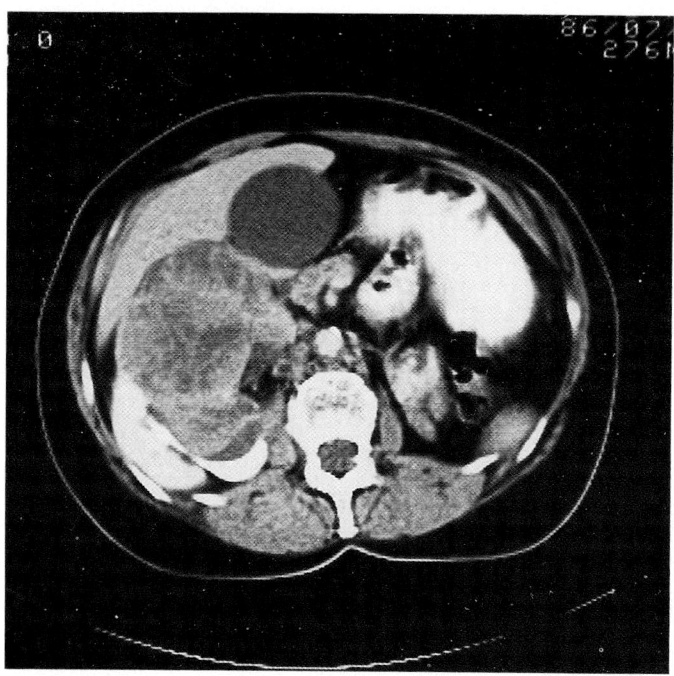

Figure 12.   Wilms' tumor in a 55-year-old patient complaining of hematuria. Left nephrectomy was performed in the past because of "pyelonephritis." Computed tomography reveals a multiloculated cystic mass involving the right kidney.

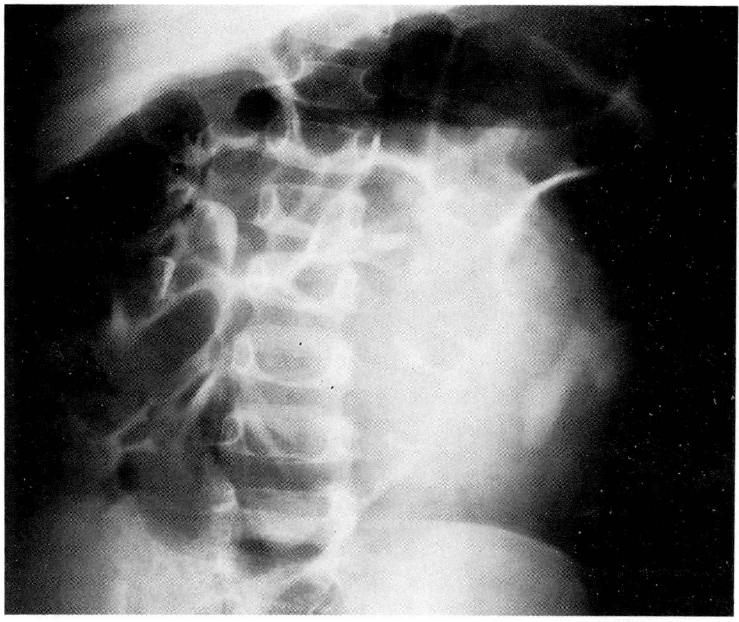

Figure 13A.   Wilms' tumor in a 3-year-old male patient. Intravenous urography shows a huge intrarenal mass stretching and displacing the collecting structures.

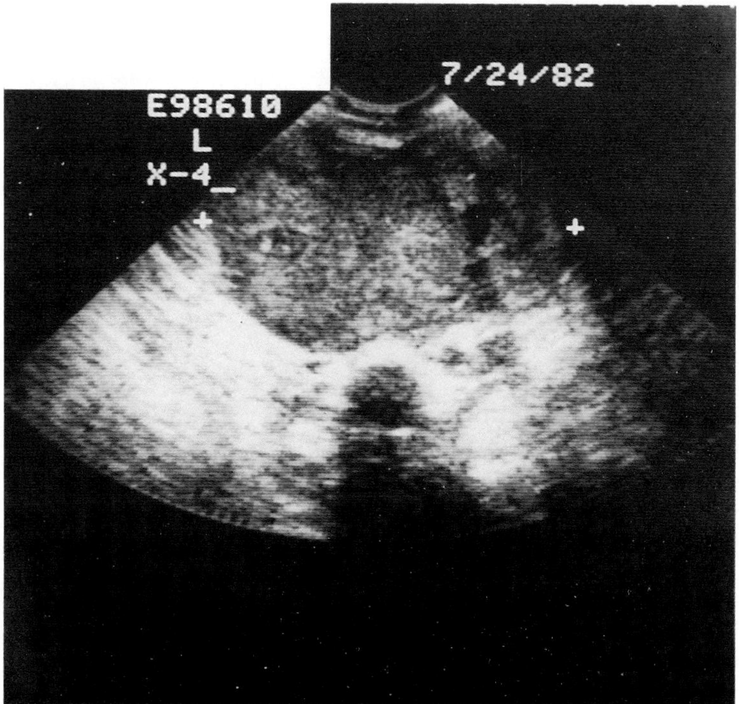

Figure 13B.   Ultrasound reveals a very echogenic intrarenal mass highly consistent with Wilms' tumor.

Tumors of the Collecting System and Ureter

The renal pelvis and ureter are lined by the same type of transitional epithelium. The tumors are classified as epithelial, mesodermal, and secondary. All epithelial tumors are, for practical reasons, considered malignant, even the so-called benign transitional cell papilloma. The mesodermal tumors, with very rare exceptions, are benign and are derived from nonepithelial elements of the walls of the pelvis, calices, and ureter (polyp).

Transitional-cell carcinoma (TCC) is the most frequent (75% to 85%) of these neoplasms and affects males more often than females in a ratio of 4 to 1. The peak incidence is between the fourth and seventh decades. The most frequent symptom is recurrent painless hematuria, especially with papillary tumors. Flank pain is usually an indication of a secondary hydronephrosis or pyelonephritis.

Multicentric and bilateral lesions, either synchronous or metachronous, occur in a significant number of instances, especially in cases of papillary tumors (about 40%). Therefore, the presence of one TCC anywhere in the collecting system mandates a thorough initial evaluation of the entire urinary system with appropriate periodic follow-up.

Very often, the diagnosis of TCC can be made easily from radiologic studies. Urography shows one or more irregular (usually) or smooth filling defects. This defect may be poorly visible when there is associated hydronephrosis. As obstruction becomes complete, the affected calix or possibly the entire kidney may not opacify (Fig. 14), and visualization of the tumor will be difficult or impossible. In such cases, the neoplasm is better demonstrated by retrograde pyelogram (Fig. 15). Urine for cytologic examination and brush biopsy can be obtained during the retrograde study.

Computed tomography plays an important role in the diagnosis of lesions that are missed or poorly visible or when radiolucent filling defects are found in the renal pelvis or ureter that cannot be distinguished from a stone or a blood clot (Fig. 16). Transitional cell carcinoma of the renal pelvis may be seen as a mass that has a density intermediate between that of urine and the normal renal parenchyma. The scan is particularly useful in demonstrating the extent of the tumor, thus aiding the surgeon in planning appropriate management. Delayed CT with the patient supine or prone may be of special benefit in defining an obstructing tumor.

Angiography does not differentiate uroepithelial tumors from inflammatory lesions or hypovascular RCCs and currently is not indicated in the evaluation of tumors. In selected cases, antegrade pyelography is useful in determining the upper margins of a tumor and to obtain material for cytologic examination.

Squamous cell carcinomas constitute 15% to 25% of all tumors of the uroepithelium. They are frequently associated with leukoplakia, calculi (50%), and chronic infections. They are usually solitary and flat with a tendency to spread diffusely into the renal parenchyma, contiguous ureter, or beyond the renal pelvis. In most patients, urography shows a filling defect in the pelvis. Hydronephrosis or absence of excretion of contrast medium occasionally occurs, in which case, retrograde pyelography is necessary to demonstrate the filling defect. The extent of invasion cannot be predicted from urographic studies, therefore, CT can be especially helpful in staging the disease. Brush biopsy of the lesion may be helpful in obtaining a sample for cytologic study; however, cytology of a urine sample is often sufficient to establish the diagnosis.

Tumors of the Bladder

Benign tumors of the bladder are rare. Nearly all (90% to 95%) of bladder tumors are uroepithelial and about 90% of the uroepithelial tumors are TCCs, which can be subdivided into papillary and nonpapillary infiltrative tumors. Adenocarcinomas are extremely rare (less than 1%) and usually originate from urachal epithelium. Squamous cell carcinoma is likewise rare (less than 5%) and is usually associated with chronic cystitis or schistosomiasis.

Most bladder tumors (about 70%) involve the posterior and lateral walls near the ureteral orifices; about 20% of the remaining tumors occur in the trigone, and about 10% in the dome. The peak age of incidence is 50 to 80 years, and the disease is 2 to 3 times more common in men than in women. The clinical picture includes painless hematuria, frequency, dysuria, and pain. The tumors are frequently multicentric and can be associated with neoplasms of the renal pelvis and ureter.

Radiologic evaluation may be complementary to cystoscopy and bimanual examination, especially in the staging of advanced malignant vesical disease.

Urographic or cystographic demonstration of a fungating or polypoid mass protruding into the lumen and causing a filling defect in the opacified bladder is almost pathognomonic of bladder tumors. On urography, lesions can be missed if radiographs of the bladder are not taken in the supine and prone positions. Oblique views of the bladder are also helpful in the detection and localization of such lesions.

Computed tomography cannot differentiate mucosal, submucosal, superficial, or deep muscular tumorous involvement, and bladder-confined disease probably is better staged by ultrasound than by CT.

Extension into the perivesical fat (Stage C) causes a localized thickening of the bladder wall and a loss of definition of the abutting perivesical fat plane, with subsequent fixation of the bladder wall, which can be demonstrated by performing CT examinations on the patient in the prone and decubitus positions. Unfortunately, postinflammatory or postoperative adhesions, and postradiation changes may give an identical image.

The diagnosis of Stage D disease rests on identification of tumor extension into adjacent structures such as the prostate, seminal vesicles, and rectum or documentation of involved lymph nodes or distant metastases (Fig. 17). Misinterpretation of loss of the fat plane between the posterior bladder wall and the seminal vesicles has been a significant cause of overstaging by CT.

The accuracy of MRI in staging bladder carcinoma appears to be at least equivalent to that of CT. Although it is too early to define the role of MRI, the ability to do sagittal and coronal scans is certainly an advantage in evaluating the dome and base of the bladder; for this reason alone, it is likely that MRI will prove superior to CT in the evaluation of carcinoma of the bladder.

Carcinoma of the Prostate

Prostatic carcinoma is the second most common cause of cancer deaths and the third most common cancer in men over 55 years of age.

To improve the clinical staging, several studies have been added to digital examination and biopsy, such as bone scans and assays for serum acid phosphatase and prostatic-specific antigen.

Sonographically, the primary lesion may have a variety of appearances. Small cancers usually are in the peripheral zone and are generally hypoechoic (Figs. 18 and 19). Cancers are usually irregular with poorly defined margins and are frequently situated adjacent to the prostatic capsule. Bulging or erosion of the capsule is indicative of a more invasive process. Lesions as small as a few millimeters can be seen. As the tumor enlarges, its echogenicity changes from the anechoic-hypoechoic nidus to a more isoechoic-hyperechoic pattern. The exact cause of these changes has not been clearly determined, but they have been suggested to be related, not only to cellular differentiation and tumor size, but also to the amount of desmoplasia and fibrosis within the tumor.

The sonographic characteristics of prostate cancer are not specific, and it must be emphasized that there is some overlap between the benign and the malignant sonographic features.

Sonography of the prostate is not a pathognomonic study, therefore, biopsy must be undertaken.

Computed tomography is rarely chosen as the primary imaging modality in the diagnosis of prostatic carcinoma because of its inability to delineate the internal gland anatomy in detail. It has been replaced by endorectal ultrasound and MRI in the evaluation of extracapsular and seminal vesicle invasion. However, its accuracy in detecting lymphadenopathy and distant metastases remains unsurpassed. It can also be useful in treatment planning and in assessing the efficacy of radiation or chemotherapy.

Magnetic resonance imaging is probably the modality of choice for staging prostatic cancer (reported accuracy of 83% to 89%). In the evaluation of capsular and periprostatic infiltration, the accuracy of MRI is similar to that of ultrasound;

however, it is superior to ultrasound in the evaluation of pelvic metastatic disease (on the 1.5T magnetic unit). Most prostatic carcinomas are hypointense compared with the normal high signal-intensity peripheral zone (where the majority of cancers arise) on long-TR (T2 weighting) pulse sequences.

Postbiopsy hemorrhage may interfere with MRI staging since the high signal emitted from blood may obscure a nearby low-signal tumor. Similarly, recent bleeding with low-signal intensity on T2-weighted images can cause a tumor to appear more extensive than it actually is. Hemorrhagic changes have been traced for as long as a month or two after biopsy.

Testicular Tumors

Testicular tumors constitute 4% to 6% of all male genitourinary tumors and less than 1% of all male malignancy. However, they are the most common neoplasm in men 25 to 30 years old. They are classified as seminomas, nonseminomatous germ-cell tumors, stromal tumors (Leydig cell and others); and secondary lesions (malignant lymphoma, leukemia, and metastatic tumors). Mixed types are common among nonseminomatous tumors. Most testicular tumors are unilateral; however, 8% or more of patients will develop a contralateral neoplasm. Most often, these tumors present as a nontender, unilateral testicular enlargement, although acute pain is not uncommon. Approximately 14% of patients with testicular neoplasm present with signs or symptoms related to metastatic disease.

Testicular neoplasms tend to metastasize to the lymph nodes accompanying the testicular veins. Therefore, metastases from the left testis tend to involve nodes in the hilum of the left kidney, while those from the right testis tend to involve nodes below the hilum of the right kidney, where the right testicular vein drains into the inferior vena cava. However, all nodes are at risk.

Imaging techniques are usually limited to ultrasonography, which is the method of choice in the diagnosis of scrotal pathology, especially in the differentiation of testicular masses. The superficial location and easy accessibility of the scrotal contents make them ideally suited for this examination. The critical clinical question is whether a lesion is intrinsic (virtually always malignant) or extrinsic (probably benign) to the testis. The advent of high-frequency, high-resolution real-time scanners and improved diagnostic skills allows this distinction to be made with an accuracy approaching 90% to 95%. Most germ-cell tumors are hypoechoic with respect to the normal tissue from which they usually are poorly demarcated (Figs. 20 and 21). They have a tendency to appear as single, focal masses; however, diffuse lesions can infiltrate the entire gland. Sonographically, seminomas usually are uniformly hypoechoic, as one would expect from their homogeneous histologic picture (Fig. 21).

Benign intratesticular tumors are rare. There are no absolute sonographic criteria for establishing benignancy. Moreover, for some lesions, such as the epidermoid cyst (Fig. 22), a benign nature cannot be assumed.

The sonographic appearance of testicular leukemia and lymphoma is nonspecific with focal hypoechoic lesions or diffuse hypoechoic enlargement of the testes.

Sonography has an important role in the detection of a primary, nonpalpable testicular lesion in patients who have presented with metastatic disease in the abdomen, chest, and neck. Occasionally, the primary tumor undergoes spontaneous regression, resulting in a calcific scar or a "burned-out" tumor. Although the sonographic finding of a highly echogenic focal lesion with shadowing is not specific for the latter lesion, this entity may certainly be strongly suggested when found in the clinical setting of metastatic disease.

Testicular abscesses are usually a complication of epididymo-orchitis, often in diabetes or tuberculosis. Sonographically, the abscess presents as a mass with hypoechoic or mixed echogenic areas. Differentiation from neoplasms can usually be made by correlation of the sonographic and clinical findings. Sarcoid can also involve the testes, resulting, usually, in a hyperechoic mass.

Testicular infarcts can be caused by torsion, trauma, leukemia, bacterial endocarditis, and polyarteritis nodosa. Sonographically, testicular infarcts may appear as focal hypoechoic masses or as a diffusely hypoechoic small testis.

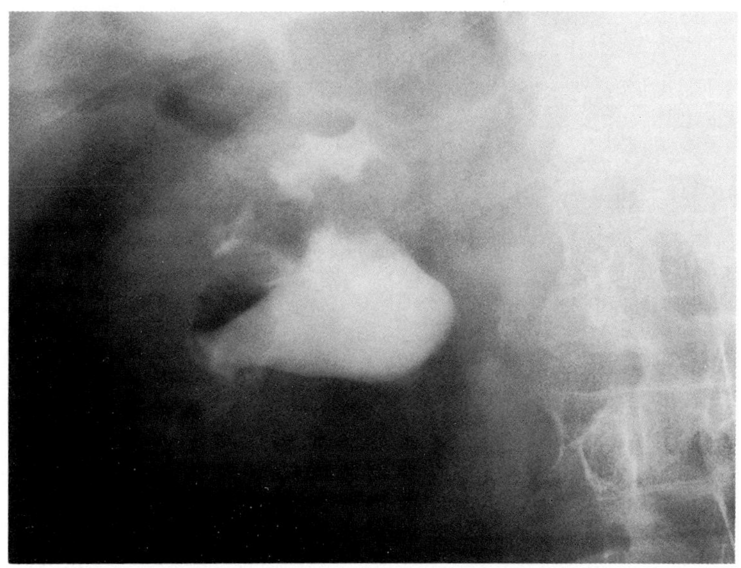

Figure 14.   Transitional cell carcinoma of the right upper infundibulum. The 15-minute IVU shows narrowing obstruction.

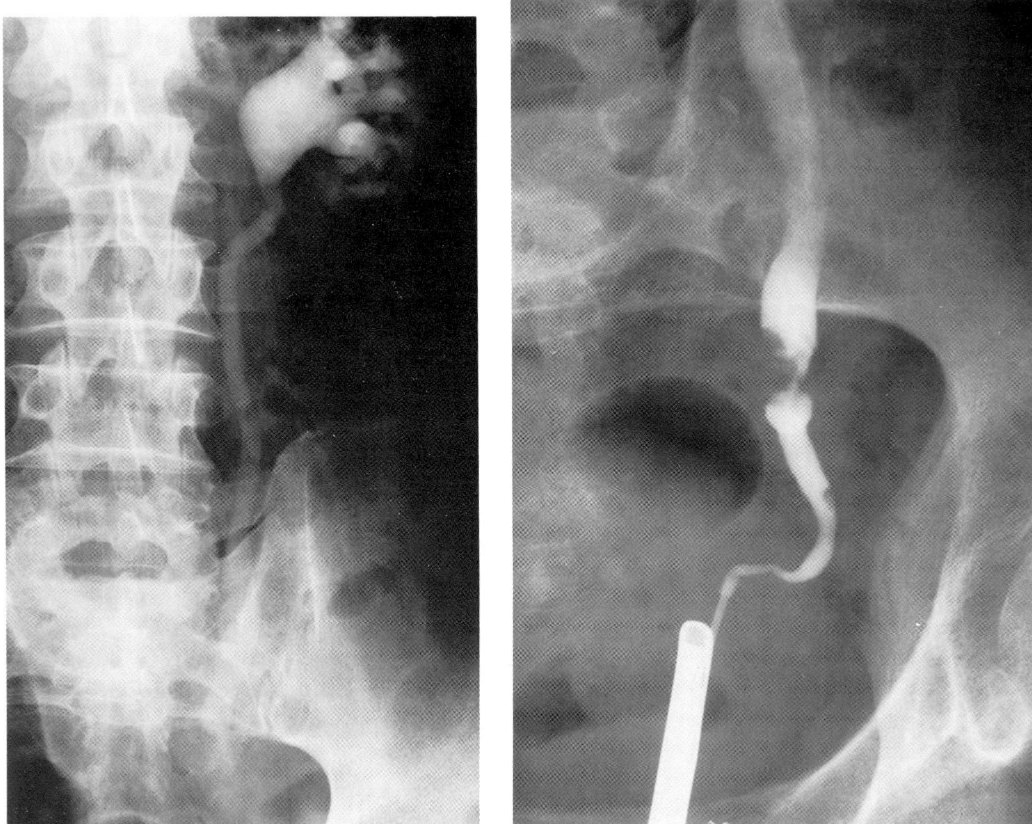

Figure 15.   Transitional cell carcinoma, distal third of the left ureter. (A, left) Urography revealed left hydroureterectasis down to the junction of the middle and distal third of the ureter, with the distal third not visible. (B, right) Retrograde pyelogram shows narrowing of the distal ureter with apple-core shape. This is most consistent with TCC.

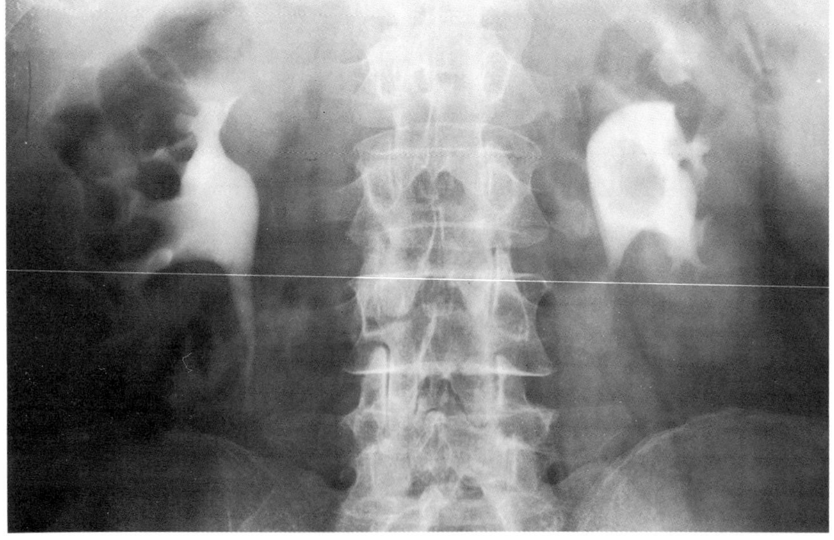

Figure 16.   Transitional cell carcinoma of the left renal pelvis. Intravenous urogram reveals a round filling defect suggesting TCC, clot, or stone.

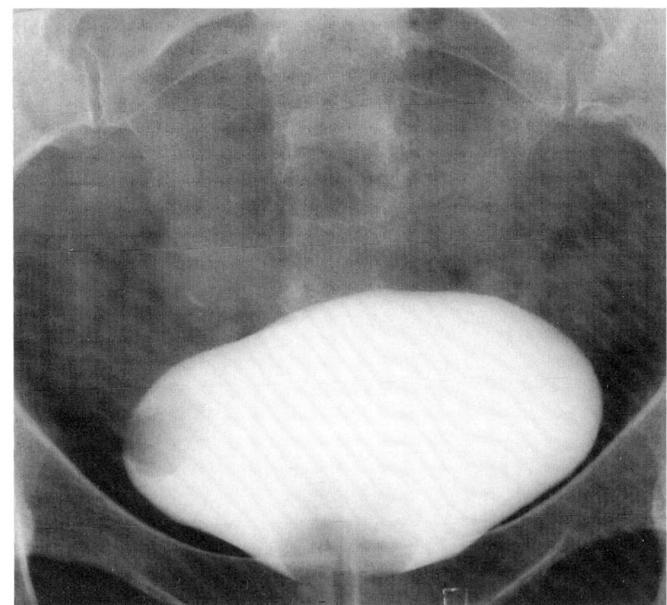

A

Figure 17. Transitional cell carcinoma of the bladder, Stage D. (A) Cystogram revealed a filling defect in the right lateral vesical wall consistent with polypoid lesion (most likely TCC).

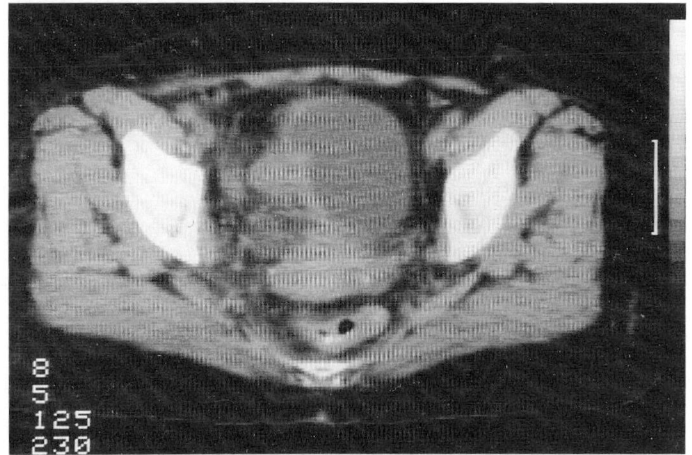

Figure 17B. CT scan with stage D TCC of the bladder shows thickening of the right lateral vesical wall with involvement of lateral iliac lymph nodes and right perivesical malignant involvement.

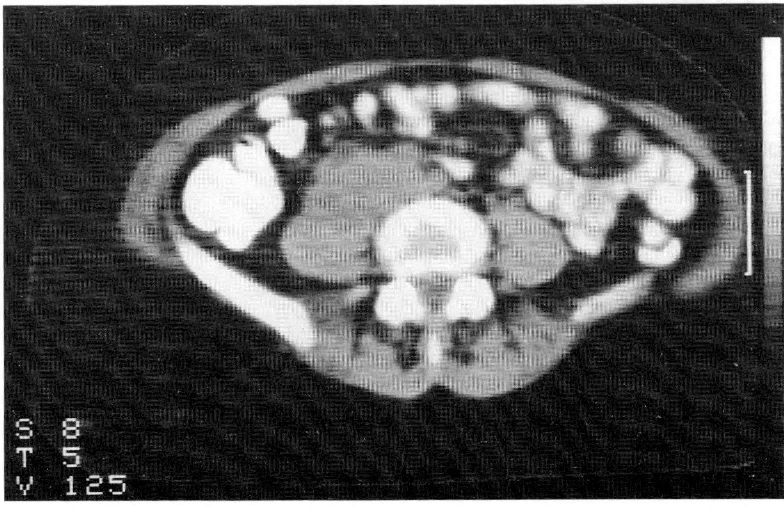

Figure 17C. Involved lymph nodes in the right paracaval area on CT with stage D TCC of the bladder.

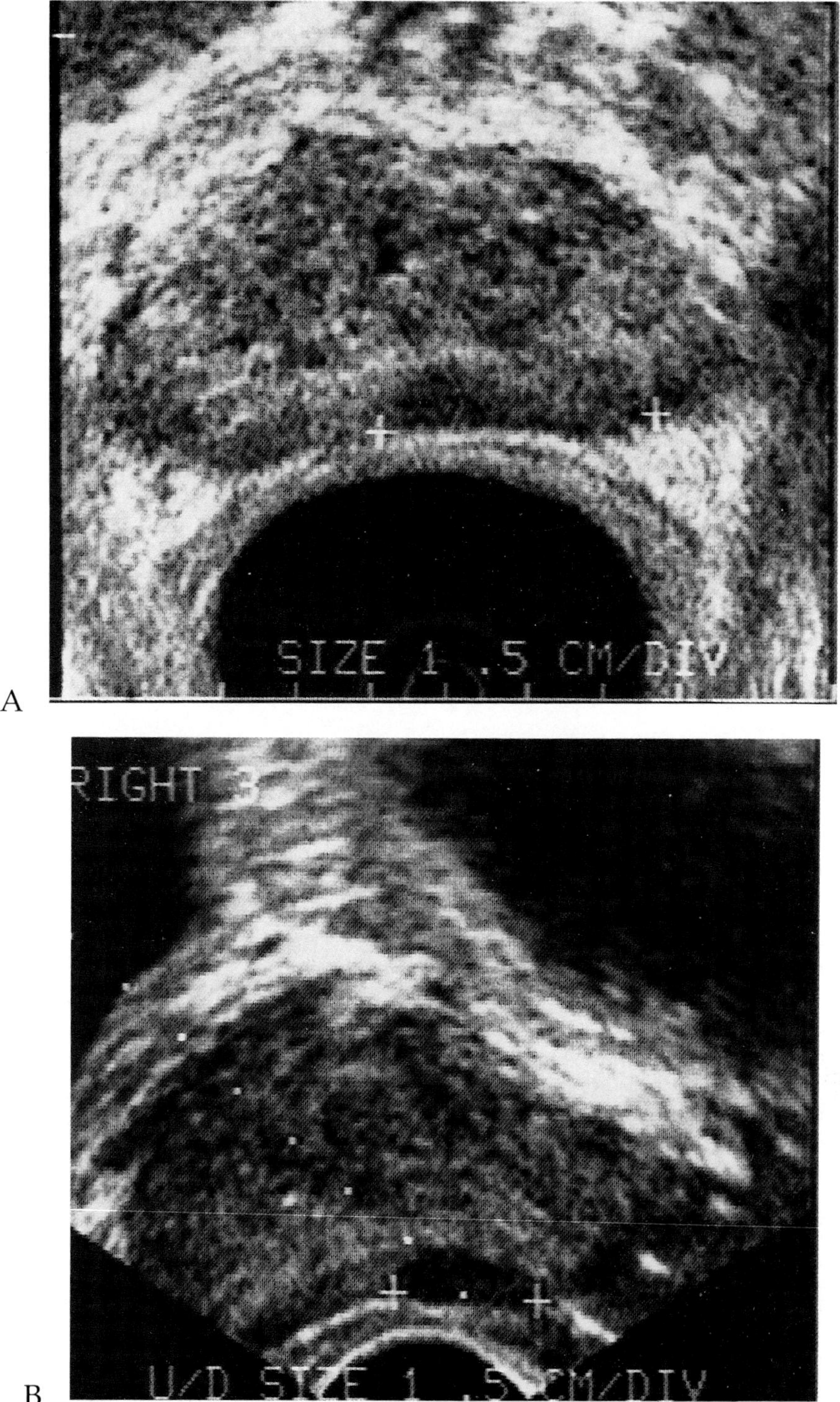

Figure 18.   Carcinoma of the prostate. Ultrasound scan shows a hypoechoic nodule on the posterior surface of the right lobe on both (A, top) transverse and (B, bottom) longitudinal scans, with biopsy guide line traversing the lesion in the longitudinal scan. Biopsy confirmed carcinoma, Gleason grade 2/3. (Courtesy of Keith Kaye, M.D.)

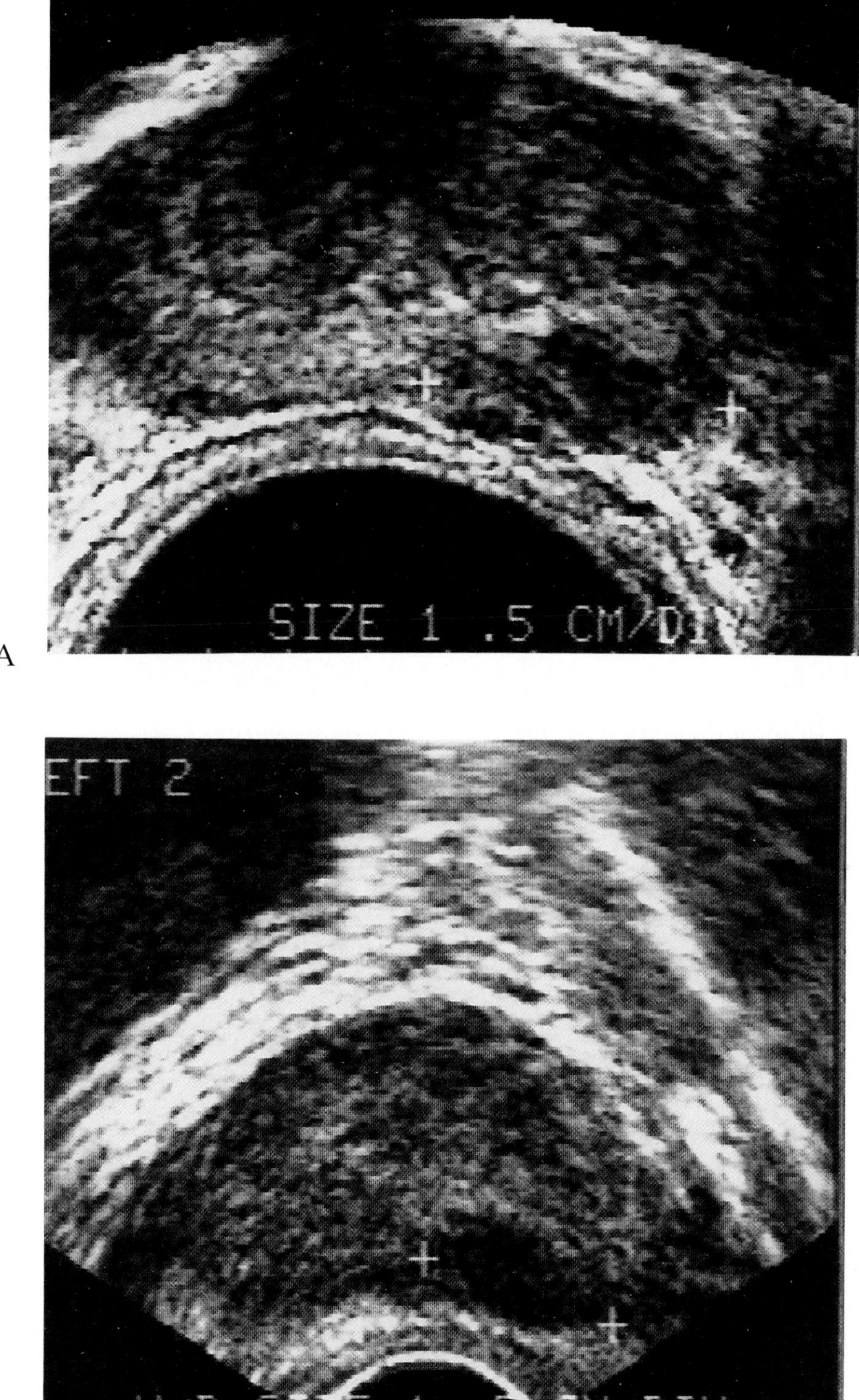

Figure 19.   Carcinoma of the prostate. Ultrasound scan depicts a hypoechoic area on (A, top) transverse scan and (B, bottom) longitudinal scan. (Courtesy of Keith Kaye, M.D.)

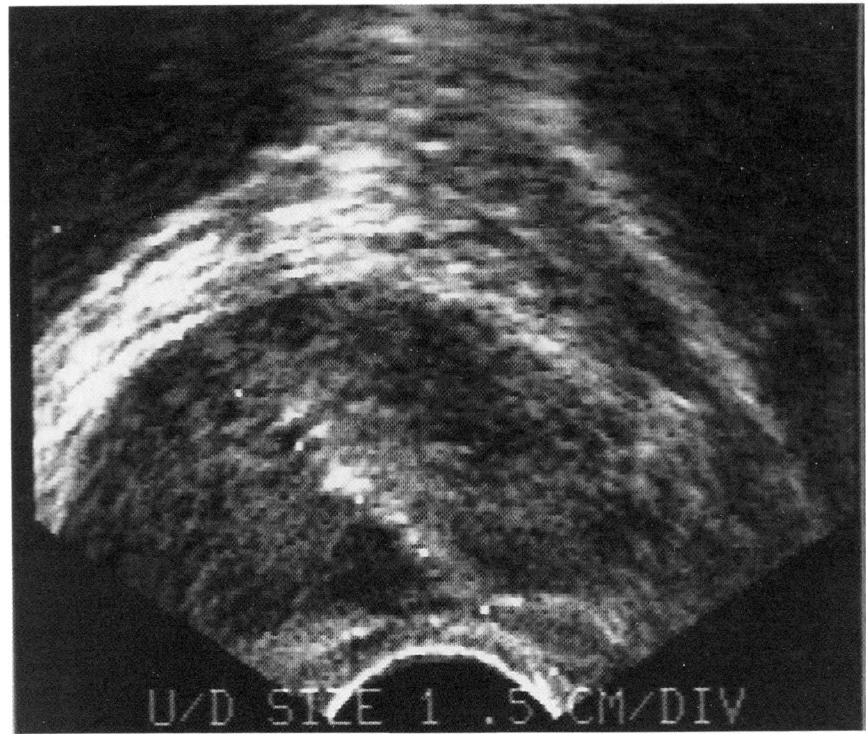

Figure 19C.   Carcinoma of the prostate. Biopsy needle transversing the lesion. Biopsy showed moderately differentiated adenocarcinoma.

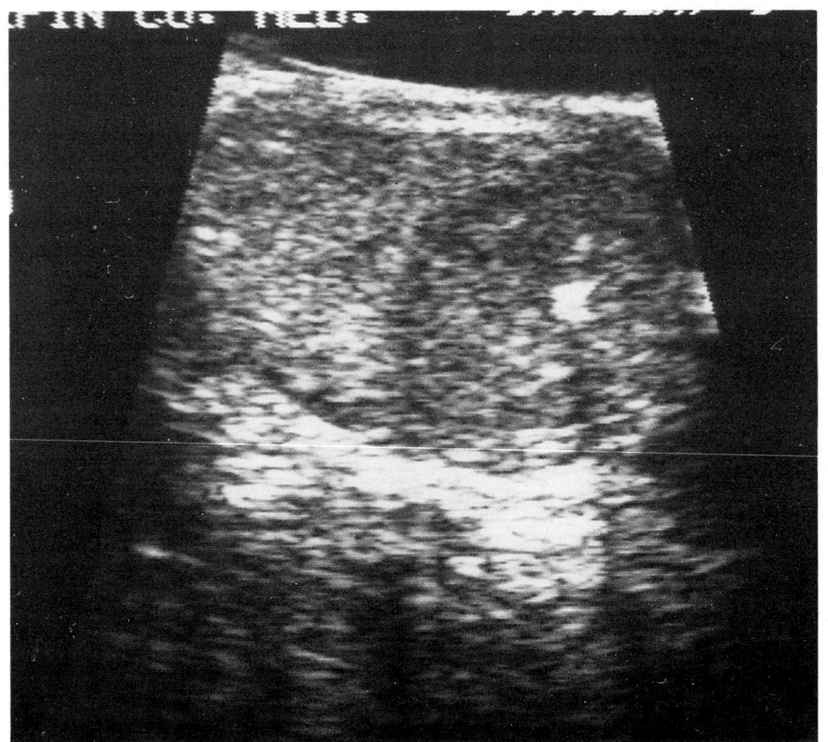

Figure 20.   Mixed testicular germ-cell tumor. Scrotal ultrasound scan shows a lower-pole mass with mixed echogenicity, including a central area of strong echogenicity representing calcification.

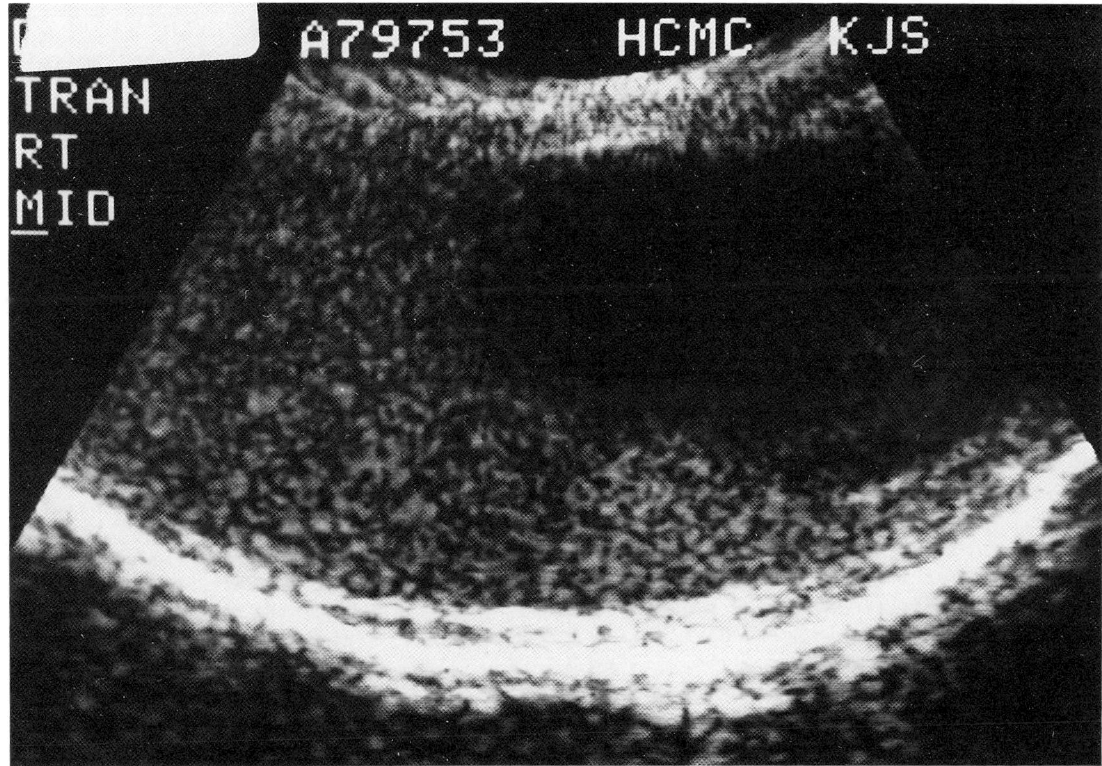

Figure 21.　Testicular tumor (seminoma). Scrotal ultrasound shows a large area of decreased echogenicity with no evidence of encapsulation.

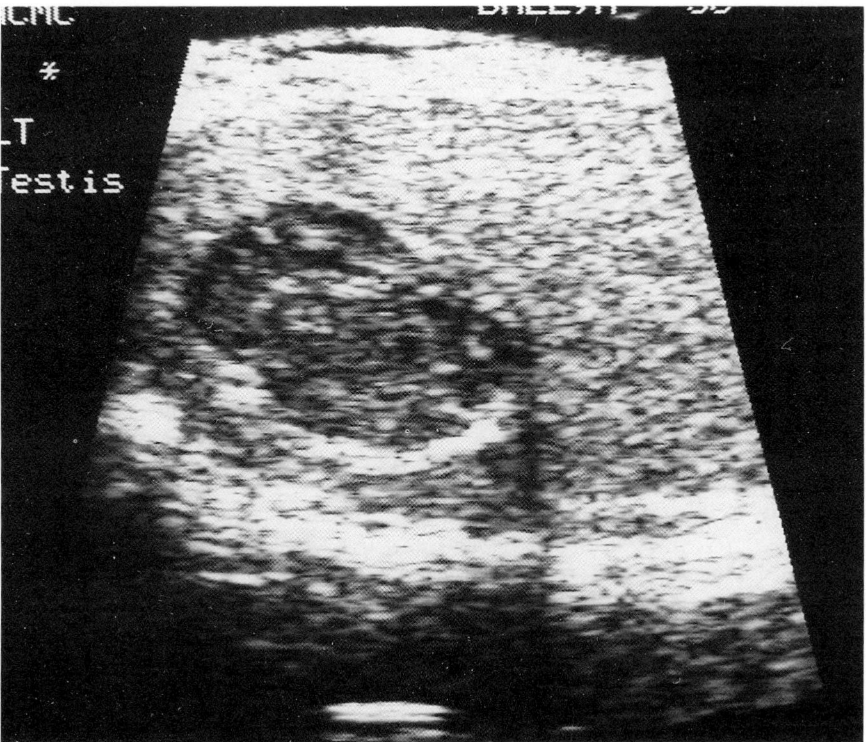

Figure 22.　Testicular epidermoid cyst. Scrotal ultrasound scan shows an oval mass medial to the upper pole and adjacent to the edge of the testis. The ultrasonic features of the mass are mixed echogenic pattern with layers of increased echogenicity.

Chapter 4

Trauma to the Urinary Tract

Joaquim Vieira, M.D. and Alexander S. Cass, M.B.B.S.

Renal Trauma

Injuries to the kidney should be suspected in any patient showing microscopic or gross hematuria after trauma, especially trauma to the abdomen or back. However, some patients with renal injury do not have any blood in the urine, including some with grave conditions such as complete avulsion of the ureteropelvic junction or traumatic thrombosis of the renal artery. It also should be emphasized that there is no correlation between the amount of hematuria and the severity of the injury.

Blunt injuries are most commonly caused by automobile accidents, sports injuries, falls, fights, and criminal assaults. Therefore, there often are significant head, extremity, or other abdominal injuries. The injury is usually the result of considerable violence, because the kidney is a mobile organ which lies in a relatively protected position.

When the extent of the renal injury appears out of proportion to the amount of trauma, pre-existing renal pathology (for instance, hydronephrosis, tumor, or congenital disorders) should be strongly suspected.

Penetrating injuries are usually the result of gunshot or stab wounds. The renal injury may be of minor importance in comparison with the other abdominal injuries, which are present in more than 80% of cases of penetrating renal injuries.

Iatrogenic injuries continue to increase in variety and frequency. They may follow renal biopsy, retrograde pyelography, percutaneous nephrostomy, and renal lithotripsy.

Renal injuries should be divided into minor, major, and severe.

Minor injuries consist of contusions, small intrarenal and subcapsular hematomas, small cortical lacerations, and segmental infarcts. In general, the renal capsule is intact. Such injuries account for 75% to 85% of the total group with blunt trauma. Patients usually have flank pain and hematuria but are hemodynamically stable. Conservative treatment is universally accepted for this category of injury.

Major injuries are deep lacerations that disrupt the capsule and extend into the collecting structures. They are usually associated with extensive perirenal and intrarenal hematomas and extravasation of urine from a deep corticomedullary laceration. This type of renal injury constitutes approximately 10% of all blunt renal trauma; it usually is associated with flank pain, hematuria, and, at times, with unstable vital signs, and a palpable flank mass. If hemodynamic instability persists, most urologists would explore and attempt to repair the kidney. However, if the vital signs do stabilize

From *Imaging of Urologic Disorders* edited by Alexander S. Cass, MBBS, © 1992, Futura Publishing Inc., Mount Kisco, NY.

most urologists will attempt to treat without surgery but will be prepared to operate should conditions deteriorate.

Severe injuries constitute approximately 5% of all blunt renal injuries and usually require immediate surgical exploration. They consist of multiple renal corticomedullary lacerations (the "shattered" kidney), renal pedicle injuries (intimal tears of the renal artery with thrombosis, renal artery avulsion, and tears of the renal vein), and disruption of the ureteropelvic junction.

The patient with a shattered kidney will generally have clinically obvious instability, an enlarging flank mass, and hematuria. The renal pedicle injuries, in contrast, may be silent; not uncommonly, there is no hematuria.

Roentgen Evaluation

Plain films of the abdomen will not demonstrate any abnormality in many patients. Fracture of the ribs or transverse processes of the spine suggest significant trauma and may be associated with renal injury. Scoliosis concave toward the site of injury and loss of psoas and renal outlines may be seen. Large hematomas may displace bowel or alter the renal axis. However, similar findings can be the result of retroperitoneal bleeding from nonrenal injuries.

The statement that all patients with suspected renal injury should undergo *excretory urography* is not as absolute as it used to be. In patients with microscopic hematuria, no shock (BP >90 mm Hg), and no associated injuries following blunt trauma, an intravenous pyelogram (IVP) is not performed since the renal injury is minor and settles with conservative management.

Minor injuries usually are adequately evaluated by properly done excretory urography (high-dose technique) and nephrotomography. More serious and severe renal injuries are not well defined by excretory urography, which should be complemented by computed tomography (CT), angiography, or both in order for an appropriate therapy to be instituted.

The most important function of the urogram is to provide information about the condition of the contralateral kidney and the presence of any

congenital malformation of the kidney that may predispose it to renal injury.

The urographic signs associated with renal trauma can be multiple.

1. Generalized decrease in nephrographic and pyelographic density with attenuation of the pelvicaliceal system;
2. Absence of excretion of contrast medium on the injured side; this finding may be seen with minor renal injury but usually indicates severe injury; frequently necessitating arteriography for further evaluation of the renal pedicle;
3. A localized nephrographic defect or lack of excretion, which indicates localized damage (contusion, intrarenal hematoma, or segmental arterial thrombosis Fig. 1);
4. A fissure in the nephrographic phase which suggests laceration of the renal parenchyma and is very often associated with perinephric hematoma, obscuring the renal outline; a defect in the nephrogram can also be attributable to a localized renal infarct;
5. Extravasation from a tear in the pelvicaliceal system with formation of intrarenal, subcapsular, or perinephric collections of urine or blood; this abnormality is usually associated with a laceration of the parenchyma and pelvicaliceal system but also occurs from laceration of the renal pelvis or ureter alone; rupture of the ureteropelvic junction or ureter must be considered in the presence of extravasation with a normal appearance of the pelvicaliceal system;
6. Renal enlargement, which can be secondary to intrarenal hematoma or edema or to thrombosis of the renal veins; reduction in renal size suggests renal artery obstruction;
7. Displacement of the kidney or loss of its outline secondary to a perirenal collection of blood or urine;
8. Caliceal or pelvic filling defects, which are highly suggestive of clots causing obstruction;
9. Displacement and distortion of the

pelvicaliceal system caused by compression by an intrarenal hematoma or by edema.

Computed tomography provides an ideal multiorgan imaging tool. Therefore, CT has assumed an important role in the evaluation of major renal trauma.

In general, precontrast images do not provide enough useful additional information to justify their routine use. However, contrast-enhanced CT has proved to be a very sensitive procedure and permits adequate identification of most types of renal injury that require specific treatment. The study is especially indicated in cases of multiple trauma or major renal trauma suspected from the clinical findings on excretory urography (Fig. 2).

The presence and magnitude of intrarenal and pararenal hematomas, parenchymal tears, corticomedullary lacerations, and fractures of the kidney with resultant extravasation of opacified urine and the viability of parenchymal fracture margins can be definitively assessed by this modality (Fig. 3).

Computed tomography, complemented by a dynamic study, can indicate the presence of renovascular injuries, which are usually associated with a nonfunctioning kidney. However, in these cases, angiography may be necessary to pinpoint the anatomic cause of the nonfunction (Fig. 4). It probably is still wise to recommend angiography in every case in which screening excretory urography shows nonfunction of the kidney.

The CT diagnostic criteria of the specific pathologic entities seen in renal trauma are as follows:

1. Renal contusion is seen on CT as delayed extravasation of contrast medium into the interstitial renal tissue.
2. Small cortical tears appear as small defects within a normally functioning kidney.
3. Corticomedullary laceration is a more extensive parenchymal tear with extension to the collecting system, subsequent extravasation of contrast-opacified urine,

and formation of a subcapsular or perinephric hematoma or both.
4. Renal fracture is a complete laceration, extending through the kidney with separation of the renal poles. The viability of the parenchymal margins of the fracture fragments can be assessed by a properly done dynamic CT study. An interposed hematoma separating the fracture fragments is also easily identified by CT.
5. The "shattered" kidney is a combination of multiple cortical and corticomedullary lacerations and renal fractures, which are usually associated with extravasation of opacified urine and perirenal and pararenal hematomas.
6. Intrarenal hematomas are seen as round or ovoid areas of decreased attenuation with poorly marginated borders; subcapsular hematomas appear as rounded or crescent-shaped masses compressing the renal parenchyma. Perinephric hematomas have a tendency to produce a streaked or bubbly appearance of the perirenal or pararenal spaces.
7. Renal artery occlusion is diagnosed by failure of the kidney to enhance. The ischemia can be segmental or total. Segmental infarcts are the most common vascular injury of the kidney after blunt trauma; a "cortical rim" of enhancing peripheral tissue may be seen in the ischemic segments, presumably because of perfusion by capsular or collateral vessels (Fig. 5). In general, the precise cause of vascular disruption cannot be determined from CT.

Angiography should be performed promptly, because within 6 to 8 hours, renal devitalization becomes irreversible (Fig. 6). The angiographic images must be of high quality in order to recognize subtle subintimal flaps that can progress to thrombosis. Intra-arterial digital subtraction angiography (IADSA) may permit a more rapid examination, reduction of catheter size and contrast volume, and simplification of film imaging sequences.

The renovascular injuries best identified by arteriography are intimal tears of the renal artery or its branches with or without arterial thrombosis (Figs. 7 and 8), renal artery avulsion, renal vein thrombosis, aneurysms of renal artery or its branches, and arteriovenous fistulae. (Fig. 9).

Sonography can be used in cases of acute renal trauma. However, it is more often utilized in the follow-up of intrarenal and perinephric collections of fluid and the diagnosis of hydronephrosis secondary to ureteral compression or stricture.

Ureteral Trauma

Injuries to the ureter are uncommon, because it is a small, mobile, elastic tube anatomically well protected by the bony spine and pelvis as well as by its surrounding musculature.

Abdominal, retroperitoneal, or pelvic operative procedures are the most common cause of ureteral injuries; these can be the result of direct surgical trauma in the form of ligation, transection, clamping, or kinking or of indirect surgical trauma associated with disturbance of the vascular supply, with subsequent delayed necrosis of the ischemic ureter.

The most common surgical causes are gynecologic operations, especially hysterectomies, either vaginal or abdominal. Posthysterectomy trauma increases in incidence if irradiation has been administered prior to surgery. Abdominoperineal resection of the colon, bladder and prostate surgery, and lumbar laminectomy at L4-L5 interspace may also result in ureteral injury.

Ureteral trauma can follow endoscopic procedures such as catheterization or instrumentation of the ureters. These injuries heal with an indwelling stent and occur most commonly near the ureterovesical junction.

Ureteral injuries caused by external trauma are rare. They may be the result of penetrating injuries (gunshot or knife wounds; Fig. 10) and blunt trauma. Because of its protected position, the ureter is injured only rarely by blunt trauma. However, occasionally, sudden hyperextension of the thoracolumbar spine associated with abrupt deceleration will disrupt the ureter at or near the ureteropelvic junction. This type of avulsion occurs mainly in children and is usually associated with massive extravasation of urine from the renal pelvis into the retroperitoneum. Very often, there is no hematuria, and physical findings in the abdomen are initially normal, which causes a delay of several days before proper diagnosis is made.

Ureteral injuries are often initially missed, since fistula with urinary extravasation may not become apparent for several days. An early diagnosis is likely to be made when there is a high index of suspicion with pain and fever and excretory urography is performed.

Excretory urography is usually well suited to demonstrate the findings characteristic of ureteral injuries such as extravasation, urinoma with ureteral displacement, stenosis, hydronephrosis, or nonappearance of the collecting structures.

Retrograde pyelography may be required to delineate the status and position of the lower ureter, to define the precise site of injury, to rule out injury to the contralateral ureter, and to clarify fistulous connections to other organs.

Sonography can be used to detect and monitor complicating hydronephrosis and to localize urinomas.

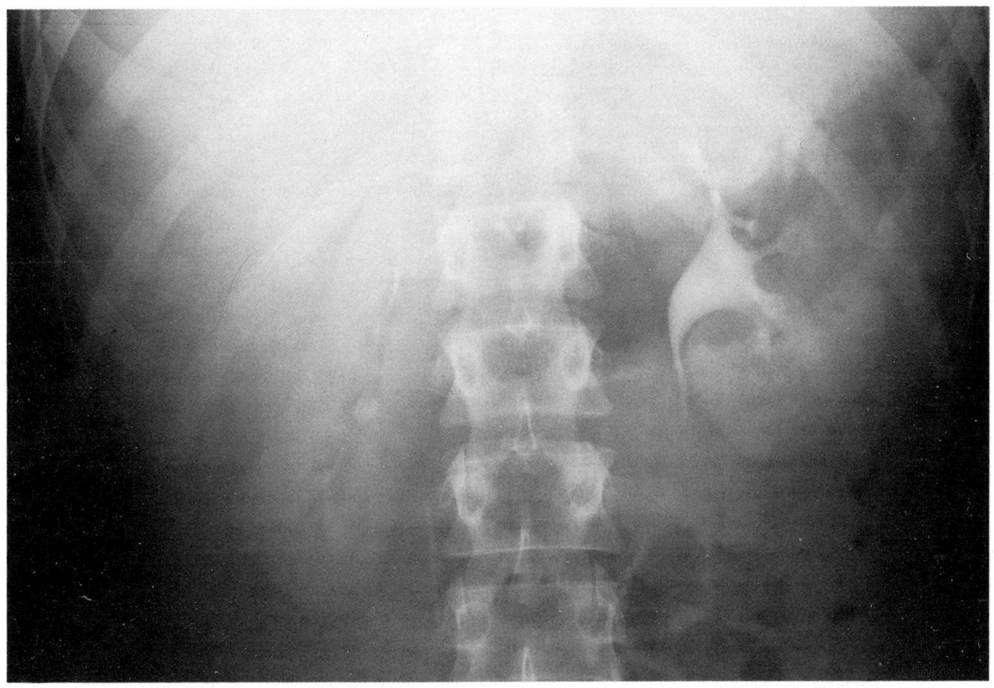

Figure 1.   An intravenous urogram; 15-minute film shows a crescentic filling defect on the lateral aspect of the right kidney consistent with a subcapsular hematoma.

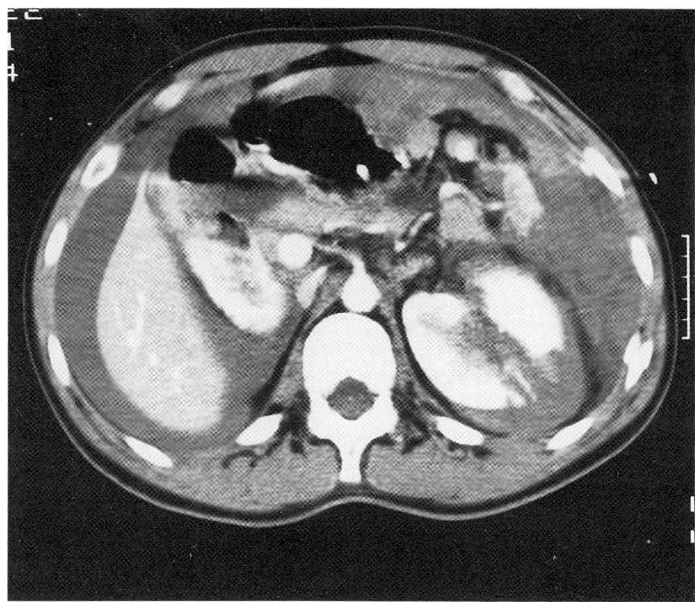

Figure 2.   Renal laceration with other injuries seen by CT. Corticomedullary laceration of the upper pole in a solitary left kidney with splenic trauma.

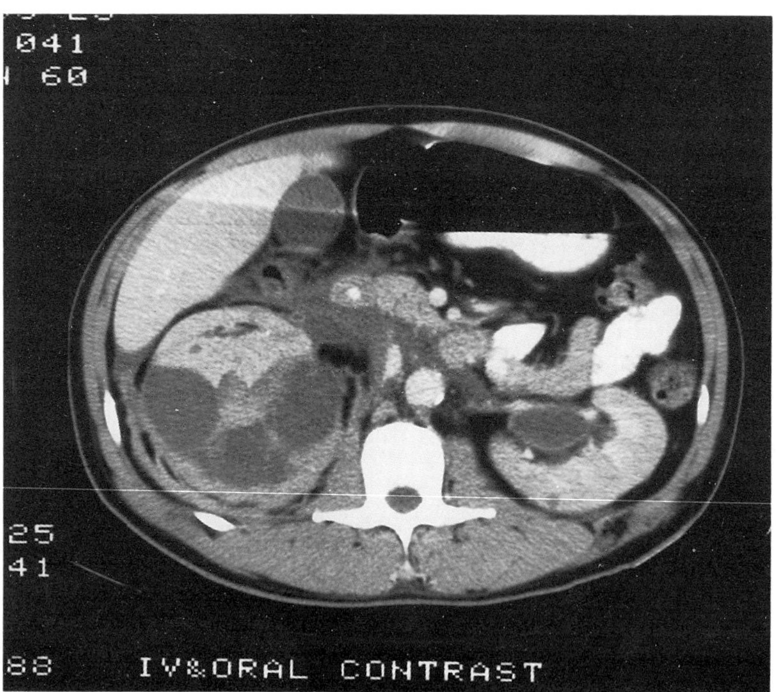

Figure 3.   Iatrogenic renal laceration in a patient with renal failure who underwent a CT-guided renal biopsy with a 3-gm hemoglobin drop. A CT scan shows a subcapsular hematoma with active bleeding into the perirenal space displacing the right kidney anteriorly.

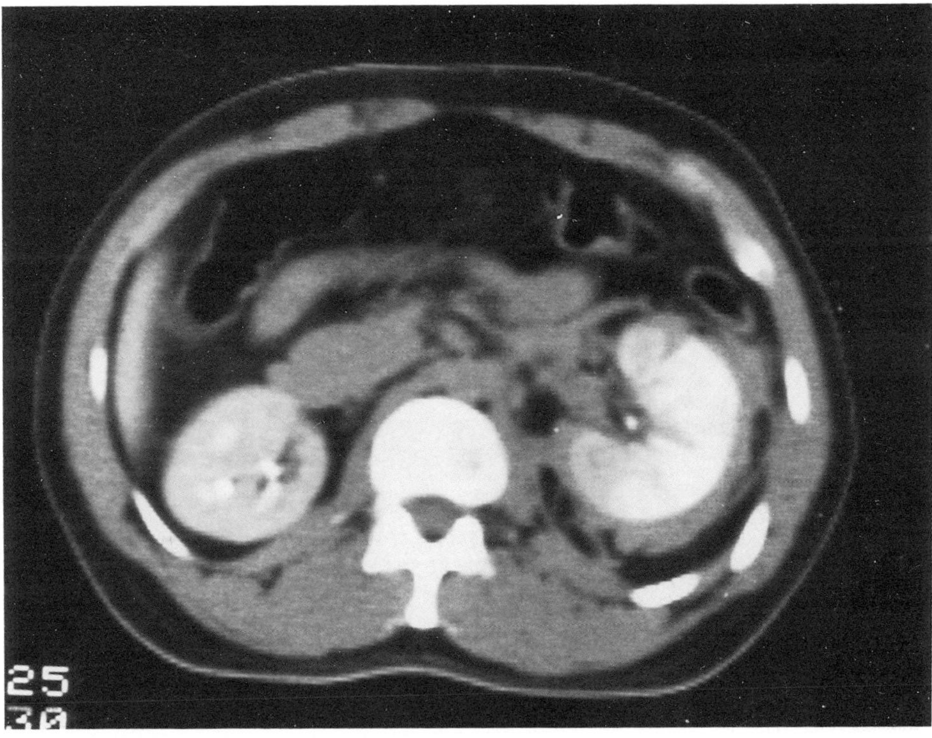

Figure 4A.   Renal laceration. The computed tomography shows a cortical laceration of the left upper pole.

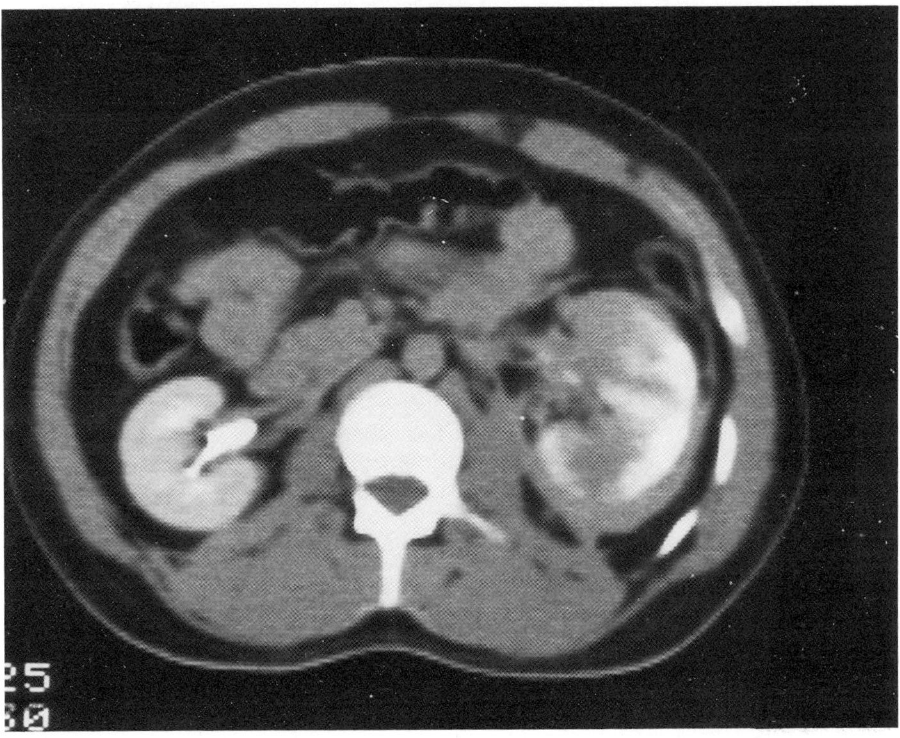

Figure 4B.   Intrarenal and perirenal hematomas, with extravasation of opaque urine.

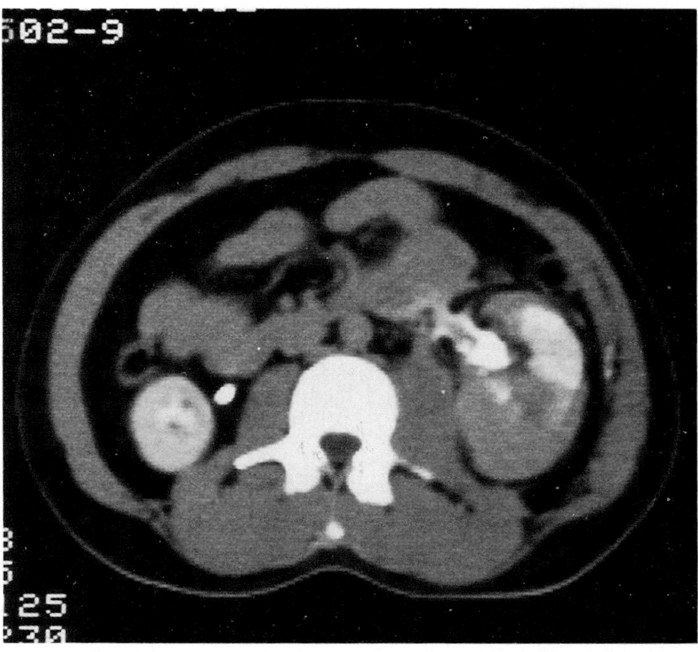

Figure 4C.   Absence of enhancement of the left lower pole characteristic of interrupted blood supply to the pole.

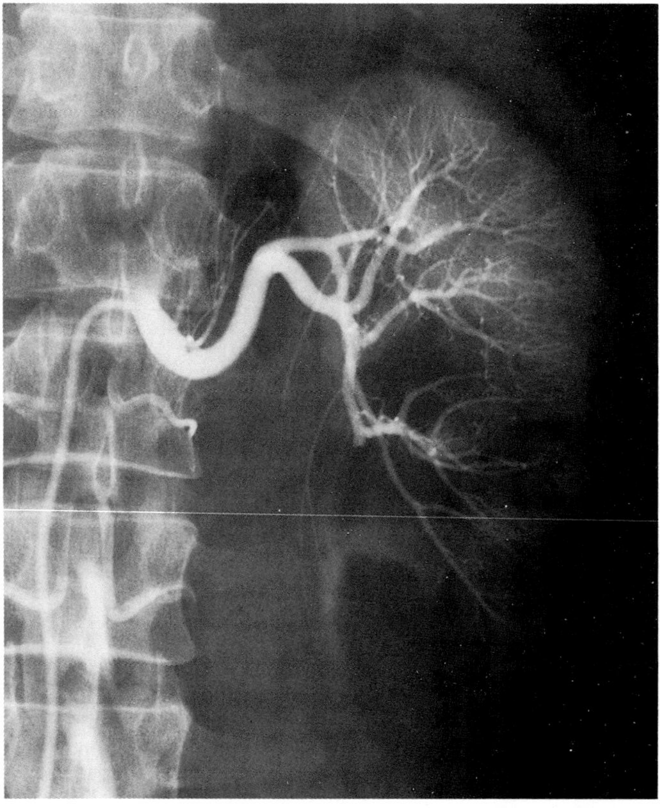

Figure 4D.   Angiography confirms the findings.

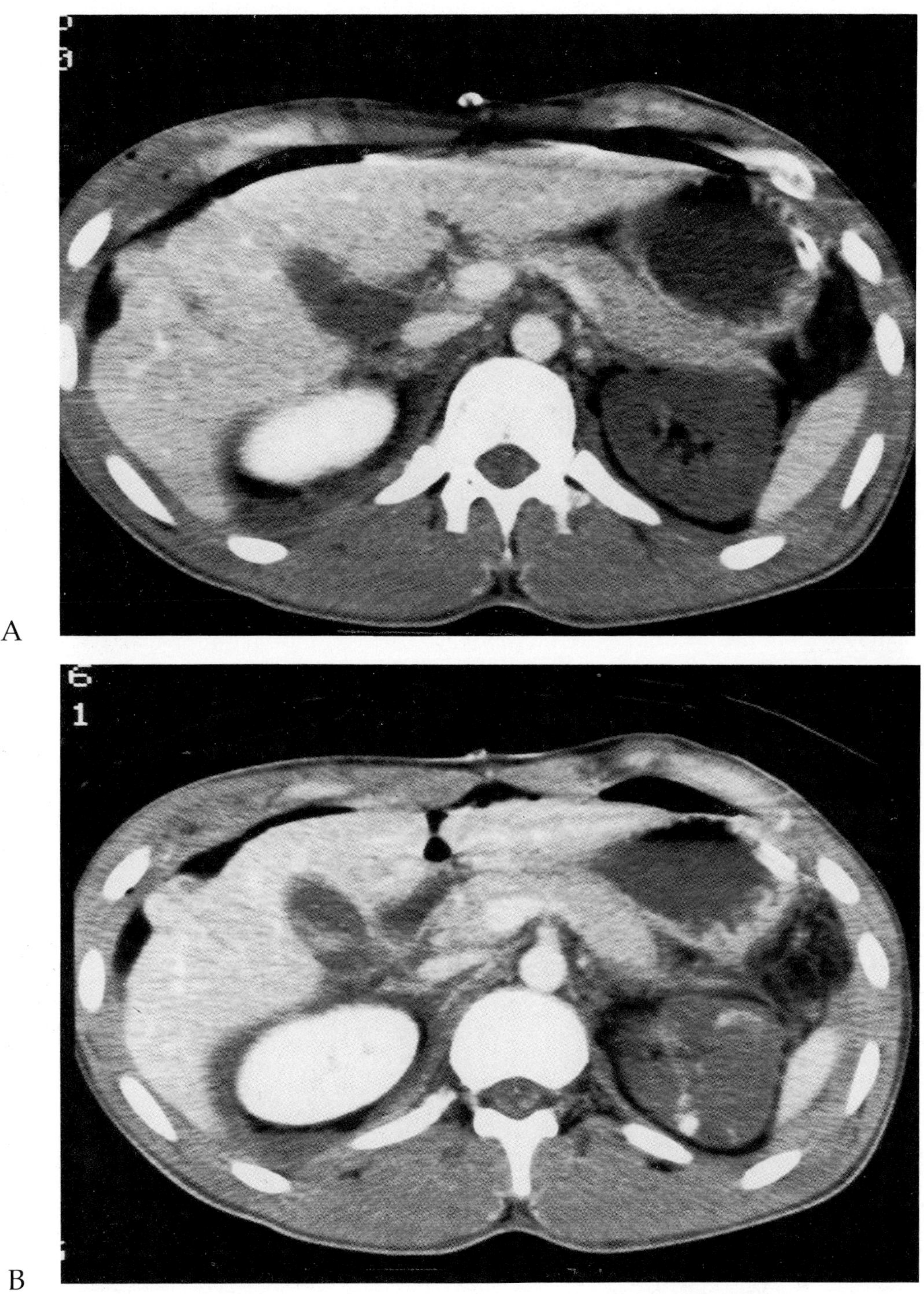

Figure 5.   Renal artery thrombosis in a 23-year-old motorcyclist who sustained multiple injuries. There were 4 to 8 RBC/HPF on the urinalysis. Intravenous urography showed no function on the left. The CT scan shows no enhancement of (A, top) the upper pole, or (B, bottom) the mid-portion of the left kidney and no perirenal hematoma. (Figure 5 continued on page 94.)

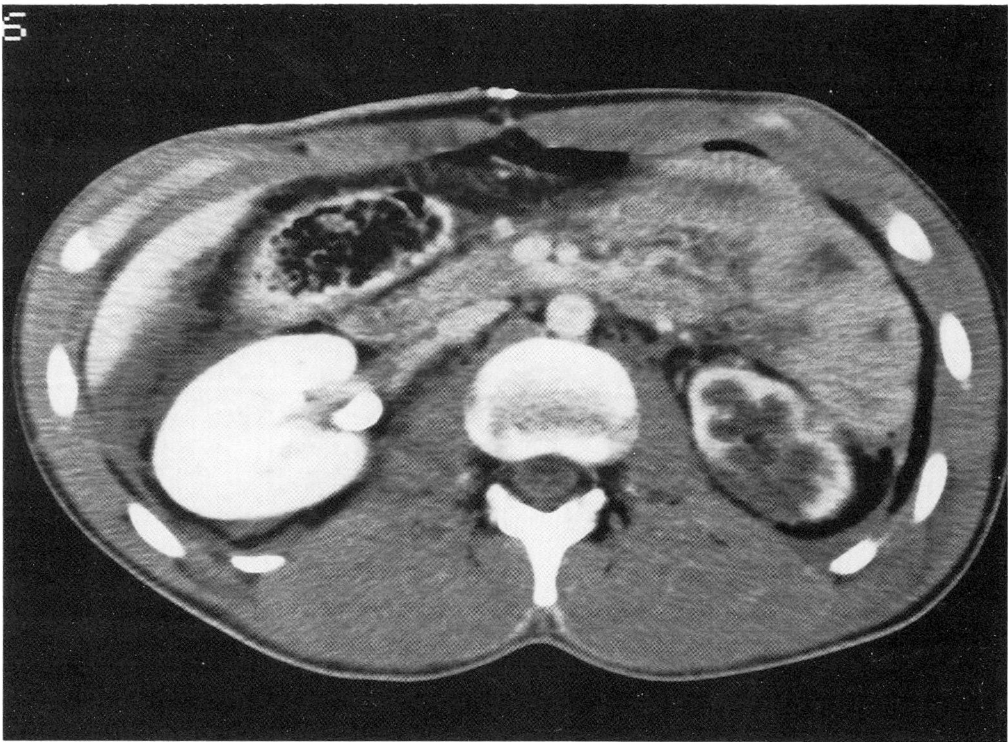

Figure 5C.   Rim sign is seen in the lower pole from collateral vascularization with renal artery thrombosis.

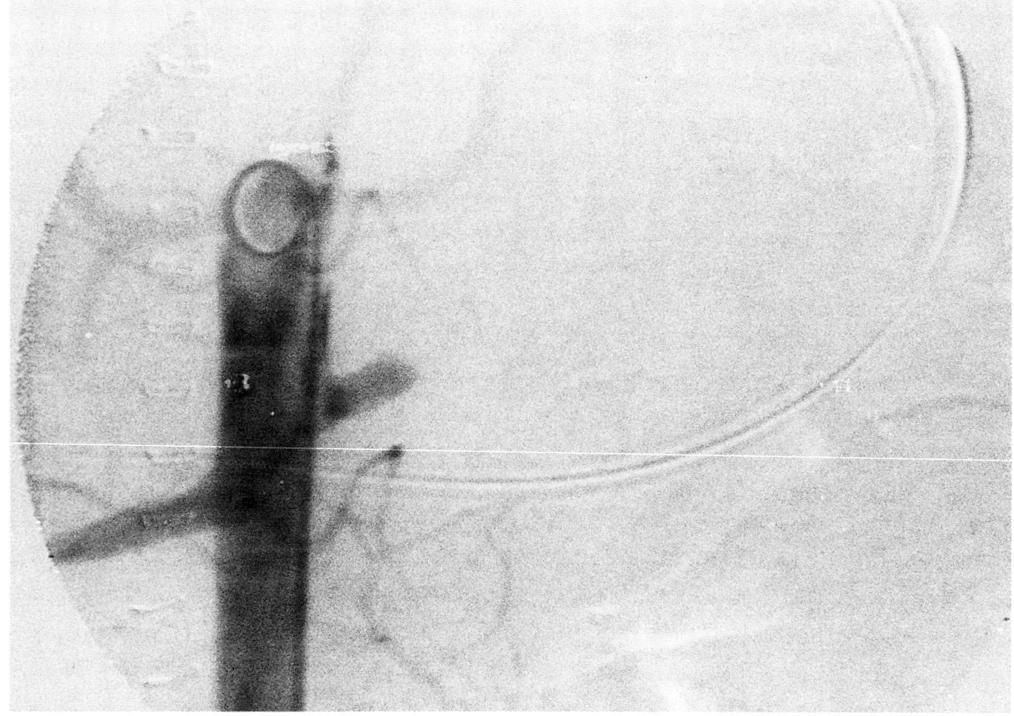

Figure 5D.   Arteriogram shows a total occlusion of the left renal artery by thrombosis. (Reprinted with permission from Cass AS, Luxenberg M: Management of renal injuries from external trauma. J Urol 1987; 138:266.)

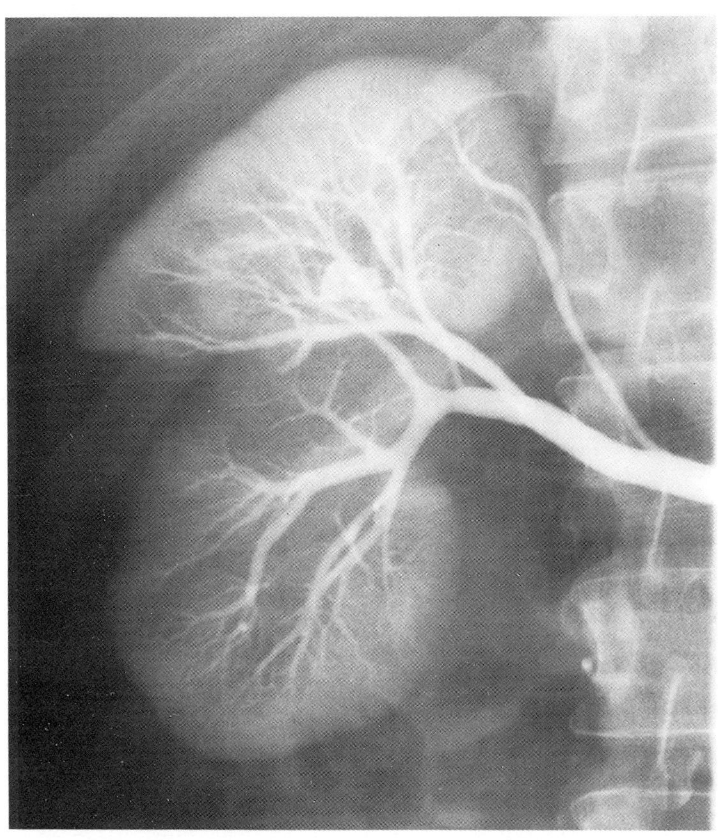

Figure 6.   Fractured kidney in a 36-year-old man involved in an automobile accident and complaining of right flank pain. Arteriography shows fractured middle third of the right kidney with medial displacement of the lower fragment and active bleeding. The patient subsequently underwent evacuation of the hematoma and suturing together of the kidney. In a clean fracture such as this, the kidney can often be saved.

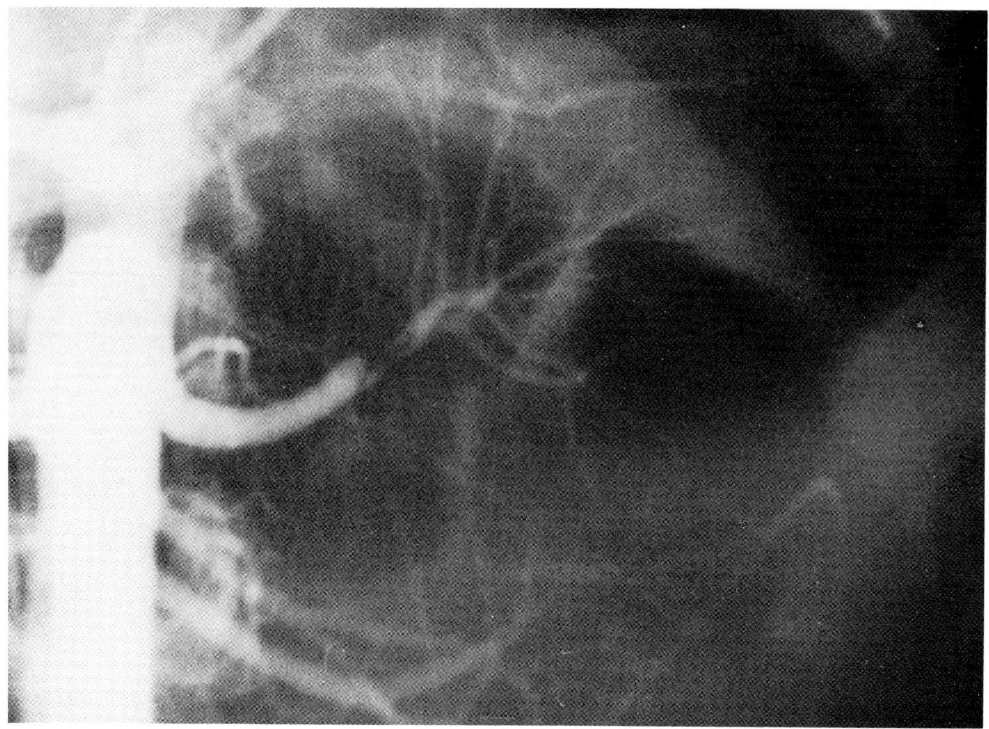

Figure 7.   Arteriogram showing thrombus of left renal artery with partial obstruction of blood flow. (Reprinted with permission from Cass AS, et al: Renal pedicle injury in patients with multiple injuries. J Trauma 1985; 25:892.)

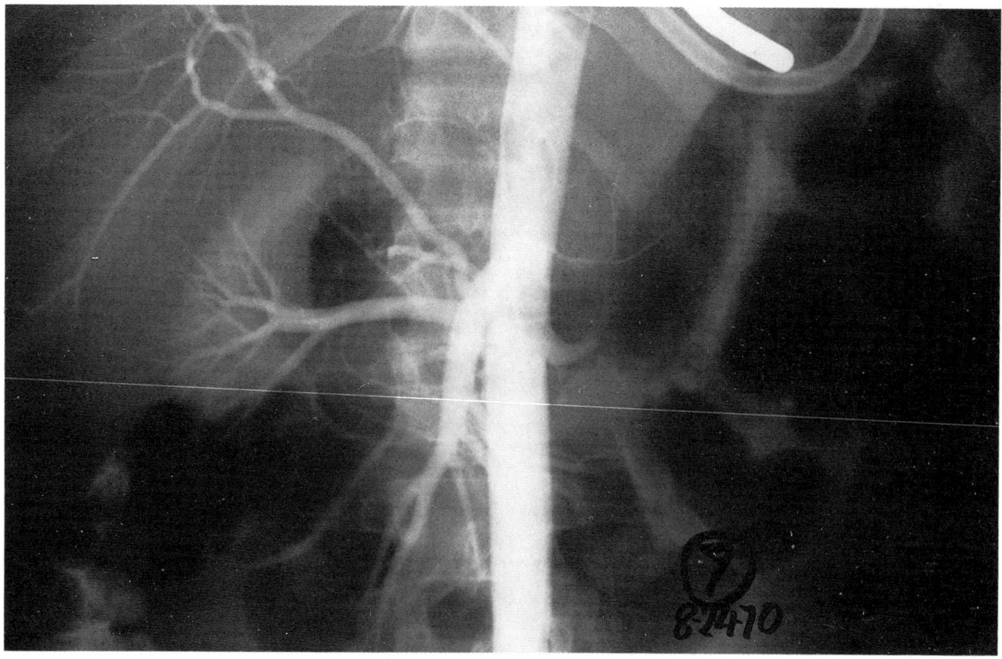

Figure 8.   Renal artery thrombosis. The arteriogram shows occlusion of the left main renal artery by an intimal tear with thrombosis.

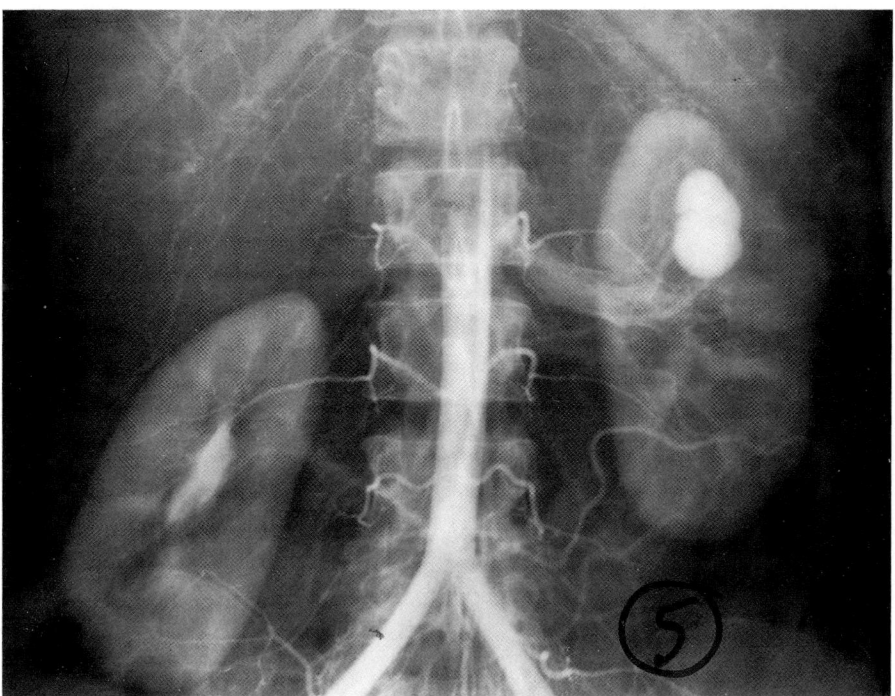

Figure 9. Traumatic arteriovenous fistula with pseudoaneurysm in a 46-year-old woman who was kicked by her husband. She complained of pain in the left lumbar region and had gross hematuria. The arteriogram shows early filling of the left renal vein and pseudoaneurysm in the left upper pole.

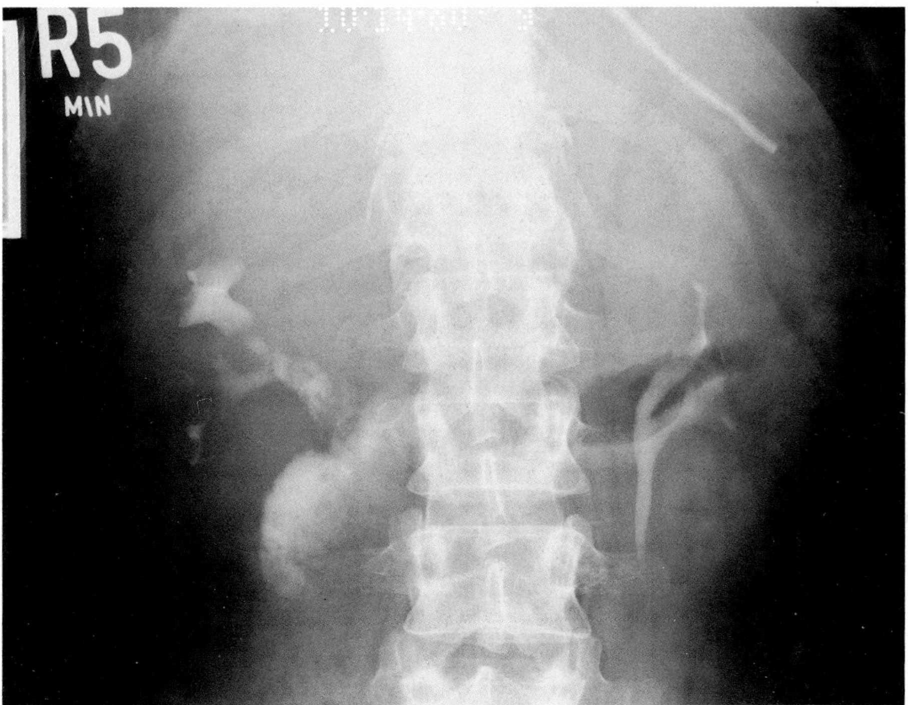

Figure 10. Rupture of the proximal right ureter secondary to a gunshot wound. The Intravenous urogram reveals extravasation of the contrast around the proximal third of the right ureter secondary to transection by a bullet. The retrograde pyelogram confirmed rupture.

Trauma to the Bladder

Injury to the bladder results most commonly from blunt trauma sustained in automobile, sports, or industrial accidents. Penetrating injuries from gunshot or knife wounds are much less common.

Iatrogenic bladder injuries are also less common and usually are associated with instrumentation (cystoscope, catheters, bougies, etc.) and surgery (inguinal hernia repair in children, gynecologic operations, obstetric procedures). These injuries are particularly prone to occur if the bladder is fixed by inflammatory or neoplastic infiltration of the perivesical tissues. Spontaneous rupture usually accompanies a serious underlying bladder lesion such as a tumor or necrotizing cystitis.

Rupture of the bladder is usually associated with pelvic fractures; of these ruptures, about 80% are extraperitoneal and 20% are intraperitoneal. The great majority of these pelvic fractures are pubic arch fractures, especially those near the symphysis. Fractures involving the pubic arch bilaterally are more often associated with serious urinary tract injury than are unilateral fractures. Most intraperitoneal ruptures result from blunt trauma to a full bladder without the presence of a pelvic fracture.

Any patient with pelvic arch fracture or a combination of severe lower abdominal trauma, pain, and inability to void should be considered as having a possible bladder injury. Hematuria is almost invariable in ruptures of the bladder. Intraperitoneal extravasation of urine generally results in signs of peritonitis, although peritonitis may not develop for 24 to 72 hours after the injury.

Bladder injuries may be classified as follows: (1) contusion; (2) intraperitoneal rupture; (3) extraperitoneal rupture; and (4) combined intraperitoneal and extraperitoneal ruptures.

1. Bladder *contusion* results from incomplete tears of the bladder, usually a mucosal bruising. As a result, the cystogram demonstrates no extravasation. Contusion of the bladder is a clinical diagnosis made by exclusion.

Perivesical hematoma is commonly present in association with pelvic fractures (Fig. 11). With these pelvic injuries, the extraperitoneal space surrounding the bladder, which is formed by loose areolar connective tissue, may be filled with hematoma causing symmetrical compression of the bladder (teardrop or pear-shaped bladder). When the hematoma is predominantly unilateral, asymmetric compression of the bladder exists.

2. *Intraperitoneal rupture* of the bladder occurs when there is a sudden rise in the intravesical pressure secondary to a blow to the lower abdomen (kick or seatbelt injuries). This increased pressure results in rupture of the weakest portion of the bladder, the dome, and as a consequence, intraperitoneal extravasation occurs. This type of injury occurs in patients who have a distended bladder and is usually not associated with pelvic fractures. Intraperitoneal rupture is more common in children, where the bladder is more an abdominal organ and thus is more susceptible to blunt trauma. Intraperitoneal rupture may also be a complication of instrumentation of the bladder such as cystoscopy or catheter manipulation.

3. *Extraperitoneal rupture* of the bladder most commonly occurs when the bladder is lacerated by a sharp, bony spicule from a fracture of the anterior pelvic arch. Most extraperitoneal ruptures occur on the anterior lateral wall close to the bladder base.

Extraperitoneal extravasation occurs within the loose tissues of the perivesical space, presenting an irregular, amorphous, and ill-defined density. Occasionally, urinary extravasation extends to the thigh, to the scrotum, or into the anterior abdominal wall.

4. *Combined intraperitoneal and extraperitoneal ruptures* are reported to occur in 9% of the cases. At times, this diagnosis is difficult because the contrast medium in the intraperitoneal portion may be obscured by the extraperitoneal extravasation.

Bladder imaging for trauma is by the retrograde cystogram. If clinical findings raise any suspicion of urethral injury (e.g., blood at the external meatus), a retrograde urethrogram should be attempted before bladder catheterization. Retrograde cystography is best carried out by instilling 400 ml of 30% concentration of contrast medium into the bladder. A postdrainage film should also be taken to avoid missing a small extraperitoneal leakage from a posterior rent, otherwise obscured by the contrast-filled bladder.

Bladder ruptures may be missed by retrograde cystography with insufficient bladder filling with dye (<400 ml) since a small tear may seal spontaneously, either by bladder wall edema and elasticity or by adherence of an adjacent loop of bowel or omentum.

When there is an intraperitoneal tear of the bladder, contrast will pool in the cul de sac and extend superolaterally into the pericolic gutters (Fig. 12). The contrast is free flowing in the peritoneal cavity and will not appear streaky. It will be seen outlining loops of bowel.

In the extraperitoneal rupture of the bladder, contrast is not free flowing and will appear as a streaky or a flame-like configuration (Fig. 13). A combined rupture will demonstrate both of these findings.

Trauma to the Urethra

Urethral injuries in females are extremely rare because of the structure's protected location and short length; however, occasionally, serious pelvic fractures result in avulsion of the urethra at the bladder neck. Direct injuries to the distal urethra may follow penetrating trauma or surgery of the urethra and vagina. Obstetric injuries, from forceps instrumentation or prolonged pressure ischemia, resulting in urethrovaginal fistulae, also have been reported.

In the male, the most common sites of blunt injury are the posterior and the bulbous urethra. Significant trauma to the pendulous urethra is infrequently encountered because the penile urethra usually moves out of the way when blunt injuries occur; injuries of the pendulous urethra are most often the result of penetrating wounds, instrumentation, and insertion of foreign bodies.

Trauma to the Posterior Urethra

Rupture of the posterior urethra is associated with fractures of the bony pelvis, especially in the region of the symphysis pubis.

At the moment of impact, the prostatic urethra is driven back along with the bladder and prostate, while the membranous portion remains fixed within the urogenital diaphragm resulting in shearing of its prostatomembranous portions by the rigid urogenital diaphragm. There is also tearing of the puboprostatic ligaments, which increases the mobility of the prostate and prostatic urethra.

Posterior urethral injuries are divided into contusion, partial rupture, and complete rupture. This classification is not dependent on the exact site of rupture, but is based rather more on the severity, as demonstrated by urethrographic patterns of extravasation.

The cardinal signs of posterior urethral injury are: (1) blood at the urethral meatus; (2) inability to void; (3) palpable bladder; (4) pelvic arch fractures; and (5) pelvic hematoma detected by rectal examination, which reveals a soft, boggy mass in the area of the prostate.

Retrograde urethrography (RUG) is the only safe and reliable method for assessing the type and severity of suspected urethral injuries. Considering the simplicity and accuracy of RUG, there is currently no role for injudicious diagnostic catheterization, which carries the risks of conversion of a partial tear into a complete rupture and of a sterile extravasation into an infected urinoma.

Retrograde urethrography is begun by inserting a No. 14 or No. 15 Foley catheter into the urethral meatus and seating the balloon in the navicular fossa with 2 ml of saline. About 25 ml of 30% contrast material is injected.

To prevent geometric foreshortening of the urethra, optimal observation and filming should be done in the steep oblique (60%) projection.

If an indwelling catheter has already been inserted it should not be removed. A RUG can be done by inserting a 16-French polyethylene catheter into the distal urethra alongside the indwelling catheter, compressing the glans penis over the catheters to obstruct the distal urethra, and injecting contrast medium. Urethral contusion or minor tear occur without evidence of extravasation. With partial rupture, the extravasation of contrast at the site of injury is limited, and contrast enters the bladder (Fig. 14). With complete rupture, the extravasation of contrast at the site of injury is large with no contrast entering the bladder (Fig. 15).

Trauma to the Anterior Urethra

Injury of the bulbous urethra most commonly results from the passage of a foreign object (catheter, cystoscope, wire, pencil, etc.), from a direct blow to the perineum (such as a kick), or from straddle-type injury (when a person falls astride a hard object). In these direct blows to the perineum or straddle-type injury, the bulbous urethra is crushed against the bony pelvis, which results in injuries ranging from a mild contusion to complete rupture.

Injuries of the pendulous urethra are most commonly caused by foreign objects. Blunt trauma to the penile urethra is rare. Penetrating trauma (e.g., stab and gunshot wounds) cause various degrees of disruption of the pendulous and bulbous urethra.

Retrograde urethrography should be performed whenever a urethral injury is suspected and identifies the site, nature (contusion and partial or complete tear), and extent of injury.

In a contusion, there is no extravasation. In a partial tear, continuity of the urethra is maintained but extravasation occurs. With a complete tear, total transection of the urethra takes place with no continuity of mucosa.

Trauma to the Testicle

Blunt trauma to the scrotum generally results from kicks, sporting events, and industrial or vehicular (especially motorcycle) accidents, in which the testicle is impacted on the pubic bone. Penetrating trauma is caused by gunshot wounds.

Blunt trauma to the testicle may result in contusion or rupture and a hematocele may be present with both types of injuries. Testicular rupture occurs when the inelastic tunica albuginea is torn, resulting in extrusion of the testicular contents and bleeding into the scrotal sac.

Injuries caused by blunt scrotal trauma are difficult to evaluate clinically if a tense hematocele is present, specifically in terms of differentiating testicular rupture from contusion.

Sonography is the diagnostic technique of choice for the evaluation of the traumatized scrotum. Sonography can identify an intact testis, thus avoiding unnecessary surgery.

If the testicle cannot be visualized or if it demonstrates ill-defined margins and inhomogeneous internal echo patterns (Fig. 16), testicular rupture is a strong possibility.

Hematoma usually accompanies testicular ruptures, producing focal hypoechoic or hyperechoic abnormalities on sonography. Although these sonographic features are very sensitive for testicular abnormality, they are not specific for the diagnosis of rupture. Hematoma can occur within the testicle (intratesticular), beneath the tunica albuginea (subcapsular), and within the tunica vaginalis (hematocele). A chronic hematocele may appear as a thick-walled fluid collection indistinguishable sonographically from a chronic hydrocele.

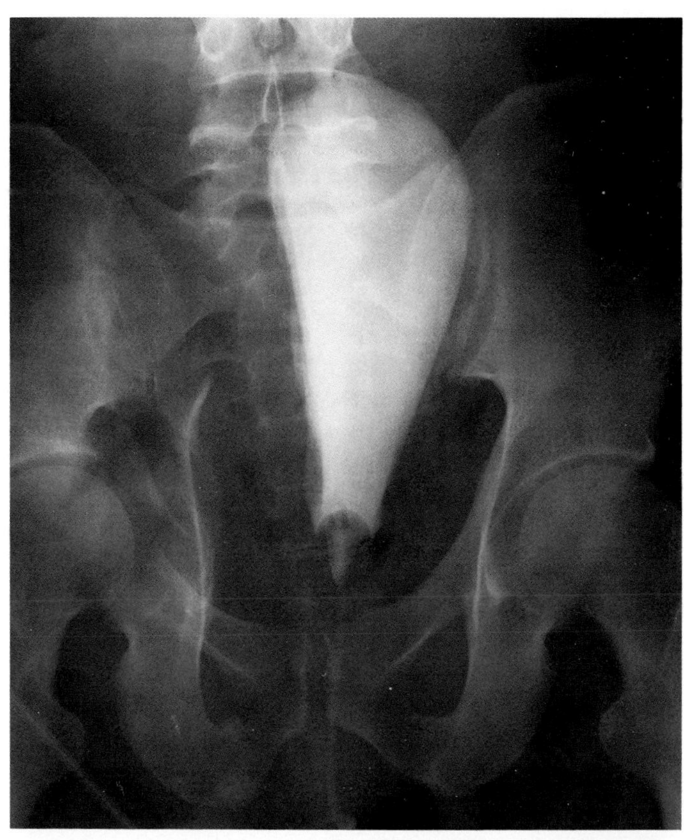

Figure 11.   Contusion of the bladder with a right perivesical hematoma. The cystogram shows a huge hematoma with a compound fracture dislocation of the right acetabulum.

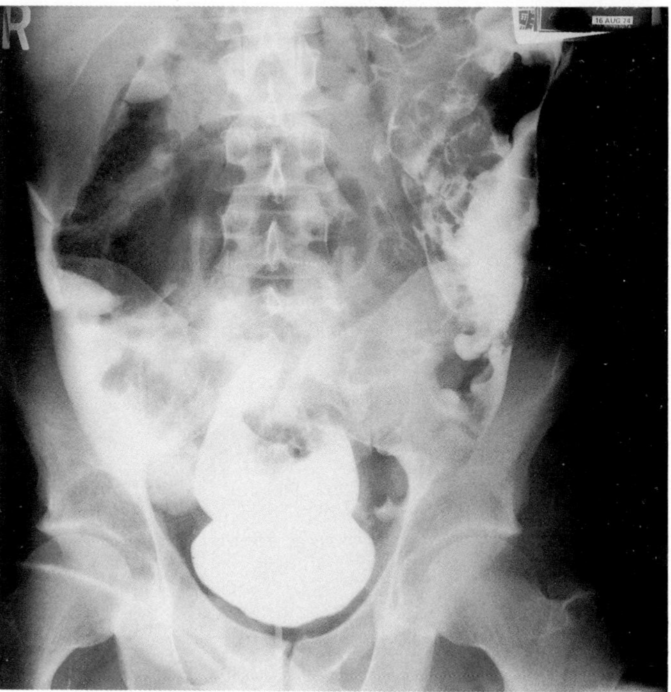

Figure 12.   Intraperitoneal rupture of the bladder. The cystogram demonstrates an accumulation of contrast medium in the cul-de-sac (hourglass appearance) and in the pericolic gutters. Note also contrast outlining several loops of bowel.

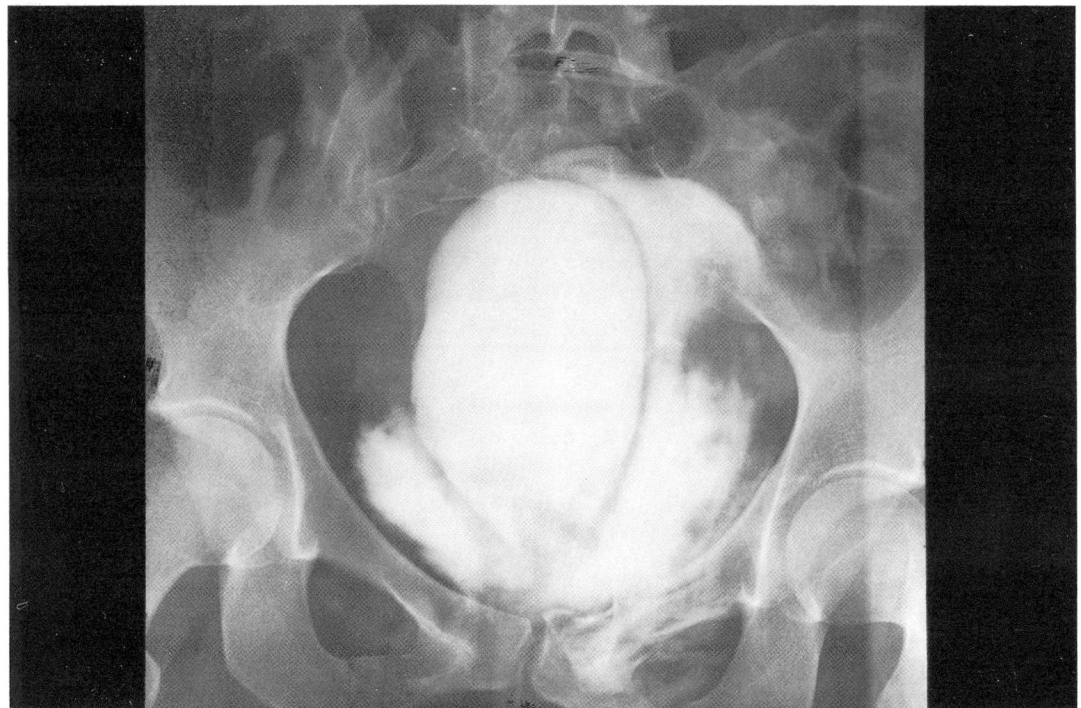

Figure 13.   Extraperitoneal rupture of the bladder. The cystogram demonstrates extravasation of contrast up the side wall of the pelvis.

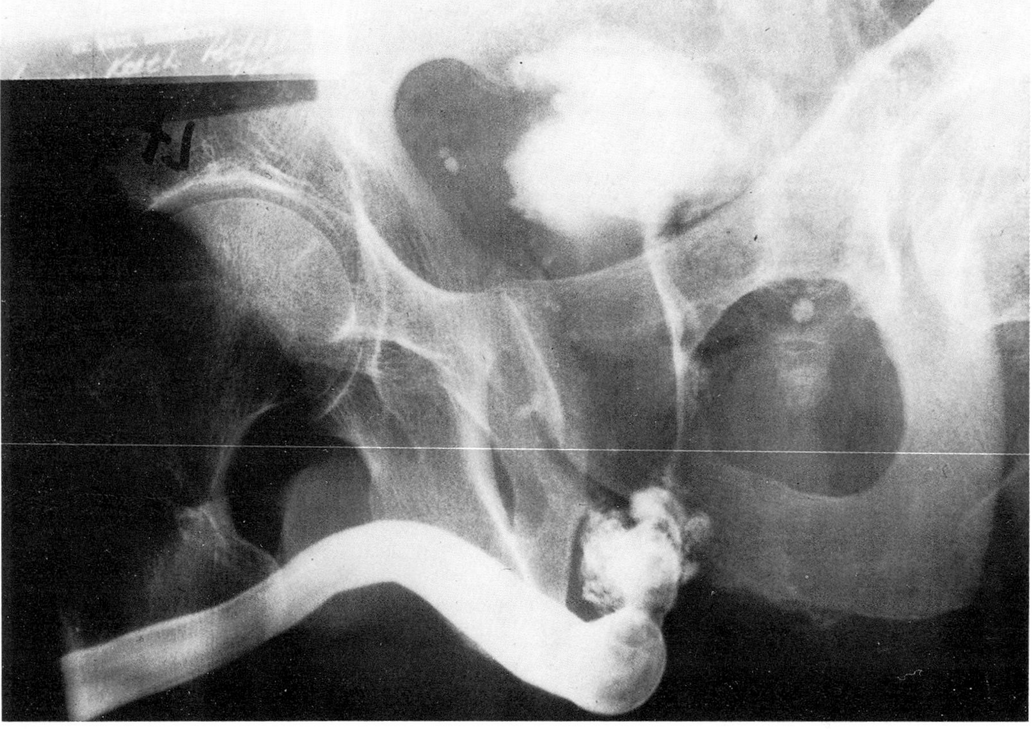

Figure 14.   Partial rupture of the urethra. The retrograde urethrography shows small extravasation at the site of the partial rupture and contrast passing up into the bladder.

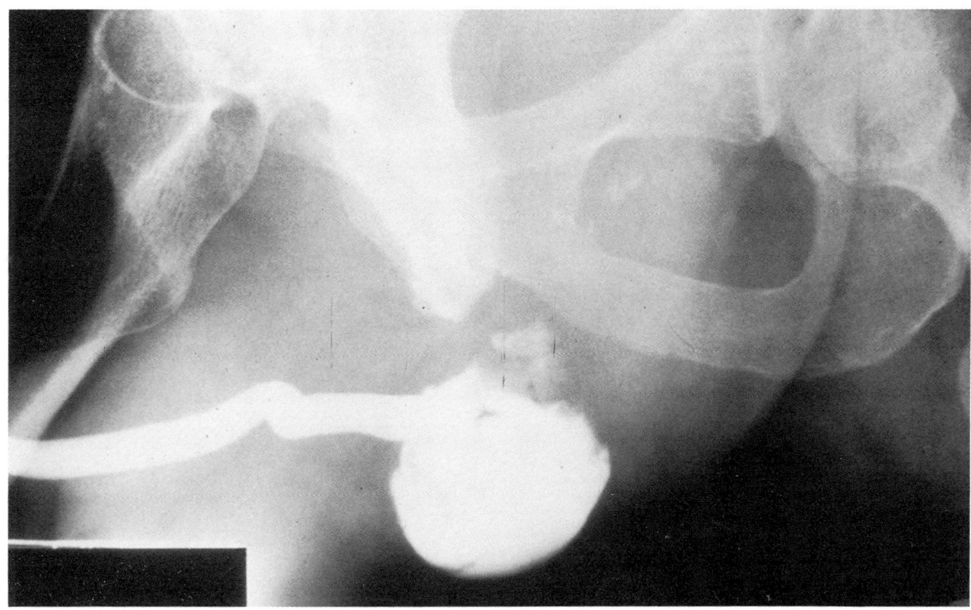

Figure 15. Complete rupture of the urethra as seen by the RUG. There is some extravasation at the site of the rupture; no contrast passes into the bladder.

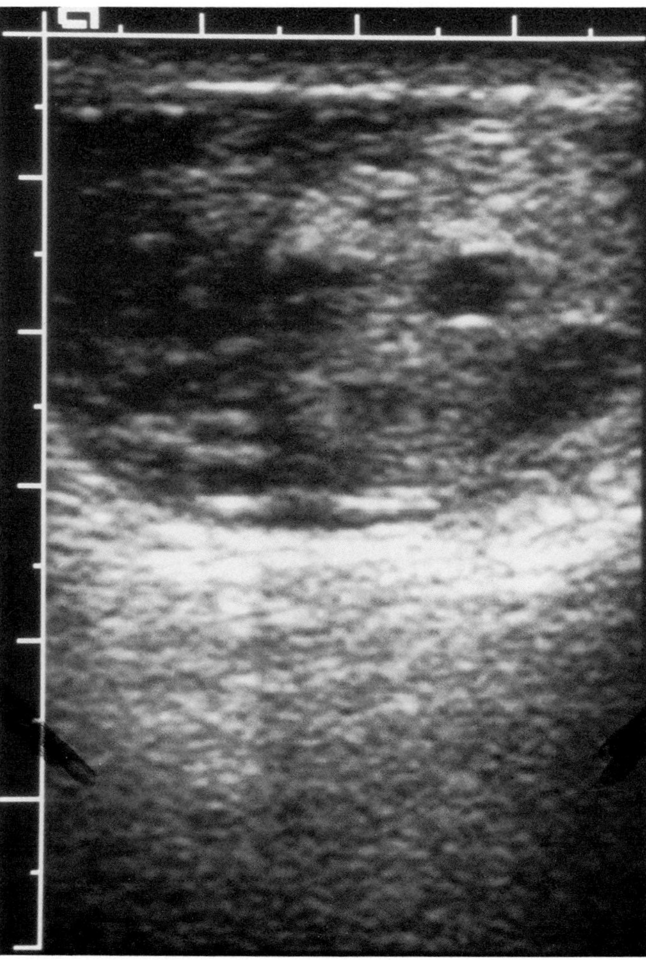

Figure 16. Testicular rupture. A scrotal ultrasound scan showing an hypoechoic area (intratesticular hematoma), disruption of tunica albuginea, and blood clot in the tunica vaginalis sac (hematocele).

Chapter 5

Calculous Disease

Charles Smith, M.D., Robert Berkseth, M.D.,
Joe Lee, M.D., and Carl Smith, M.D.

Radiologic imaging is essential to the diagnosis, management, and monitoring of nephrolithiasis. In the patient with ureteral colic, imaging confirms the diagnosis of stone disease and aids in decision making regarding management. In the asymptomatic patient, imaging is the only way to make the diagnosis. Medical management of nephrolithiasis is aimed at the prevention of stone formation or growth and, in some cases, at stone dissolution. Radiologic monitoring is the only acceptable means for judging the adequacy of such therapy. This chapter reviews current imaging modalities to aid the clinician dealing with nephrolithiasis.

Plain Film

The visibility of a stone on a plain film of the abdomen is dependent on its size, radiopacity, and location (Fig. 1). Bowel gas, fecal material, and other opacities such as gallstones, calcified lymph nodes, medications in the intestinal lumen, and phleboliths may interfere with visualization.

The size required for visibility on a plain film of the abdomen is interdependent with radiopacity and interfering factors. With good-quality radiographs and no significant interference, a stone as small as 1 to 2 mm can be seen. Table 1 shows which stones are considered radiopaque and which are radiolucent. Radiopaque stones make up approximately 90% of all stones. Cal-

cium phosphate stones tend to be the most radiopaque and struvite the least. Cystine stones are radiopaque, although they are not as opaque as calcium-containing stones.

The location of the stone can also influence its recognition. Stones in the ureter or overlying the bony pelvis may be particularly difficult to see. Stones in the lower ureter are frequently difficult to differentiate from phleboliths and may require oblique films. The most reliable way of differentiating these calcifications is by outlining the ureter with contrast. Plain films are used to diagnose ureteral stones in patients with ureteral colic and to diagnose intrarenal stones (Fig. 2).

The sensitivity of the plain film for radiopaque stones is unknown. Studies have reported that stones are visible on plain films in from 39% to 60% of patients presenting with renal colic. Some of the stones not seen were radiolucent, but many were radiopaque. A true-positive rate of 33% to 45% and a true-negative rate of 19% to 60% have been found in patients with ureteral colic, with false-positive and false-negative rates of 0.9% to 27% and 27% to 36%, respectively. Such data have lead to the conclusion that the plain film is of limited value. This view is probably true in the patient who has flank or abdominal pain, in whom the question to be answered is whether there is a ureteral stone. However, it should not detract from the benefits of the plain film in diagnosing intrarenal stones.

From *Imaging of Urologic Disorders* edited by Alexander S. Cass, MBBS, © 1992, Futura Publishing Inc., Mount Kisco, NY.

Table 1. Radiopacity of Calculi

Radiopaque	Radiolucent
Calcium phosphate	Uric acid
Calcium oxalate	Ammonium acid urate
Cystine	Xanthine
Struvite	2, 8-Dihydroxyadenine
	Matrix

Studies have shown that the plain film can detect intrarenal stones in 85% to 90% of patients. Stones easily seen on plain films can be monitored by this modality during medical therapy instead of by more expensive procedures.

In conclusion, although the plain film of the abdomen may have limited value in the determination of the cause of abdominal pain, it is an important modality to diagnose intrarenal stones and monitor them during medical therapy.

Linear Tomography

Imaging of stones by linear tomography is less influenced by overlying bowel gas, fecal material, or rib shadows. This study has been found to be more sensitive than the plain film in detecting renal stone disease when no calcifications are seen on plain films or in identifying additional calcifications beyond those seen on plain films. This study can be accomplished without bowel preparation and can detect stones as small as 1 mm. It has been suggested that three to four films be taken 1.0 to 1.5 cm apart using a linear or circular motion.

Tomography is the most sensitive method for detecting intrarenal calcifications (Fig. 3). It is also the most effective method of monitoring patients under medical management for stone growth or new stone formation.

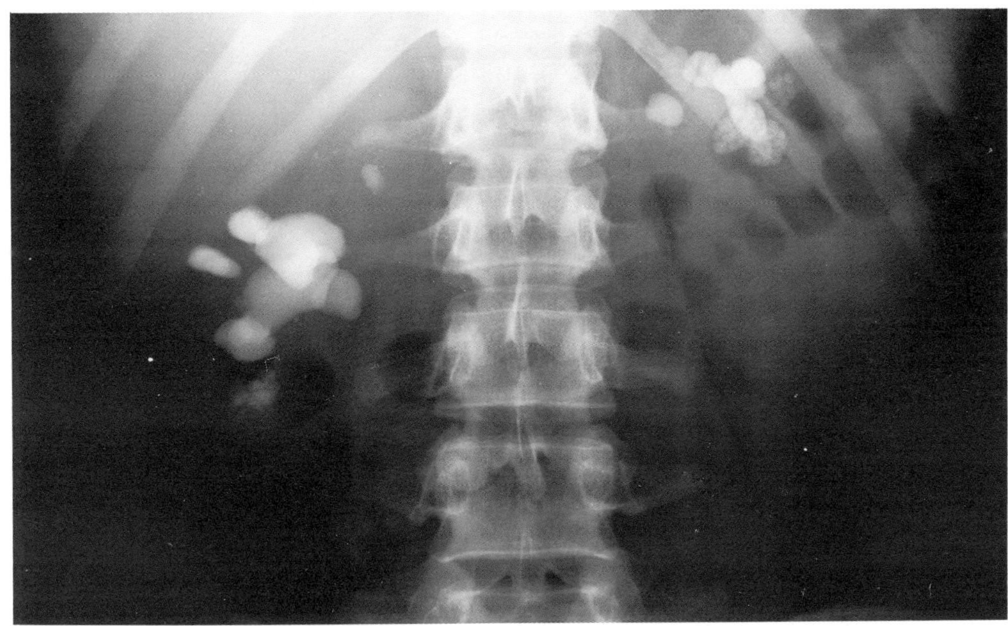

Figure 1. Plain film showing bilateral staghorn calculi.

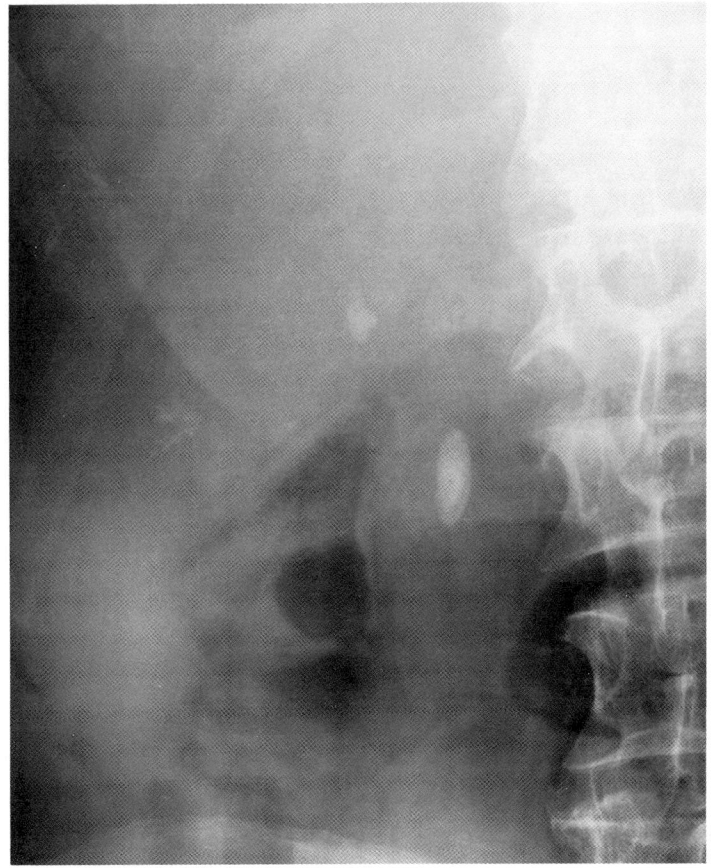

Figure 2. Plain film revealing stones in the ureter and in the lower pole of the kidney.

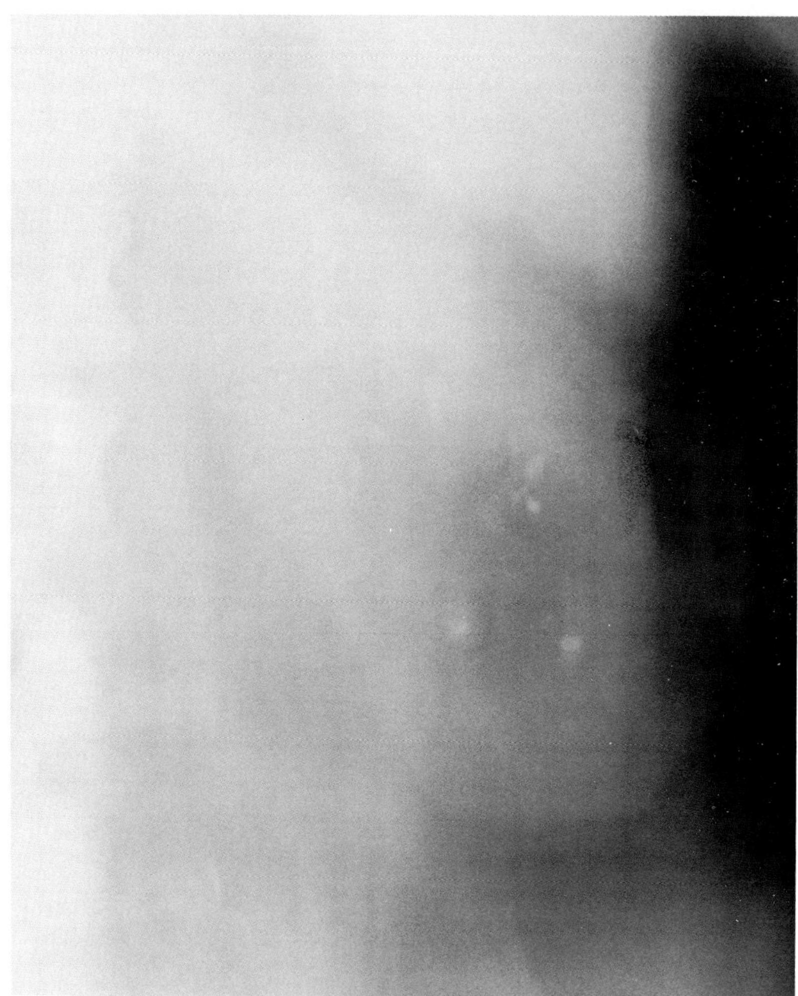

Figure 3.   Tomography of left kidney showing many small calculi.

Intravenous Urography

The role of intravenous urography is diagnostic in the patient with suspected renal colic and in those with radiolucent stone disease. In the patient with the clinical picture of renal colic, intravenous urography is the imaging modality of choice.

There should be a systematic approach to reviewing the films. The plain film should be reviewed first for calcifications overlying the kidneys, the course of the ureters, and the bladder because once contrast has been administered, most opaque calculi will no longer be visible. Findings after contrast administration include a delayed but frequently intense nephrogram on the involved side. Appearance of the contrast in the collecting systems can also be delayed (Fig. 4). Pyelocaliectasis and ureteral dilatation down to the point of obstruction confirm the diagnosis. It is important to do the study as soon as possible after the onset of pain. Studies done during pain have revealed the etiology of obstruction in 68% to 86% of patients, whereas when the studies were done within 7 days of the pain, only 48% were positive, and the yield fell to 24% if the studies were done more than 7 days after the pain.

Not all ureteral calculi result in dilatation of the ureter. The radiopacity of the contrast in the ureter on the side with the stone may be less than on the uninvolved side, and this may be the only finding suggesting a ureteral stone.

Arguments have been put forth that intravenous urography is not necessary in all patients with suspected ureteral stones because the diagnosis can be made with a great deal of certainty on the basis of clinical presentation and hematuria. This view tends to ignore the other benefits of the study: intravenous urography determines the site and degree of obstruction, the size of the stone, and the status of the contralateral kidney. This information will assist in formulating a plan of management. Stones less than 0.5 cm in diameter, no matter where they are located, will likely pass spontaneously. Stones between 0.5 and 0.8 cm will usually migrate into the distal ureter and pass spontaneously. Stones larger than 0.8 cm are much less likely to pass spontaneously, and stones greater than 1.0 cm and located in the middle to upper-third of the ureter are unlikely to pass and usually dictate a more aggressive surgical approach.

Occasionally, the intravenous urogram is negative in the face of symptoms suggestive of renal colic. Possible explanations include a small and nonobstructing stone that therefore is not seen, passage of the stone prior to the study, or a cause of the symptoms other than a ureteral stone. "The larger the pile of films of negative intravenous and retrograde pyelograms, the lower the probability that a patient's symptoms are due to stones."[1]

Retrograde Pyelography

Retrograde pyelograms are indicated when the intravenous urogram is equivocal, nondiagnostic, or contraindicated. The advantage of the study is that the technique does not rely on the renal excretion of contrast medium. Thus, unless there is an anatomic abnormality such as complete obstruction, the direct injection of contrast can usually demonstrate the lesion and the collecting system. Contrast allergies are not usually seen with retrograde pyelograms. Even in high-risk male cardiac patients, the retrograde pyelogram may be performed under local anesthesia with contemporary flexible cystoscopes.[2] The disadvantage of the retrograde pyelogram is that it does require instrumentation, which can result in ureteral edema, obstruction, perforation, submucosal injection, extravasation, or bacteremia. Therefore, extreme care should be used when performing this procedure.

Retrograde pyelography is an integral part of endourologic procedures for ureteral stone manipulations, ureteroscopy, ureteral stenting, and percutaneous nephrolithotomy. Retrograde pyelograms may also be performed intraoperatively during extracorporeal shock-wave lithotripsy to localize small or radiolucent renal calculi. Thus, the retrograde pyelogram is an important adjunct in the management of urinary calculous disease.

Computed Tomography

Computed tomography's greatest role in urolithiasis is in the evaluation of radiolucent filling defects in the urinary tract. Computed tomography (CT) gives greater density discrimination than does routine radiography or linear tomography: differences of 0.5% can be detected with CT, whereas a difference of 5.0% is required with routine radiography.

There is an extensive list of possible causes of filling defects, but the most common are radiolucent stones, tumor, blood clot, and papillae. By CT, radiolucent stones appear densely opaque (Fig. 5), whereas tumors, blood clots, and papillae appear as soft-tissue densities. The exception to this high attenuation is a matrix stone, which has low attenuation value and can still be confused with other soft-tissue lesions.[3] The most common radiolucent stone is composed of uric acid. This stone can be dissolved with alkali treatment, and CT has been used to monitor dissolution therapy.

Stones as small as 2 mm can be seen by CT.[4] It can also detect nephrocalcinosis, which cannot be seen on plain radiographs or with linear tomography.[5–6]

Studies have examined the possibility of using CT attenuation values for analysis of stone composition. However, because of the small size of most stones, partial volume averaging can affect the attenuation value. Probably of more importance, stones are seldom composed of a single substance. The extensive variety would predictably make identification of stone composition by density determination unreliable.

Ultrasonography

Ultrasonography (US) can detect opaque or nonopaque stones, and matrix material. It is therefore a valuable procedure in the patient with a radiolucent filling defect. The advantages of this imaging modality are the absence of radiation exposure, its usefulness in the patient with reduced renal function, and the absence of need for contrast injection. The sensitivity of US for renal calculi has been determined to be 91%, with most of the stones missed being 2.5 mm or smaller, but with a false-positive rate of 11%.[7] It may be possible to monitor stone dissolution therapy with US.

Detection of stones is dependent on finding an echogenic focus with an acoustic shadow (Fig. 6). The demonstration of the acoustic shadow is,

in turn, dependent on the size of the stone, the amount and type of intervening tissue, and the focal zone placement of the transducer. The differential diagnosis of an acoustic shadow is limited to stones and intrarenal gas.

Ultrasonography has been studied as a diagnostic imaging modality in patients with acute flank pain. Findings include the detection of the calculus or the presence of hydronephrosis. Compared with intravenous urography, US is not as sensitive in this setting,[8] primarily because of the absence of dilation of the collecting system proximal to the site of obstruction. Small stones located at the ureterovesical junction can be diagnosed more often with US than with intravenous urography, but stones are missed by both modalities. In the patient with symptoms of distal ureteral stone but a negative intravenous urogram, US is a valid alternative to proceeding to retrograde pyelography. It is the modality of choice in the pregnant patient and may also be the best procedure in children where the classic intravenous urographic changes of adults frequently are not seen.[9]

Ultrasonography is a sensitive method to detect nephrocalcinosis. Early nephrocalcinosis appears as an echogenic focus without an acoustic shadow. At this stage of development, it will not be seen on plain radiographs or with linear tomography, although it will be seen with CT. When the calcification is dense enough to be seen on plain radiographs, it will be associated with an acoustic shadow. The differential diagnosis of an echogenic focus without a shadow includes blood clots, tumor, focal scarring, abscesses containing microbubbles, renal parenchymal disease, and angiomyolipoma. However, it is now accepted that when the echogenic foci are limited to the renal pyramids, nephrocalcinosis is the most likely diagnosis.

Intraoperative Localization of Renal Calculi

The goal of open surgery for renal stone disease is the removal of all stone material. This is especially important in infection stone disease, where each fragment contains bacteria and the rate of recurrence of clinically significant stone disease has been reported to be 65%. Residual fragments can occur in 36% of operations, but with intraoperative radiography, this figure has been reduced to 10%.

Intraoperative contact radiography has been used for a number of years. Plastic-coated and sterile film is placed into the operative wound with the kidney on top of the film. Mammography film has been reported to give better resolution.

Contact radiography has facilitated the localization and removal of retained fragments. However, it gives two-dimensional information. Ultrasonography has been used intraoperatively, and there are several possible advantages over contact radiography. For example, US will detect radiolucent stones. The exploratory needle used as a guide for a nephrotomy incision can be placed under ultrasonic guidance, adding a third dimension to the procedure. Also, the procedures can be done repeatedly without any radiation exposure.

Other Modalities

Magnetic resonance imaging has not found a place in the radiologic assessment of stone disease. The elements in stones do not resonate easily and consequently appear as dark structures not easily separated from other poorly resonating substances.

Renal stones have been labeled with radioactive material in vivo.[10] This technique has potential as a stone localization procedure intraoperatively, but further evaluation needs to be done.

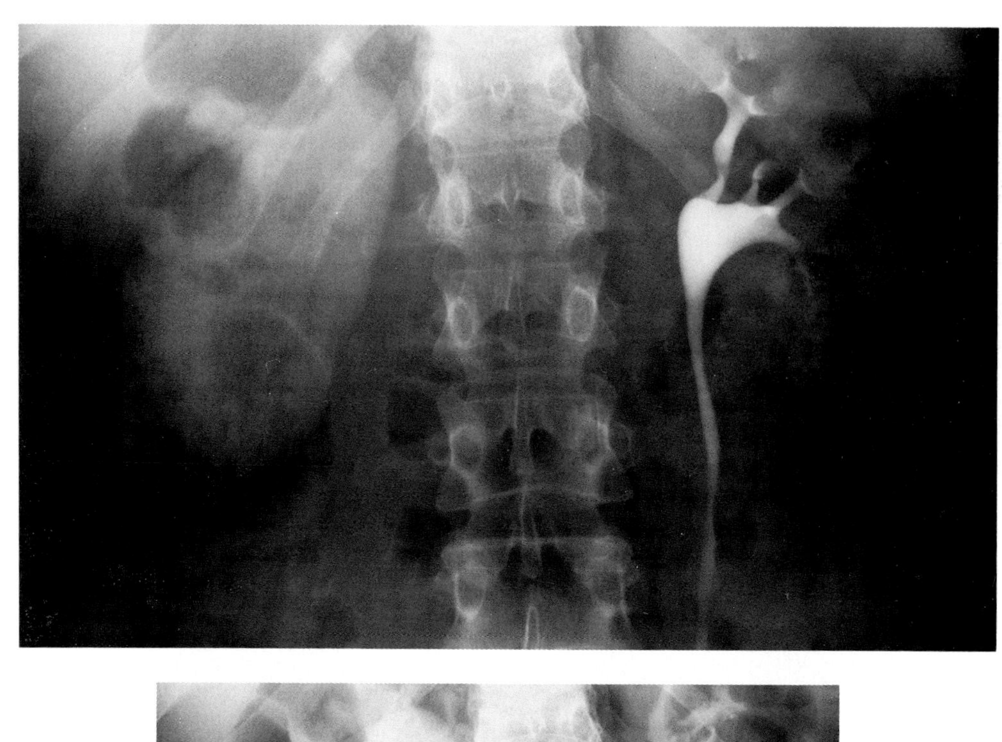

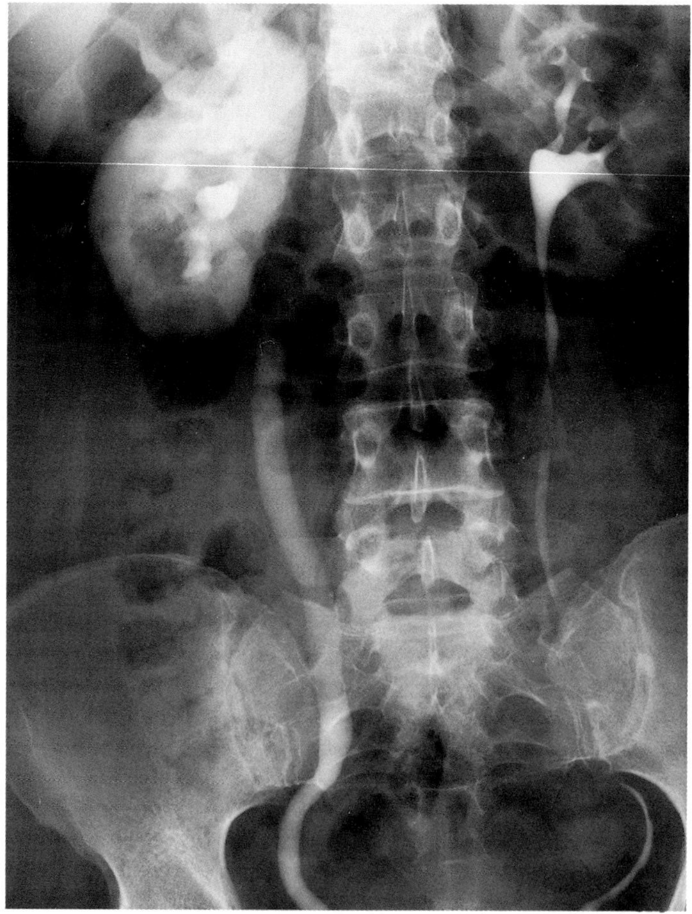

Figure 4. Intravenous urogram demonstrated delayed appearance of contrast medium in the obstructed right kidney in the (A, top) 10-minute film and (B, bottom) 45-minute film with intense nephrogram.

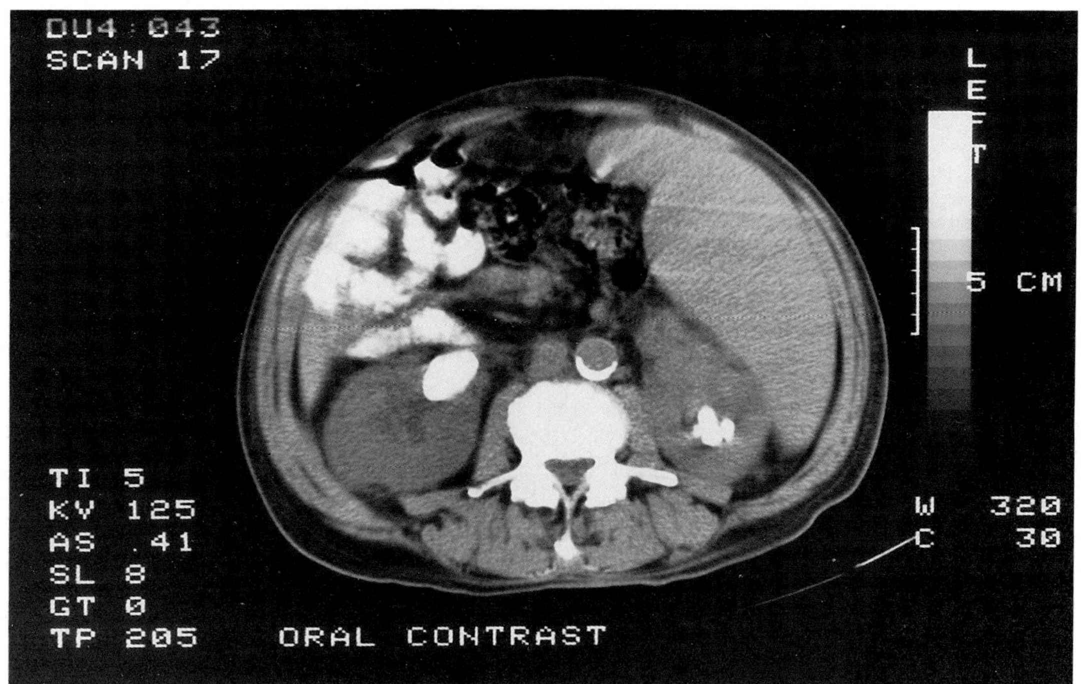

Figure 5.   Noncontrast enhanced CT scan revealed bilateral dense opaque renal stones which were composed of uric acid.

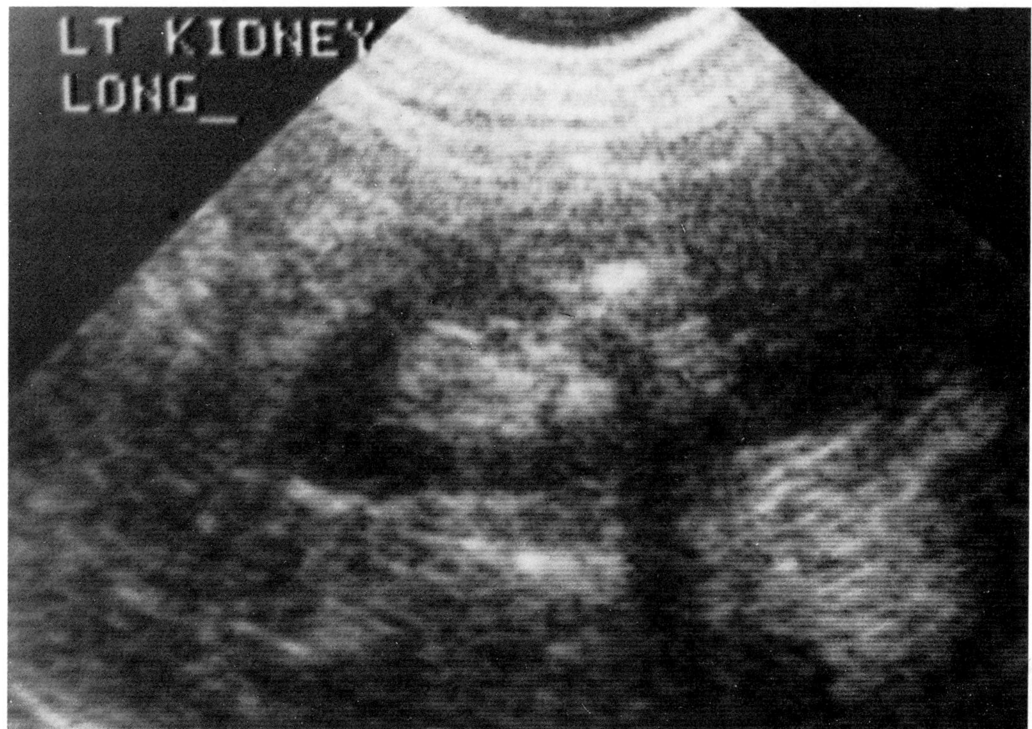

Figure 6.   Renal ultrasound showing a stone as an echogenic focus with an acoustic shadow.

References

1. Posen S: Some problems concerning urinary calculi. Practitioner 1971; 207:600.
2. Reddy PK, Hulbert JC: Retrograde pyelogram using the flexible cystoscope. J Urol 1986; 136:1283.
3. Sheppard PW, White FE: Demonstration of a matrix calculus using computed tomography. J Radiol 1987; 60:1028.
4. Parienty RA, Ducellier R, Pradel J, et al: Diagnostic value of CT numbers in pelvocalyceal filling defects. Radiology 1982; 145:743.
5. Afschrift M, Rachtegade P, Van Rattinghe R, et al: Nephrocalcinosis demonstrated by ultrasound and CT. Pediatr Radiol 1983; 13:42.
6. Manz F, Jaschke W, VanKaick G, et al: Nephrocalcinosis in radiographs, computed tomography, sonography and histology. Pediatr Radiol 1980; 9:19.
7. Middleton WD, Dodds WJ, Lauson TL, et al: Renal calculi: sensitivity for detection with US. Radiology 1988; 167:239.
8. Hill MC, Rich JI, Mardiat JG, et al: Sonography vs. excretory urography in acute flank pain. AJR 1985; 144:1235.
9. Breatnach E, Smith SEW: The radiology of renal stones in children. Clin Radiol 1983; 34:59.
10. Barker MCJ, Noble R, Williams RE: *In vivo* labelling of renal calculi with technetium JJM methylenine diphosphonate. Br J Radiol 1982; 55:39.

Chapter 6

Obstruction and Dilatation, Reflux, and Neuromuscular Bladder Dysfunction

Evan J. Kass, M.D. and Alexander Cacciarelli, M.D.

Just a few short years ago, intravenous urography (IVU) and voiding cystourethrography (VCUG) were the primary imaging options employed for the evaluation of children with urinary tract infection, hydronephrosis, vesicoureteral reflux, or neuropathic bladder dysfunction. Today, ultrasonography and nuclear scintigraphy have become an integral part of the routine imaging protocol for these common pediatric urologic problems. It is essential that urologists learn to interpret these "other" studies and understand how to best incorporate them into the imaging algorithm.

Sonography of the urinary tract has virtually replaced the IVU as the preeminent imaging modality in children because: (1) there is no contraindication to its use; (2) it is noninvasive; (3) it can be performed repeatedly at no additional risk to the child; (4) it provides simultaneous information about other intra-abdominal organs, such as the liver, spleen, uterus and ovaries, and great vessels; and (5) it permits the evaluation of renal and perirenal abnormalities that excrete contrast poorly or not at all. With experience, it will become obvious that an IVU adds little to the ability to describe a normal kidney ultrasonographically (Fig. 1) and to distinguish it from a hydronephrotic kidney (Figs. 2A,B), or a duplex collecting system. (Fig. 2C)

Perhaps less obvious is the ability of ultrasound to evaluate bladder wall thickness and emptying in children with disorders of micturition (Fig. 3) and to identify ureteroceles (Fig. 4), bladder calculi, or urachal abnormalities,[1] as well as to screen for urinary tract involvement in a child with nonspecific voiding symptoms (Fig. 5).

Radionuclide scintigraphy has assumed an increasingly important role in children because it is the only imaging study capable of providing significant renal functional information, it is relatively noninvasive, and the radiopharmaceuticals pose no risk to the patient, since hypersensitivity reactions are virtually nonexistent. Nuclear medicine imaging techniques allow one to measure both total and individual renal function (glomerular filtration rate; GFR),[2] evaluate upper urinary tract obstruction (diuretic renography),[3] and identify renal parenchymal injury (cortical imaging).[4] Several radioisotopes are available, and while it is not the purpose of this text to provide an in-depth review of their pharmacology, it is important to understand the specific use of each isotope as well as its advantages and disadvantages.[5]

Technetium-99m diethylenetriamine pentaacetic acid (Tc-99m DTPA) is the isotope we prefer for diuretic renography as well as for measuring total GFR. This radiopharmaceutical

From *Imaging of Urologic Disorders* edited by Alexander S. Cass, MBBS, © 1992, Futura Publishing Inc., Mount Kisco, NY.

is excreted primarily by glomerular filtration and is not secreted or reabsorbed by the renal tubules. The images produced, although not as anatomically detailed as those of an IVU, are adequate to determine the location of the obstruction (ureterovesical vs. ureteropelvic junction) and to allow one to compare the degrees of hydronephrosis over time (Fig. 6). Both total and individual kidney GFR can be determined by measuring the rate of disappearance of the radiotracer from the blood without the need for ureteral catheterization or urine collection. This ability to monitor individual kidney function serially is of critical importance in any child with hydronephrosis or vesicoureteral reflux whether or not corrective surgery is performed.

I-131 Orthoiodohippurate (I-131 Hippuran) is not a good agent for pediatric renal imaging because the I-131 nuclide delivers an unacceptably high absorbed radiation dose and therefore must be administered in very small quantities. As a result, renal images cannot be obtained, and an additional renal scanning agent is required in order to derive anatomic information as well as to help localize the kidney in order to obtain a renogram curve. I-123 Hippuran is superior to the I-131 form in that it results in significantly less radiation exposure and produces satisfactory renal images. However, it is relatively expensive and difficult to obtain, often contains some I-131 impurities, and, in our opinion, does not have any significant advantage over Tc-99m DTPA.

Recently, another renal radiopharmaceutical, Tc-99m Mercaptoacetyltriglycine (MAG3) has been shown to produce images superior to those of Tc-99m DTPA and may very well become the agent of choice for diuretic renography. However, it cannot be used to measure GFR because it is cleared primarily by tubular secretion.[6]

Tc-99m Dimercaptosuccinic acid (Tc-99m DMSA) is the agent of choice for determining individual renal function.[5] The majority of the tracer remains bound to the proximal renal tubules in the cortex for 12 to 24 hours, and there is little activity within the collecting system or other background organs to interfere with the calculation of differential renal function (Fig. 7). The amount of Tc-99m DMSA fixed to the renal cortex closely correlates with the amount of functioning renal mass. This agent is especially helpful when evaluating a poorly functioning kidney with only a thin rim of parenchyma (Fig. 8). In as many as 90% of children with acute pyelonephritis, an area of decreased localization of the radionuclide within the cortex of the kidney is observed (Fig. 9A). This change often appears prior to any detectable anatomic deformities on either ultrasound or IVU and when seen in a child with a urinary tract infection is very specific for acute pyelonephritis. After successful treatment, these defects often resolve (Fig. 9B); unchanging deformities of the cortical outlines indicate permanent renal scarring.

Tc-99m glucoheptonate is both excreted by glomerular filtration (Fig. 10A) and bound to the renal cortex (Fig. 10B). It cannot be used for diuretic renography but is useful to evaluate individual kidney function and enlargement of the collecting system in a child with hydronephrosis. It is an acceptable alternative to Tc-99m DMSA in a child with acute pyelonephritis.

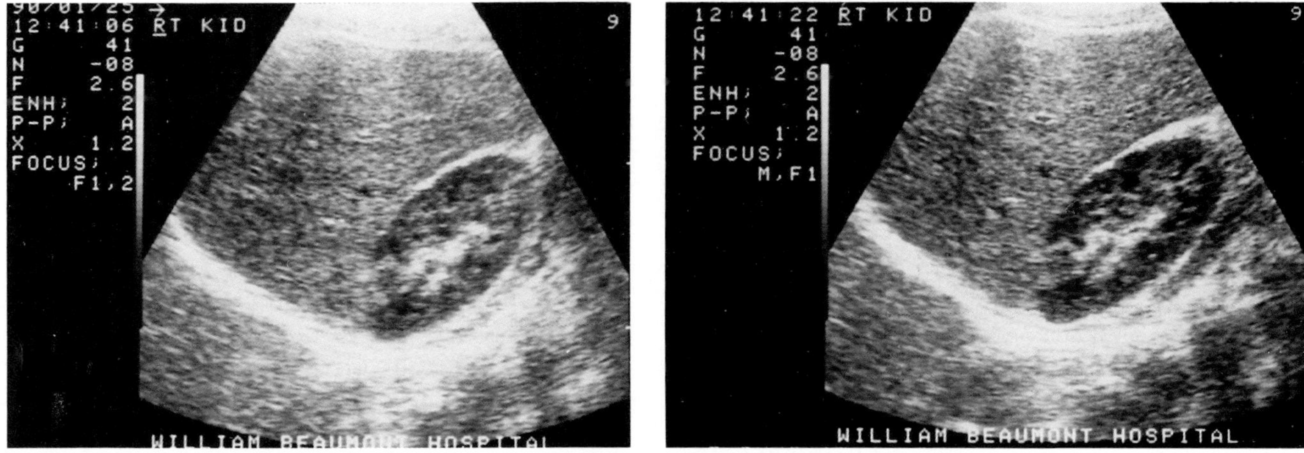

Figure 1.   Normal renal ultrasound scan. Central echo complex is normally hyperechoic. In infants, the renal pyramids are normally hypoechoic and should not be confused with cysts or dilated calices.

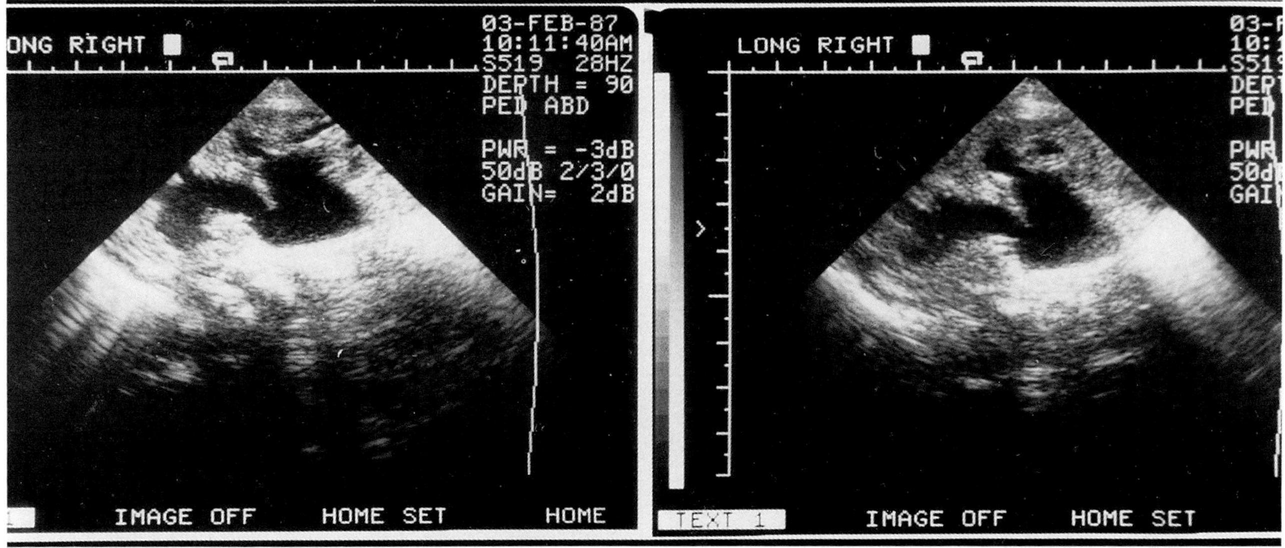

Figure 2A.   Ultrasonic picture of hydronephrosis in a child with urinary tract infection (UTI). Central echo complex is hypoechoic. The renal pelvis and calices are enlarged. Ureteral dilatation was not seen. Ureteropelvic junction (UPJ) obstruction was diagnosed.

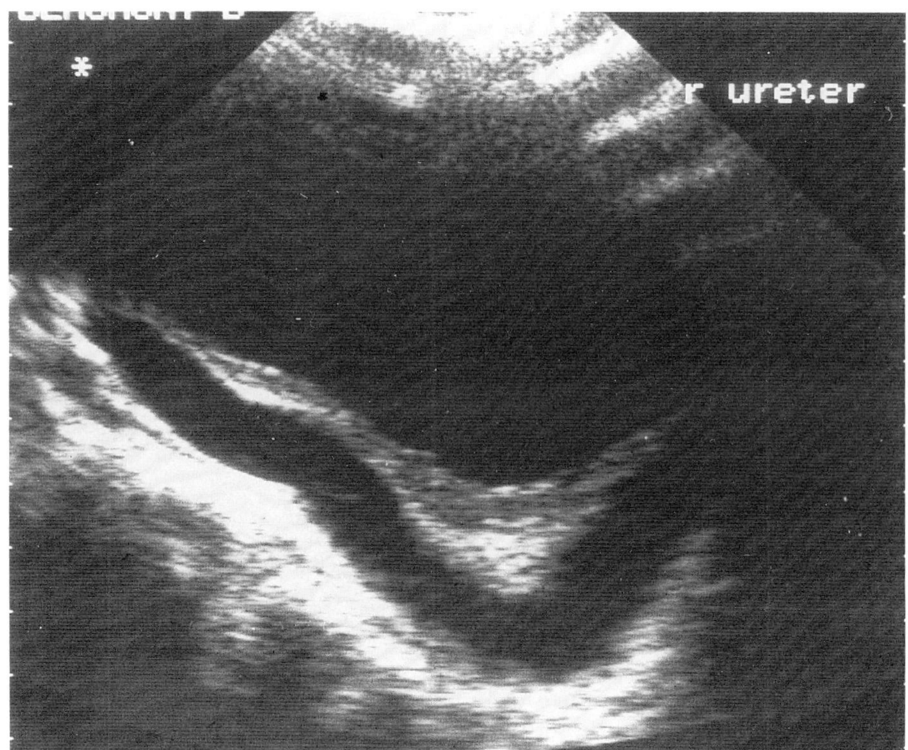

Figure 2B. This girl presented with UTI. Ultrasound scanning demonstrated hydronephrosis as well as a significantly dilated ureter behind the bladder. Ureterovesical junction (UVJ) obstruction was diagnosed.

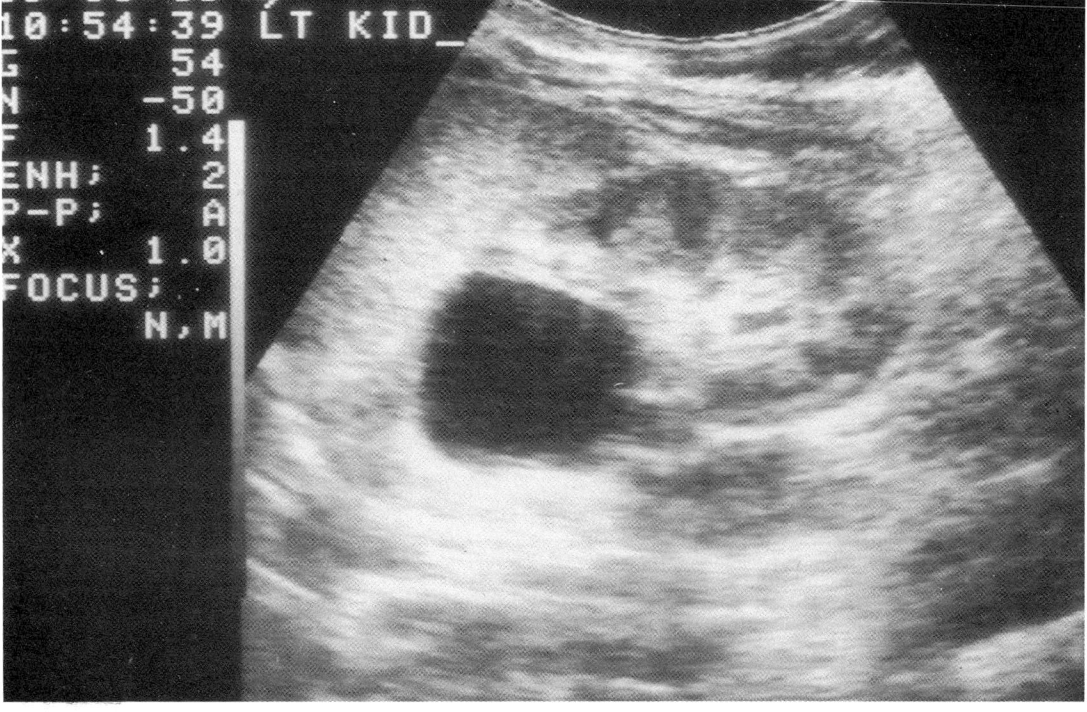

Figure 2C. This infant presented with febrile UTI. Ultrasound scan demonstrates a double collecting system with normal lower-pole and a markedly hydronephrotic upper-pole system with virtually no overlying parenchyma.

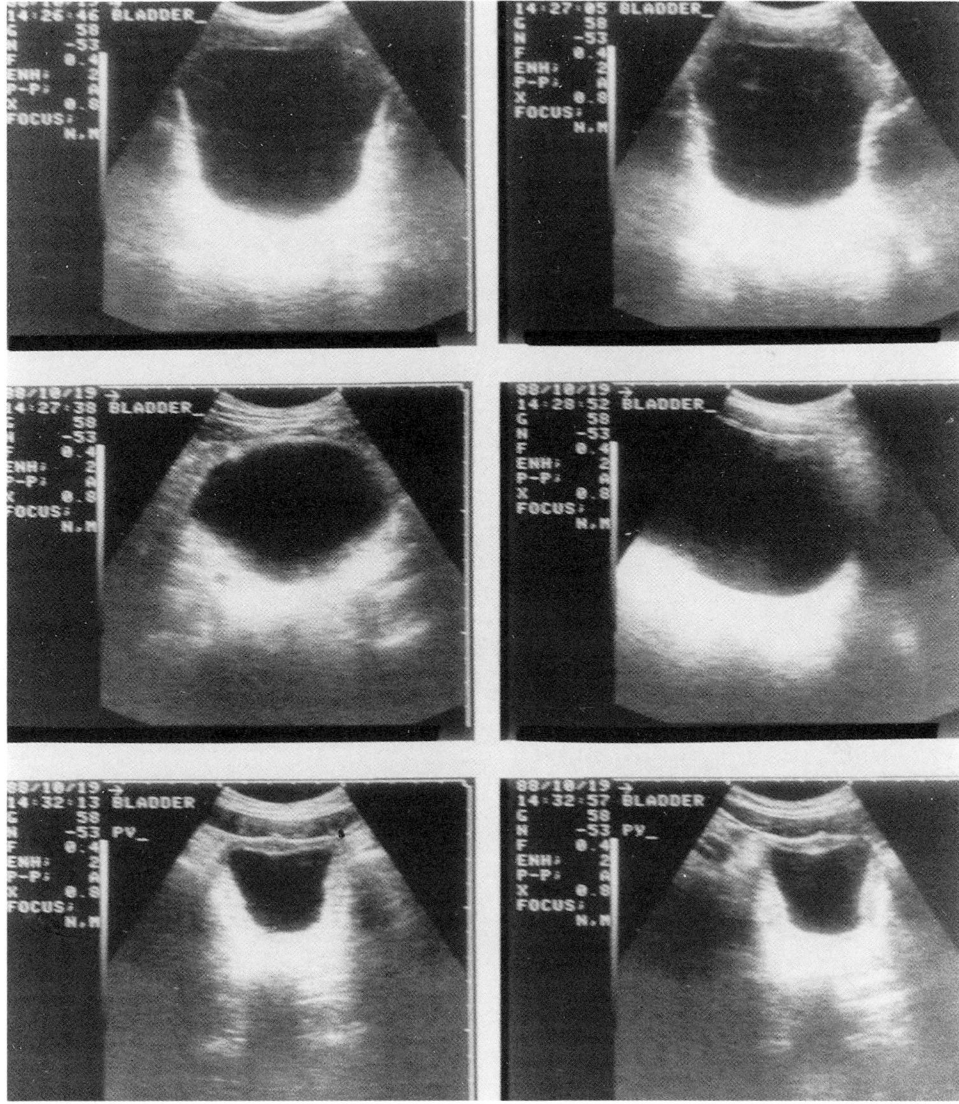

Figure 3A.   Evaluation of bladder wall thickness by ultrasound. Scan of a normal urinary bladder. The outline is smooth, and the muscular wall is almost imperceptible when the bladder is full. With emptying, the bladder wall thickness increases, but the outline remains smooth. It is important not to overinterpret thickening of the bladder wall in a child with a partially full bladder.

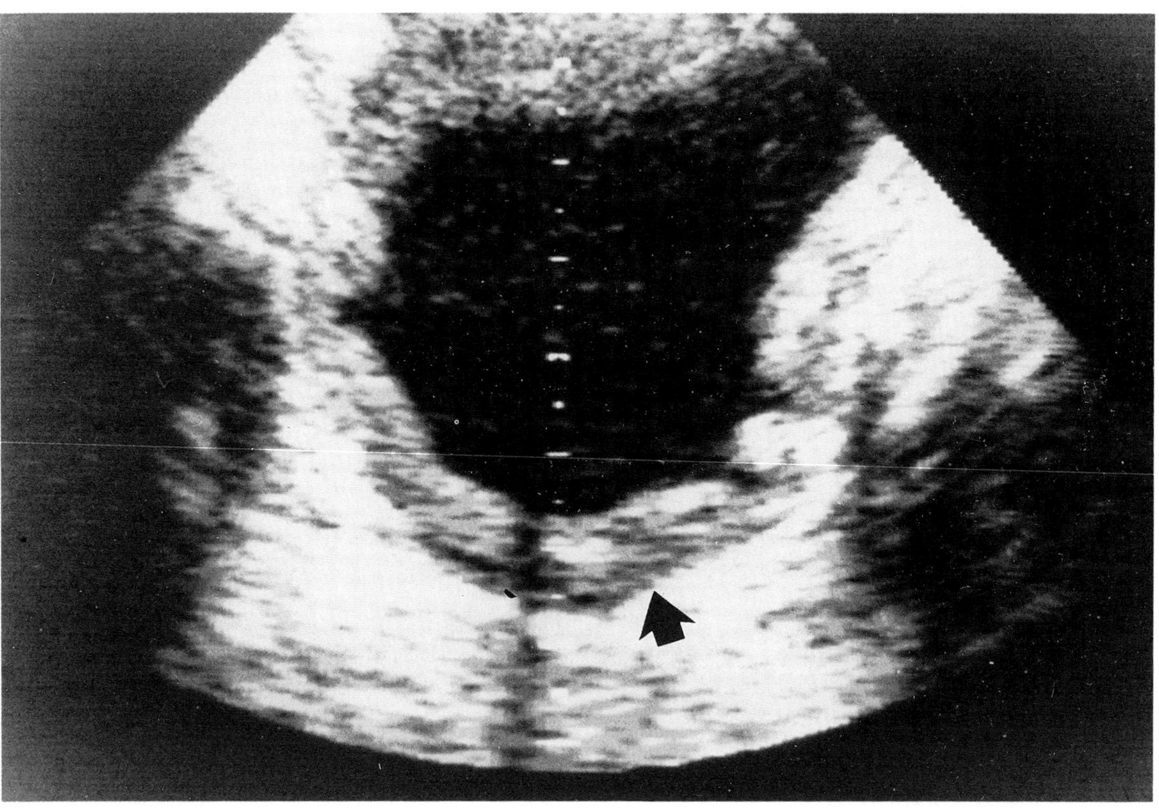

Figure 3B.   This child has a markedly thickened bladder wall (arrow) with an irregular outline consistent with bladder outlet obstruction (posterior urethral valve) or voiding dysfunction.

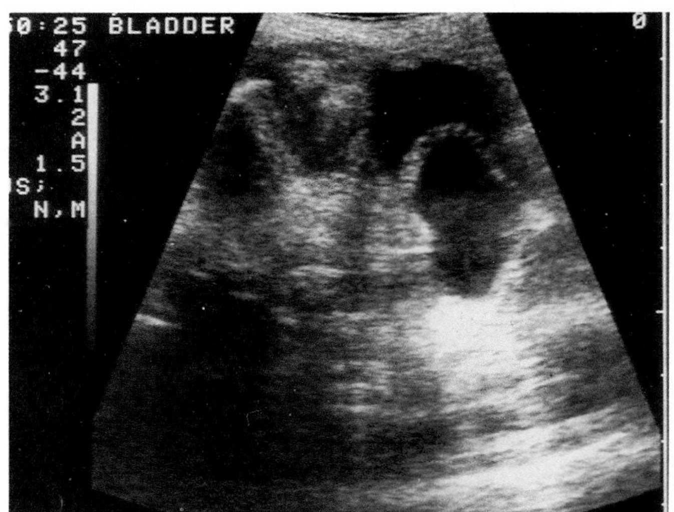 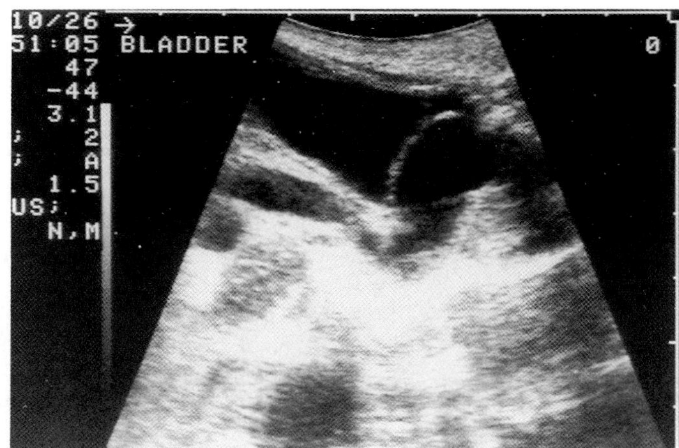

Figure 4A. Identification of ureterocele by ultrasound. Scan of the bladder demonstrating an obvious ureterocele and a dilated ureter. Renal images showed a normal left lower-pole collecting system and a hydronephrotic upper-pole segment (see Fig. 2C).

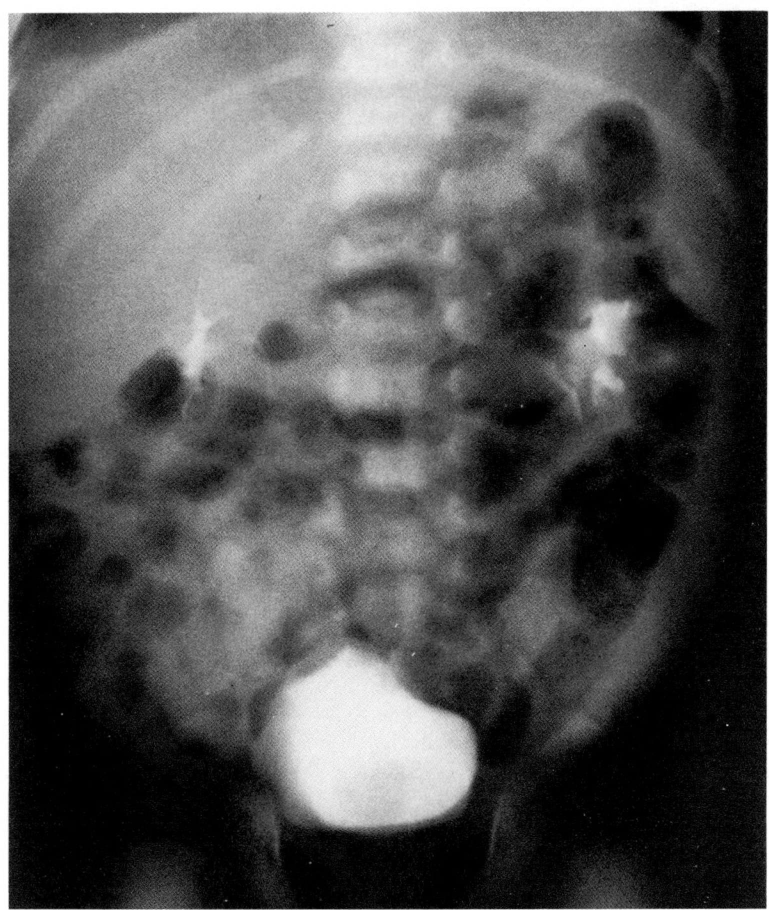

Figure 4B. Intravenous urogram in the same child. Hydronephrotic left upper-pole does not opacify, but a filling defect in the bladder from ureterocele can be seen. In this circumstance, ultrasound scanning provided more clinically useful information than IVU.

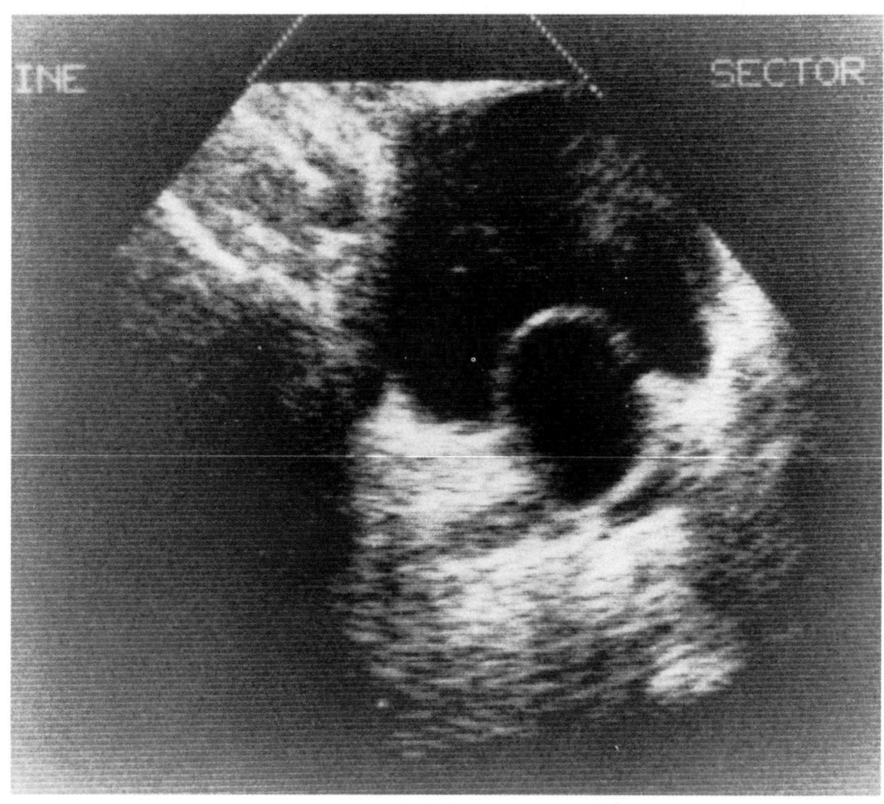

Figure 5. Ultrasound scan in a 16-year-old boy with difficulty voiding shows a cystic structure behind the bladder. The left kidney was not seen and there was compensatory hypertrophy of the right kidney. At surgery, an atrophic left kidney with its ureter entering a seminal vesical cyst was identified.

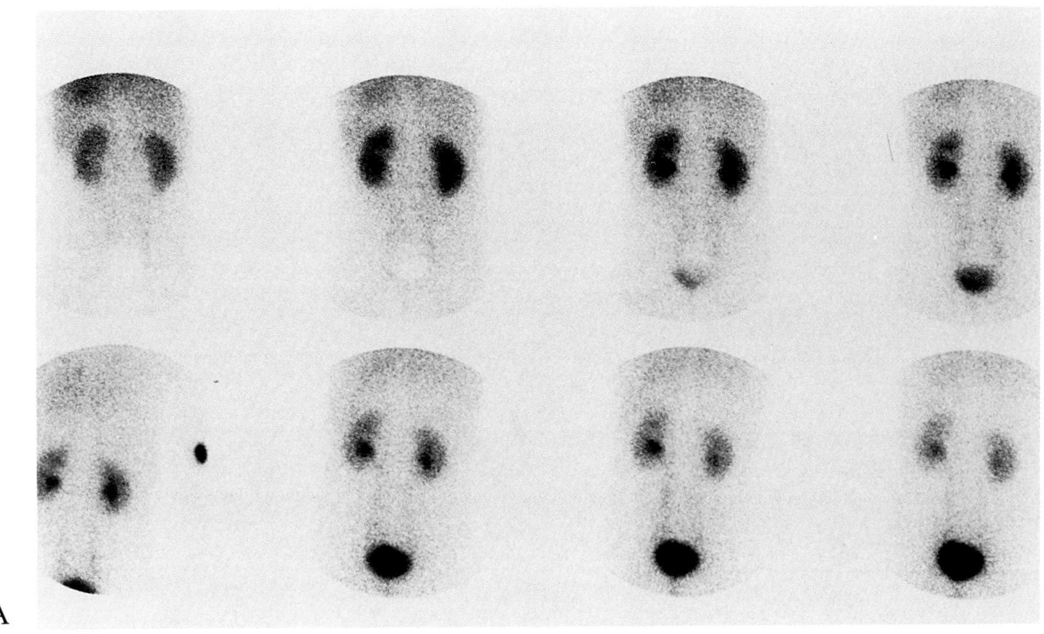

Figure 6.   Use of Tc-99m DTPA in renal scanning. (A) Normal scan. Prompt and equal excretion of the radiopharmaceutical is seen bilaterally. The kidneys are similar in size and shape. Note that the normal ureter is only faintly imaged.

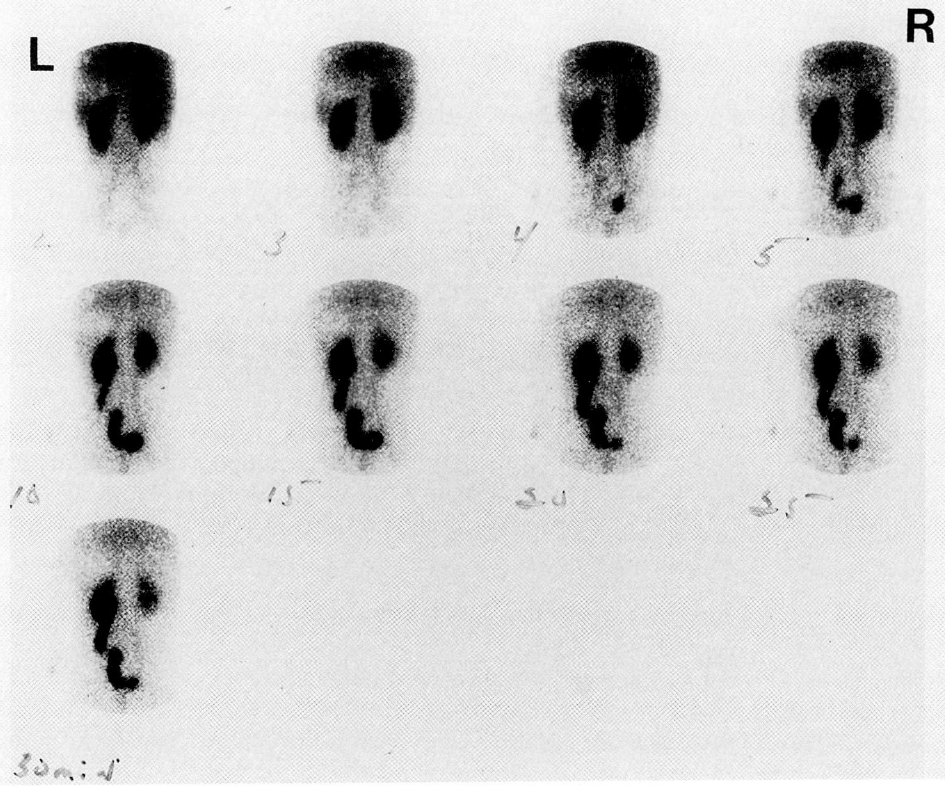

Figure 6B.   TC-99m DTPA renal scan in a 1-year-old child with left hydroureteronephrosis. Enlargement of the left ureter is clearly delineated.

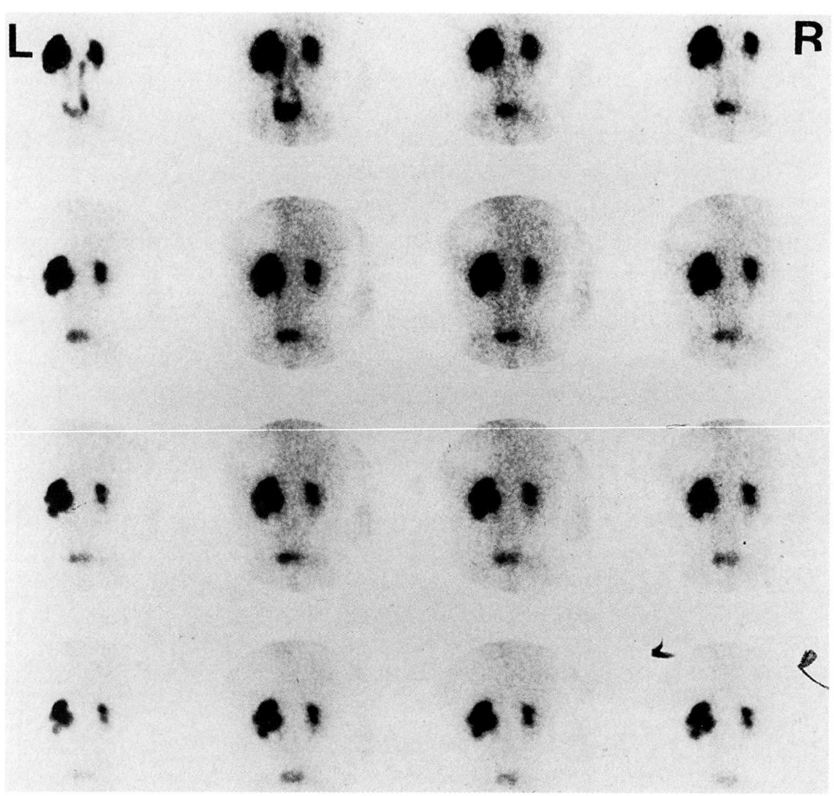

Figure 6C.   TC-99m DTPA renal scan in a child with left hydronephrosis suggestive of UPJ obstruction. There is obvious enlargement of the left upper collecting system compared with the right. Note: Distinguishing a UPJ obstruction from a UVJ obstruction on these studies is relatively straightforward.

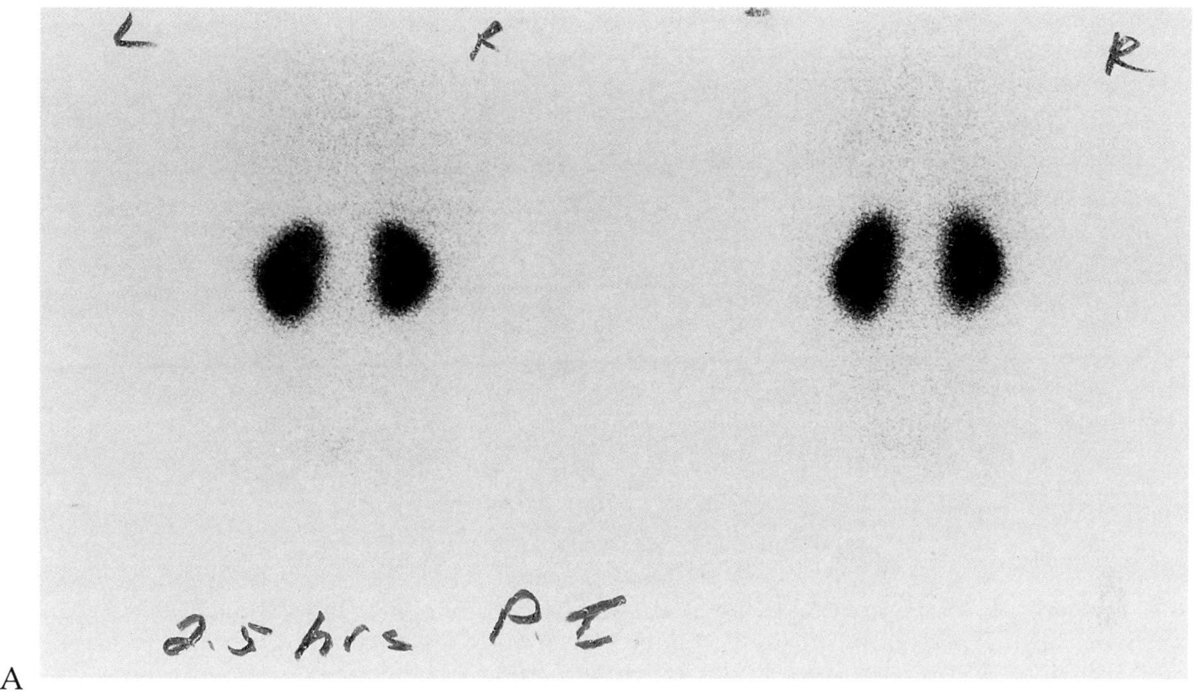

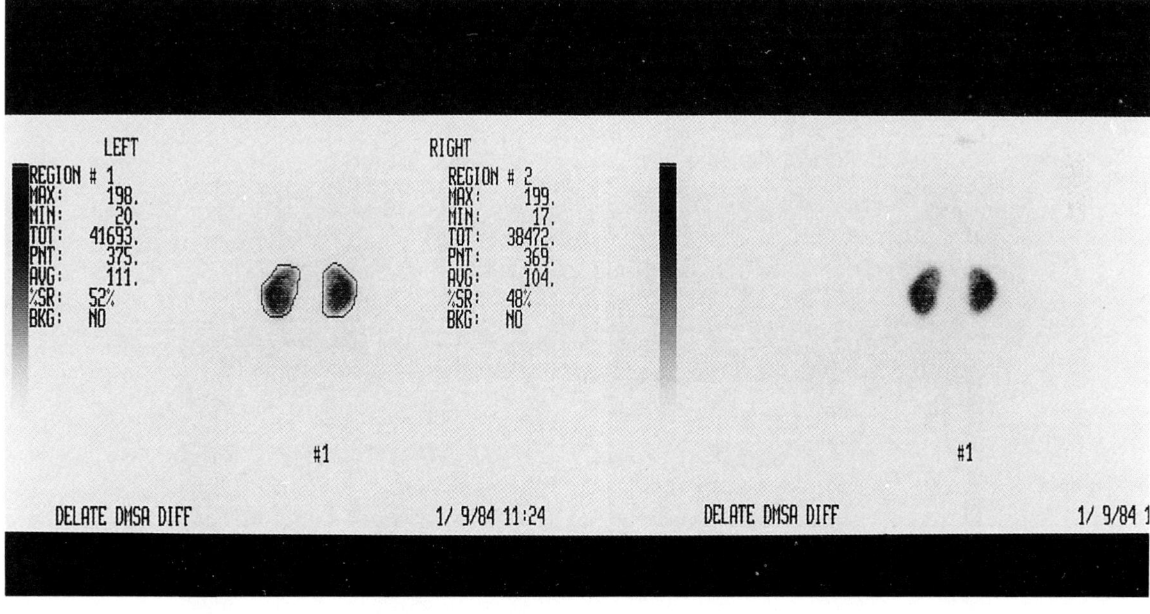

Figure 7.   Calculation of function of individual kidneys with Tc-99M DMSA renal scanning. (A, top) Normal scan. Note that virtually all the radiopharmaceutical remains attached to renal cortex; there is little background activity in other organs compared with what is seen in Tc-99m DTPA renal scans. In addition, no activity is noted within the collecting system. (B, bottom) Calculation of differential renal function is simplified because there is no need to subtract tracer activity in the collecting system or other background organs.

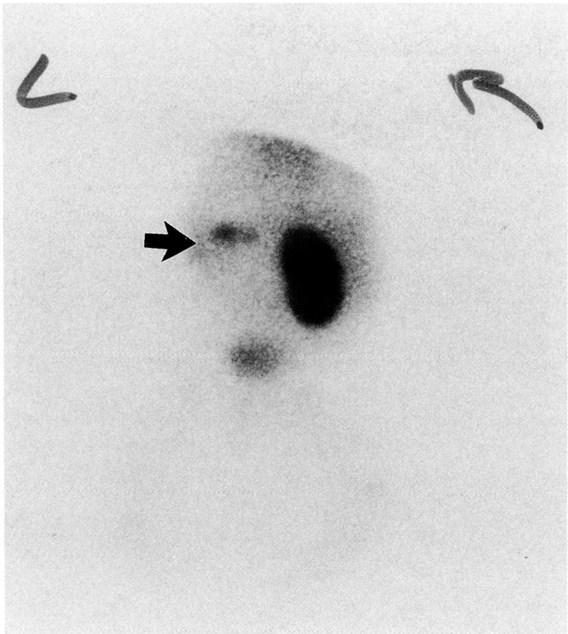

Figure 8. A Tc-99m DMSA scan in a child with severe left hydronephrosis. Only a small island of functioning renal parenchyma (arrow) is present on the left side, representing less than 10% of total renal function. At surgery, only a small nubbin of renal parenchyma was found, and a nephrectomy was performed.

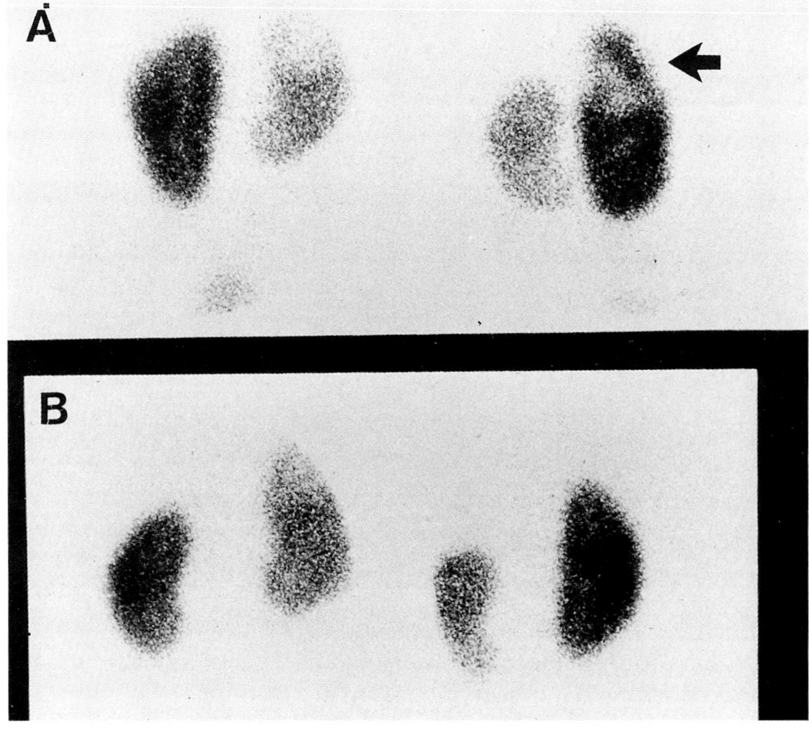

Figure 9. Scanning with Tc-99m DMSA in acute pyelonephritis. (A) Renal scan in a girl with acute pyelonephritis involving the upper pole of the right kidney (arrow). (B) After successful treatment, a repeat scan shows complete resolution of the inflammatory process without residual parenchymal scarring.

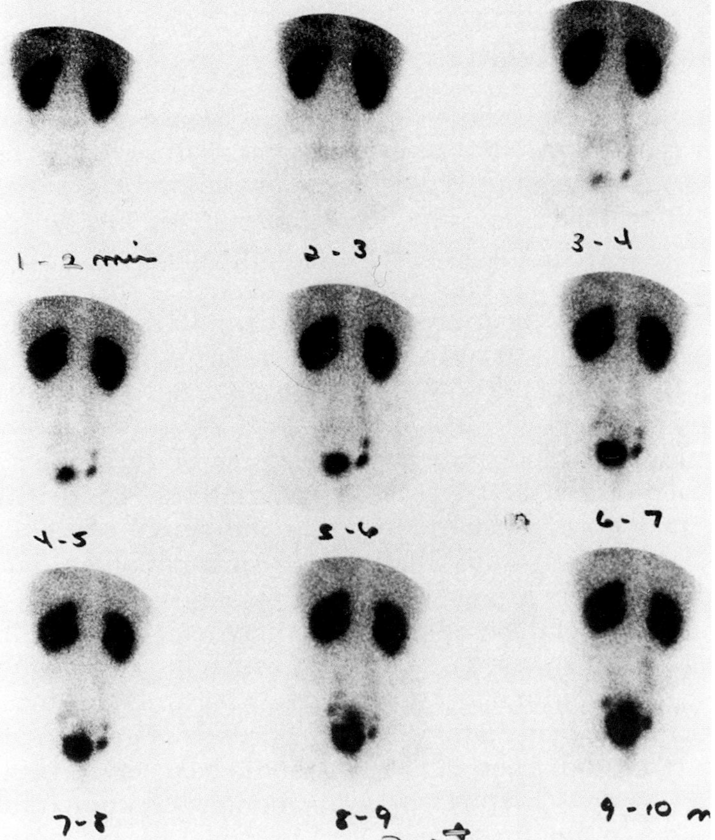

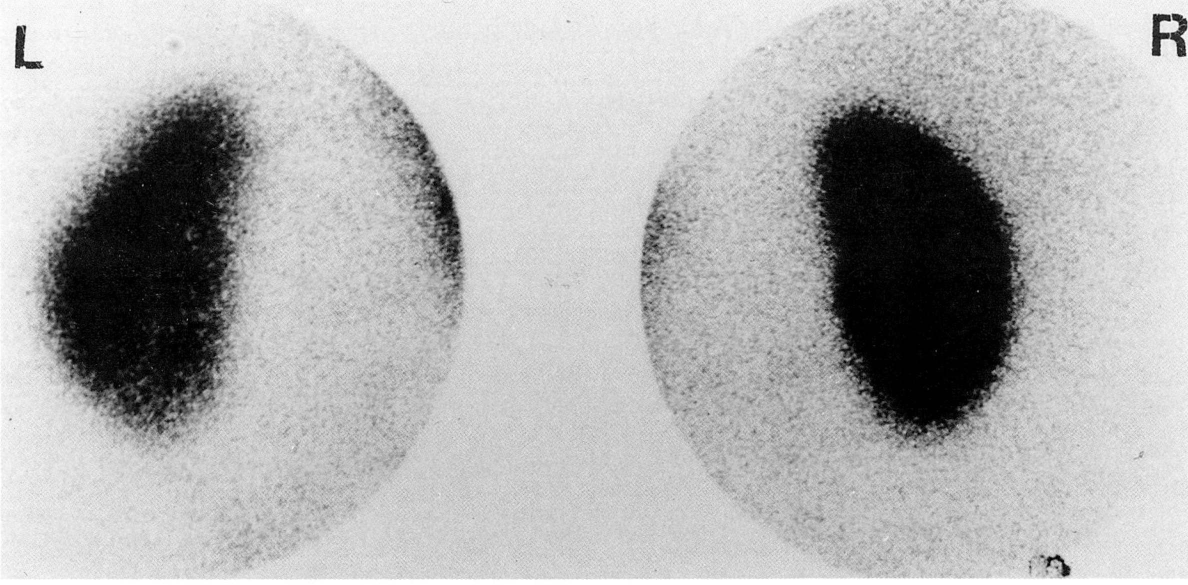

Figure 10.   Examples of Tc-99m glucoheptonate renal scans. (A, top) Early images of the collecting system are similar to those obtained with Tc-99m DTPA. Because some tracer remains bound to the renal cortex, this agent cannot be used for diuretic renography, but in a child with hydronephrosis, it is useful in following renal function and degree of hydronephrosis. (B, bottom) Late images of the left and right kidney are similar to those of Tc-99m DMSA, as is ability to measure individual kidney function and identify acute pyelonephritis or renal parenchymal scarring.

Integrated Imaging for Urinary Tract Infection and for Reflux

The combination of renal ultrasound scan and a VCUG are the usual imaging studies performed in children after their first documented urinary tract infection (UTI). The studies can be performed as soon as the urine culture is sterile and the child is clinically well: it is not necessary to wait another 4 to 6 weeks to perform a VCUG.[7] The argument that it is better to wait because some children demonstrate transient insignificant reflux either during or soon after an acute infection is not valid, because it is the reflux of infected urine that is responsible for renal scarring. Therefore, transient reflux that occurs only during an acute infection is just as important as reflux that occurs all of the time in a child who is only periodically infected. The antimicrobial therapy usually is continued until after the imaging studies are completed and the need for long-term prophylaxis has been determined. In children with simple cystitis, no additional imaging studies are routinely performed when the VCUG and renal ultrasound scan are normal. Certainly, minor degrees of renal scarring and simple duplications may be missed with this protocol (Fig. 11), but rarely would these findings significantly alter the clinical management.

It is important to consider whether a standard VCUG or an isotope cystogram is preferable as the initial screening study. The VCUG provides images of the urethra, (Fig. 12A,B) allows one to grade the magnitude of the reflux precisely (Figs. 13A,B) and to detect other anatomic abnormalities such as duplex collecting systems (Fig. 13C), bladder trabeculation (Fig. 14A), bladder diverticula (Fig. 14B) and abnormalities of the lumbosacral spine (Fig. 14C). The isotope cystogram is simply a test to determine the presence or absence of vesicoureteral reflux and typically does not provide any other anatomic information (Fig. 15). In female patients, urethral obstruction does not exist. Therefore, nuclear cystography, with its lower radiation exposure and greater sensitivity for the detection of reflux, would in theory, seem preferable to the VCUG. Certainly, most urologists and radiologists

would agree that isotope cystography is the preferred study for following patients with known reflux. However, nuclear cystography is a less attractive alternative to the VCUG as the initial study, even for females. First, it is difficult to grade the vesicoureteral reflux accurately, yet grade is often the principal determinant of whether medical or surgical management is to be employed. Performing a VCUG when the isotope study demonstrates reflux simply to grade the reflux is, in our opinion, unduly traumatic for the child. Second, the isotope cystogram may not detect other significant bladder abnormalities (see Figs. 14A, B) that may be the first indication of significant bladder dysfunction. Third, unless an abdominal scout film is obtained routinely, the combination of a nuclear cystogram and renal ultrasound scan may fail to detect significant lumbosacral abnormalities (see Fig. 14C). Therefore, in our opinion, a VCUG should be the initial study performed to evaluate any child with a UTI regardless of gender, and the nuclear cystogram should be reserved primarily for the follow-up of patients with known reflux.

When a child presents with a febrile UTI, a different imaging algorithm is employed.[8] In these children, a renal ultrasound scan is often performed within 24 to 48 hours of presentation in order to identify significant structural abnormalities that may require early intervention (Fig. 16) and a VCUG some days later when the child is clinically well and the urine culture sterile. Additional imaging studies are often recommended for this subgroup of children even when the VCUG and renal ultrasound scan are normal because it is unusual for the IVU or renal ultrasound scan to be abnormal in children with acute pyelonephritis[9] (Fig. 17), even when there is significant renal parenchymal injury, and because an isotope cystogram may demonstrate reflux that was missed on the VCUG (Fig. 18). In practice, a Tc-99m DMSA scan is performed as soon as is practical in order to provide confirmatory evidence of the upper urinary tract infection, measure individual kidney function, and define preexisting renal parenchymal scarring. When the scan demonstrates an upper tract injury (acute or chronic), vesicoureteral reflux is strongly suggested, and, even if the VCUG is normal, nuclear cystography should be performed. The Tc-99m DMSA technique is preferable to an IVU because it provides a precise measure of individual kidney function as well as a superior definition of renal parenchymal injury (Fig. 19).

Imaging studies are performed annually in children with known vesicoureteral reflux to assess status of both the reflux and the upper urinary tracts. We routinely obtain an annual isotope cystogram and renal ultrasound scan in children with known reflux, the end-point being resolution of the reflux (Fig. 20).

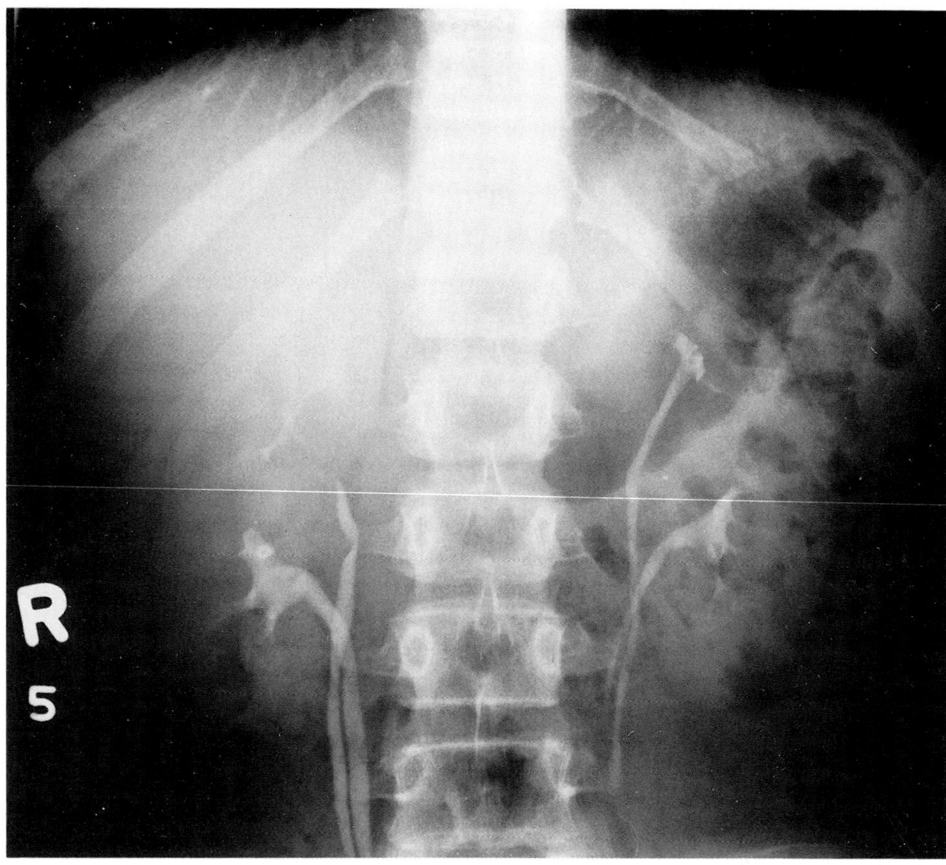

Figure 11. Intravenous urogram demonstrating bilateral duplications of no clinical significance. Renal ultrasound scan in this child was within normal limits. Presence of duplex collecting systems did not alter the management protocol.

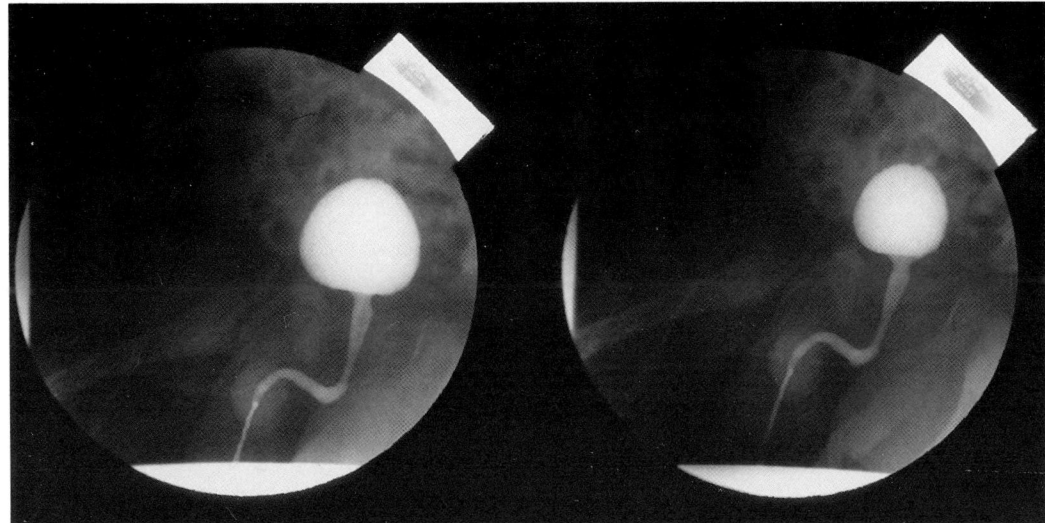

Figure 12A. Utility of VCUG. Normal study in a boy with UTI. In a male patient, it is necessary to exclude vesicoureteral reflux and urethral obstruction.

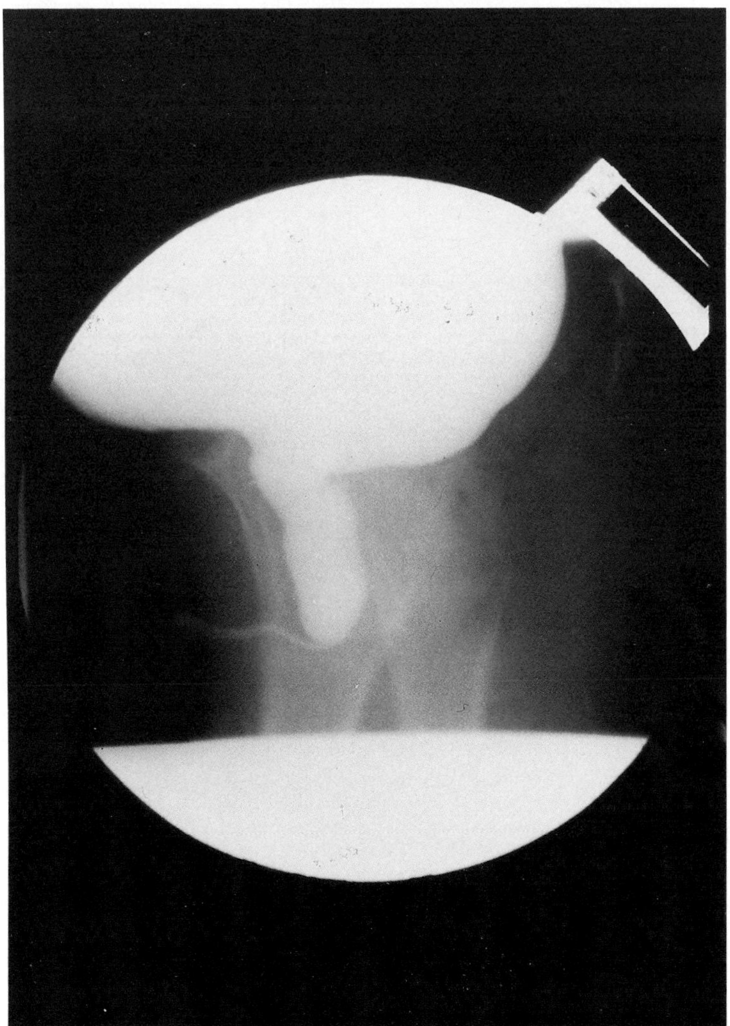

Figure 12B. Voiding cystourethrogram in a male with posterior urethral valve.

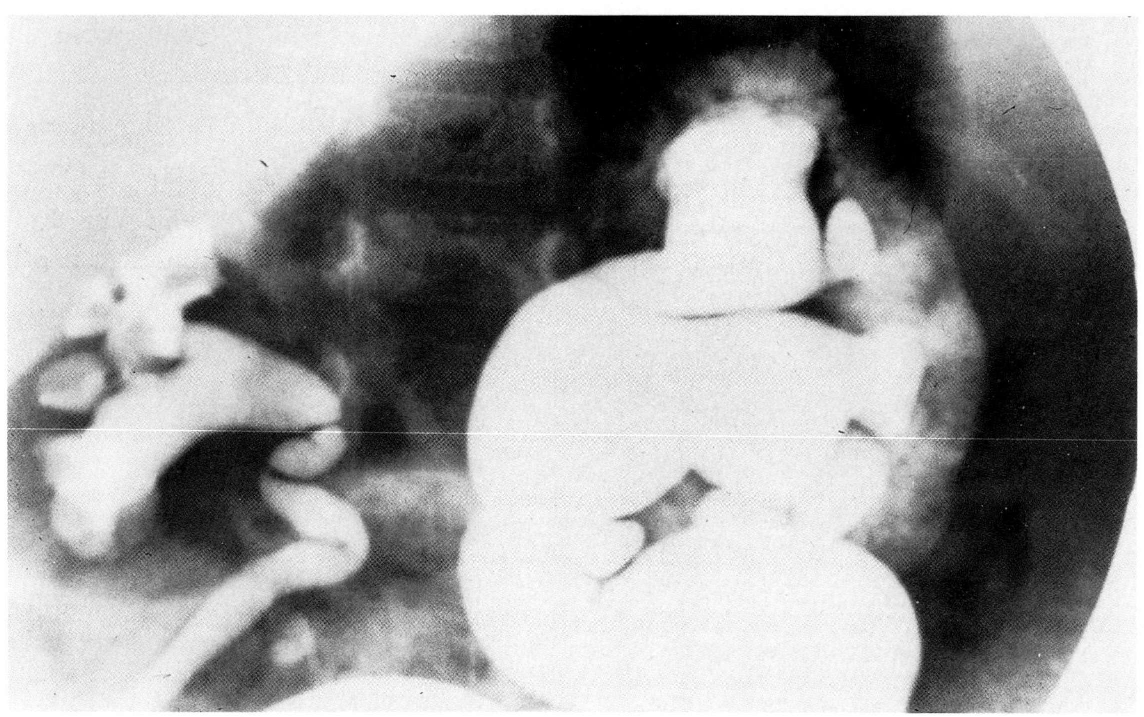

Figure 13A.   Evaluation of reflux with VCUG. (A) An infant with bilateral reflux. There is grade 5 reflux with associated intrarenal reflux on the left side. The right side demonstrates grade 3 reflux. Such precise grading is not possible with nuclear cystography.

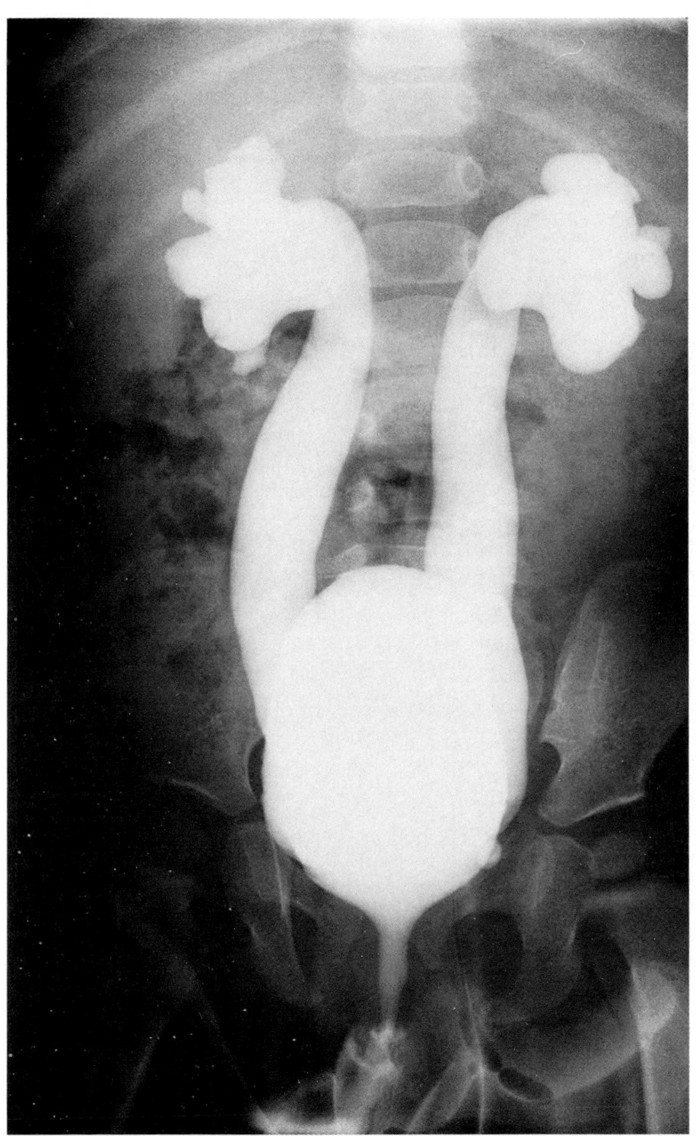

Figure 13B. VCUG study in a child with bilateral grade 5 reflux. It is unlikely that reflux of this degree will resolve.

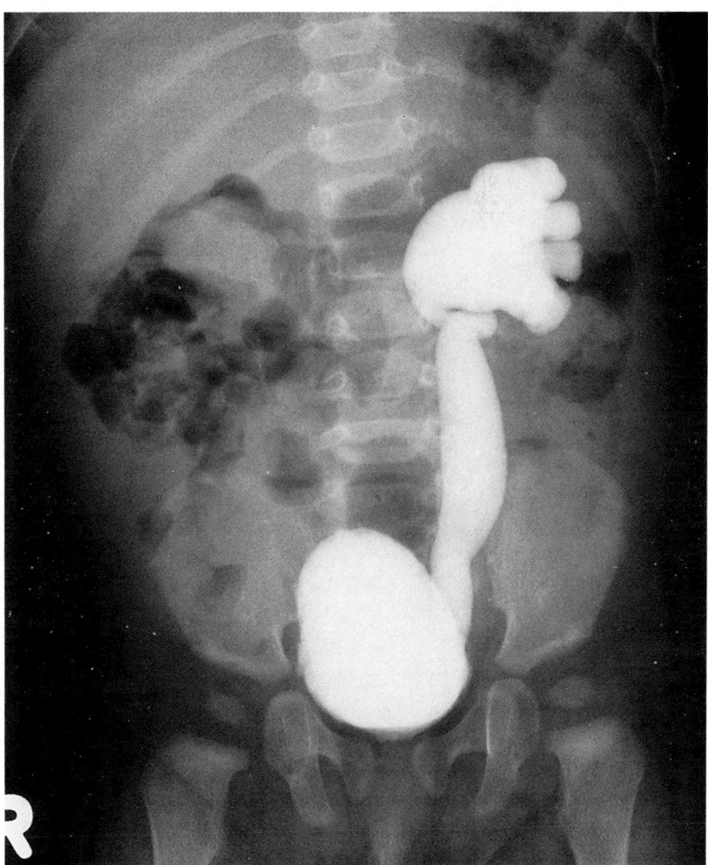

Figure 13C. VCUG in a child with high-grade left vesicoureteral reflux into the lower pole of a duplex system.

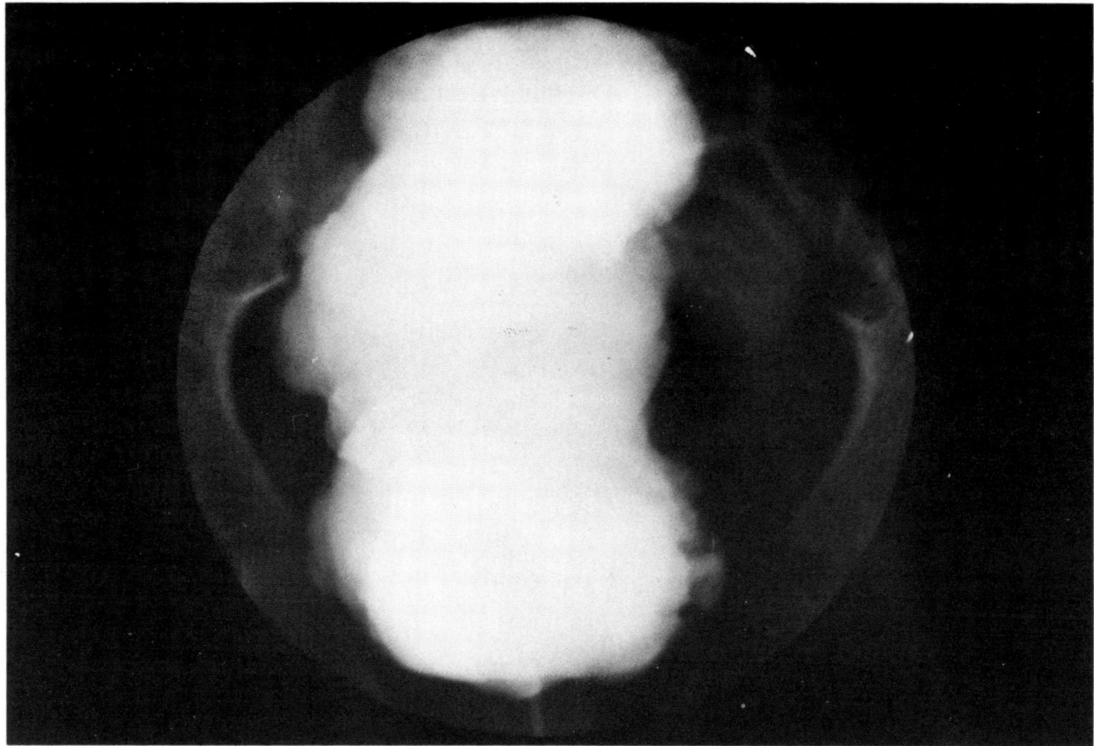

Figure 14A.   Voiding cystourethrogram demonstrating significant elongation and trabeculation of the bladder in a child with urinary tract infection and enuresis. These findings may have been missed with isotope cystography.

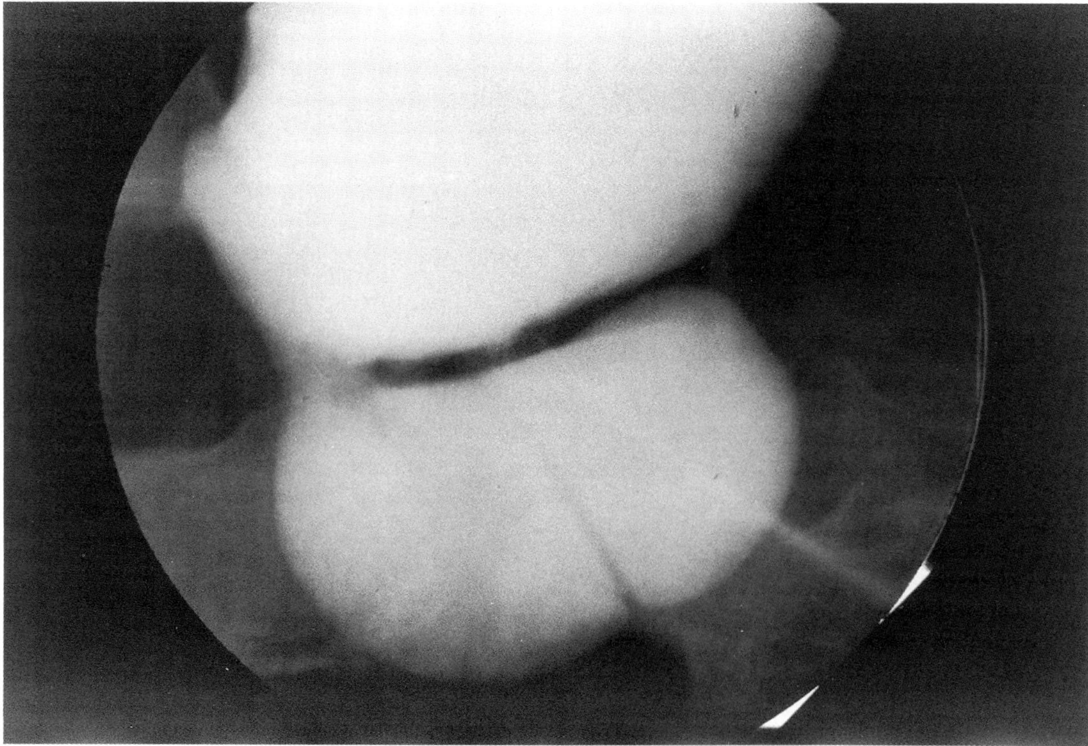

Figure 14B.   VCUG in a child with a large posterior bladder diverticulum that may have been missed on a nuclear cystography.

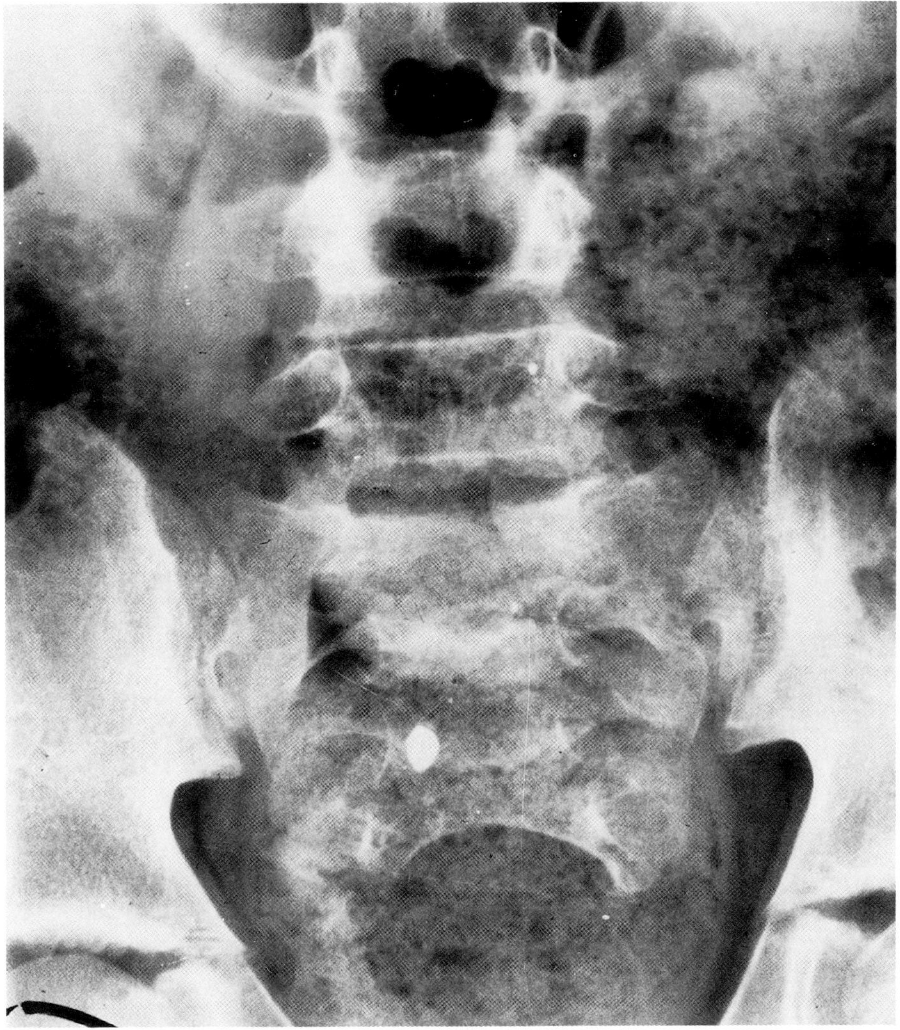

Figure 14C. This child presented with day and night enuresis without a urinary tract infection. The physical examination was normal. Absence of lower sacral spines might have been missed if nuclear cystography and renal ultrasound alone had been used to evaluate this problem.

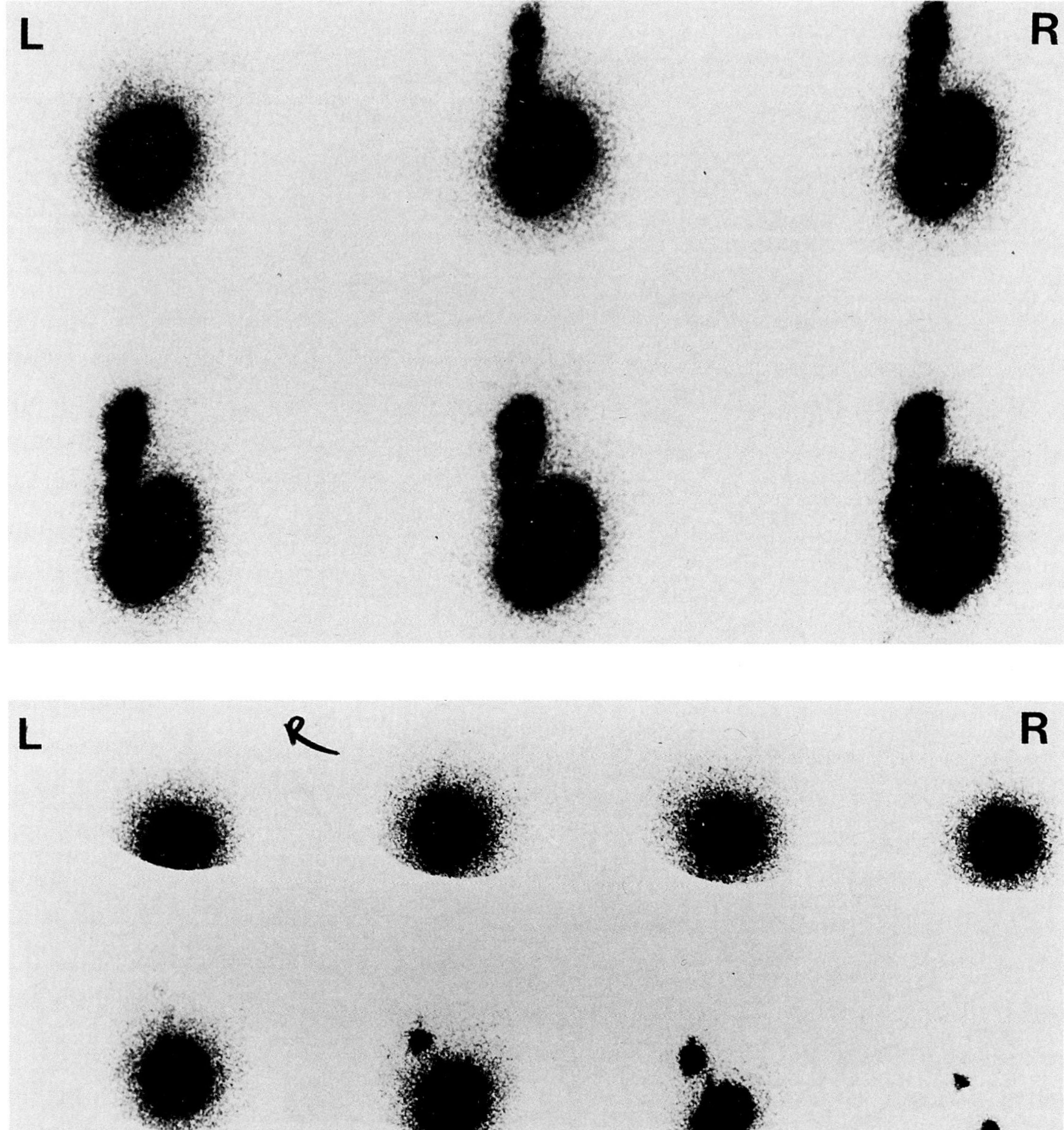

Figure 15.   Features of nuclear cystogram. (A, top) The study demonstrates a high-grade vesicoureteral reflux on the left side; however, there is no suggestion on this study that the reflux is into the lower pole of duplex system (see Fig. 13B). (B, bottom) In addition, a nuclear cystogram does not allow precise grading of vesicoureteral reflux, which is often important in deciding whether medical or surgical management is preferred. This child had a grade 2 vesicoureteral reflux on a standard VCUG.

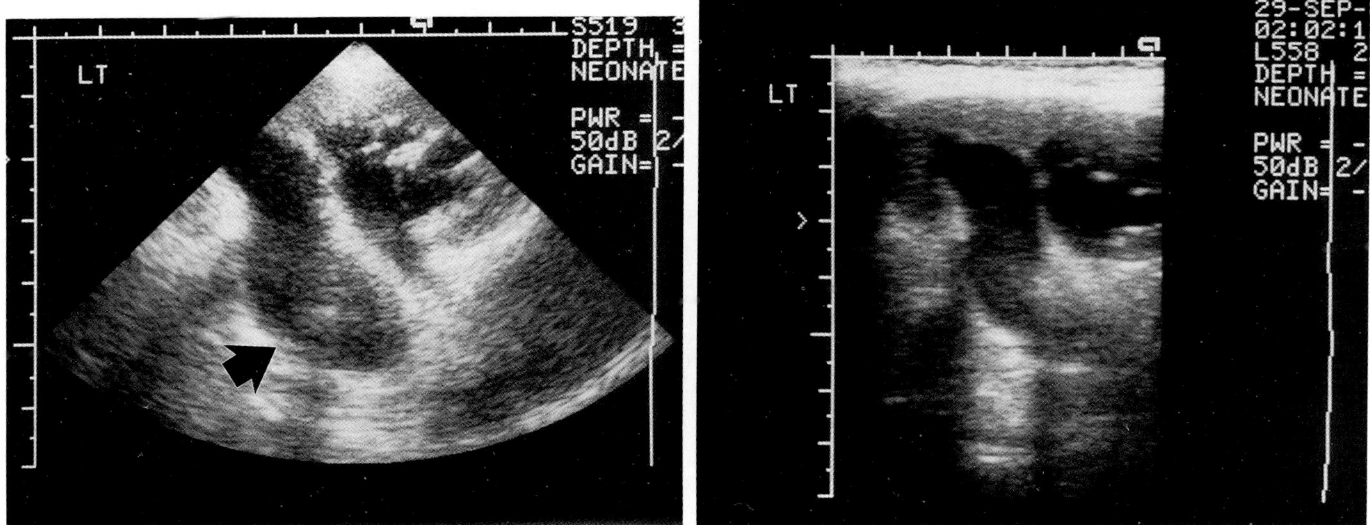

Figure 16A. Evaluation in a child with a febrile UTI. Renal ultrasound scan in a 1-year-old girl presenting with urosepsis secondary to an obstructed upper-pole segment in a duplex system. Scan performed shortly after admission demonstrates a markedly enlarged ureter filled with echogenic material consistent with pyohydronephrosis (arrow).

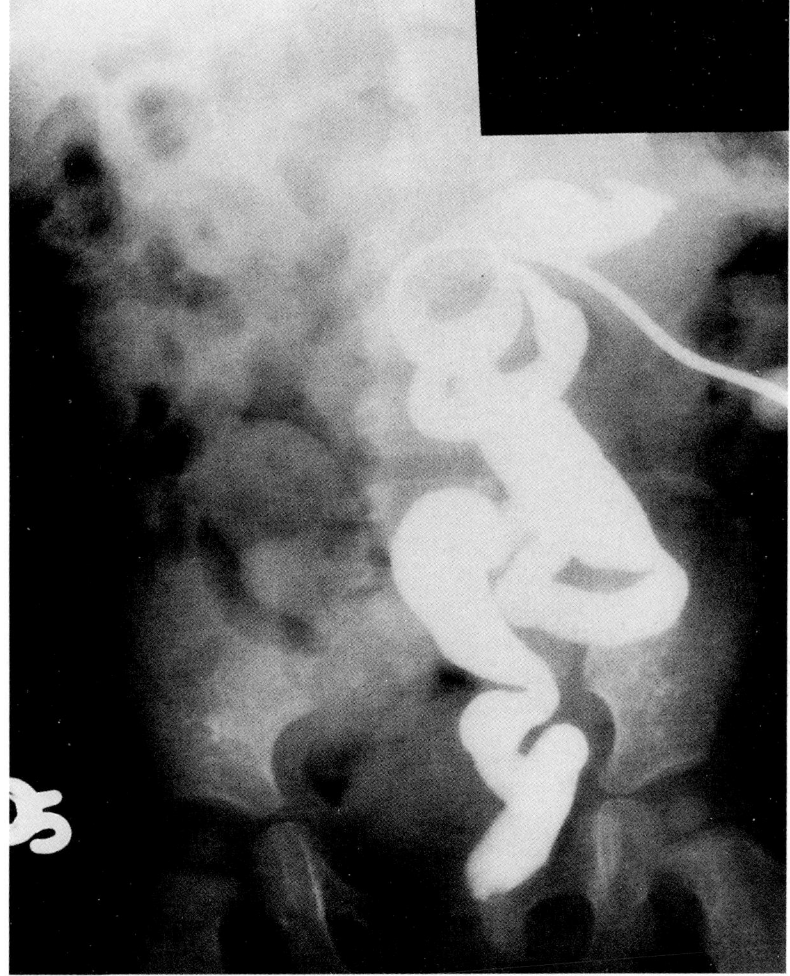

Figure 16B. A percutaneous nephrostomy tube was inserted into this dilated system, allowing drainage of purulent material. After resolution of the infection, an upper pole nephroureterectomy was curative.

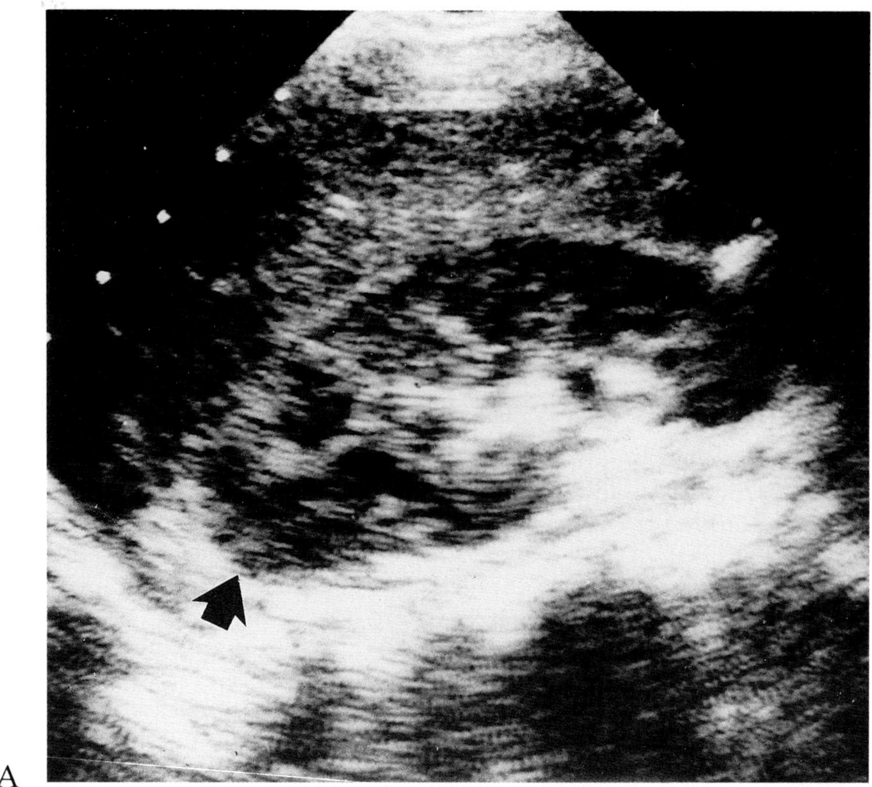

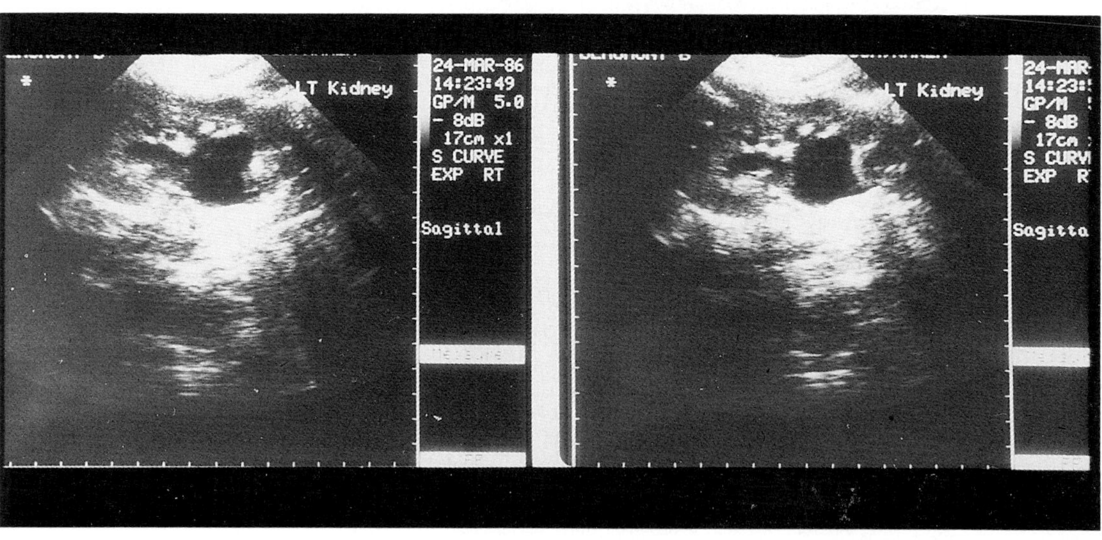

Figure 17. Other examples of workup in a child with acute pyelonephritis. (A, top) Ultrasound scan demonstrates loss of distinct corticomedullary junction, as well as a relatively hyperechoic area in upper pole (arrow). These findings, although nonspecific, are consistent with acute pyelonephritis. However, typically, the ultrasound picture is normal in children with acute pyelonephritis. (B, bottom) Renal ultrasound scan in a 2-month-old infant with acute pyelonephritis reveals moderate hydronephrosis that disappeared completely after treatment.

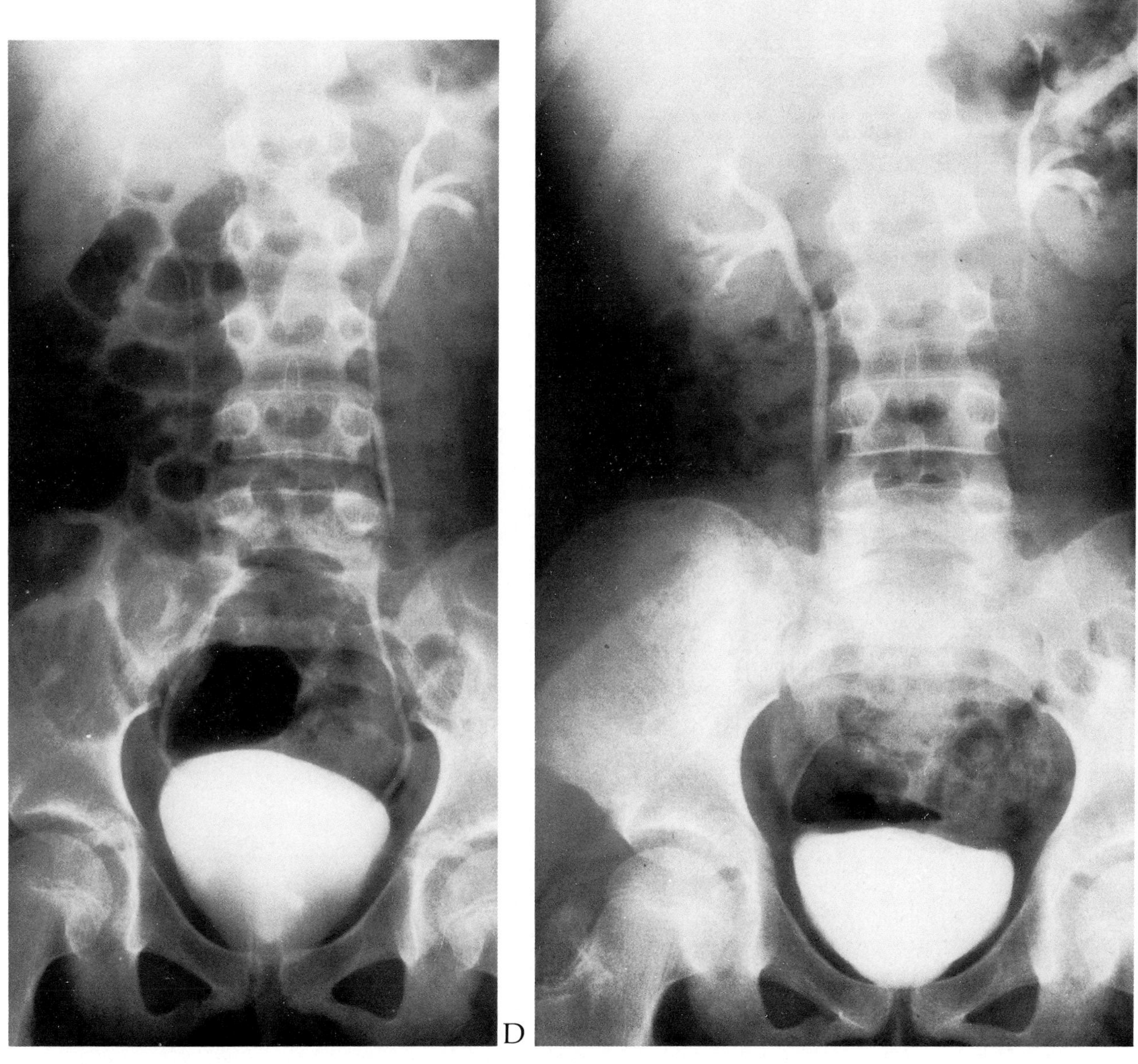

Figures 17C,D. (C, left) An IVU in a child with acute pyelonephritis demonstrates decreased contrast excretion and generalized parenchymal swelling of the right kidney. (D, right) After treatment, the IVU is normal.

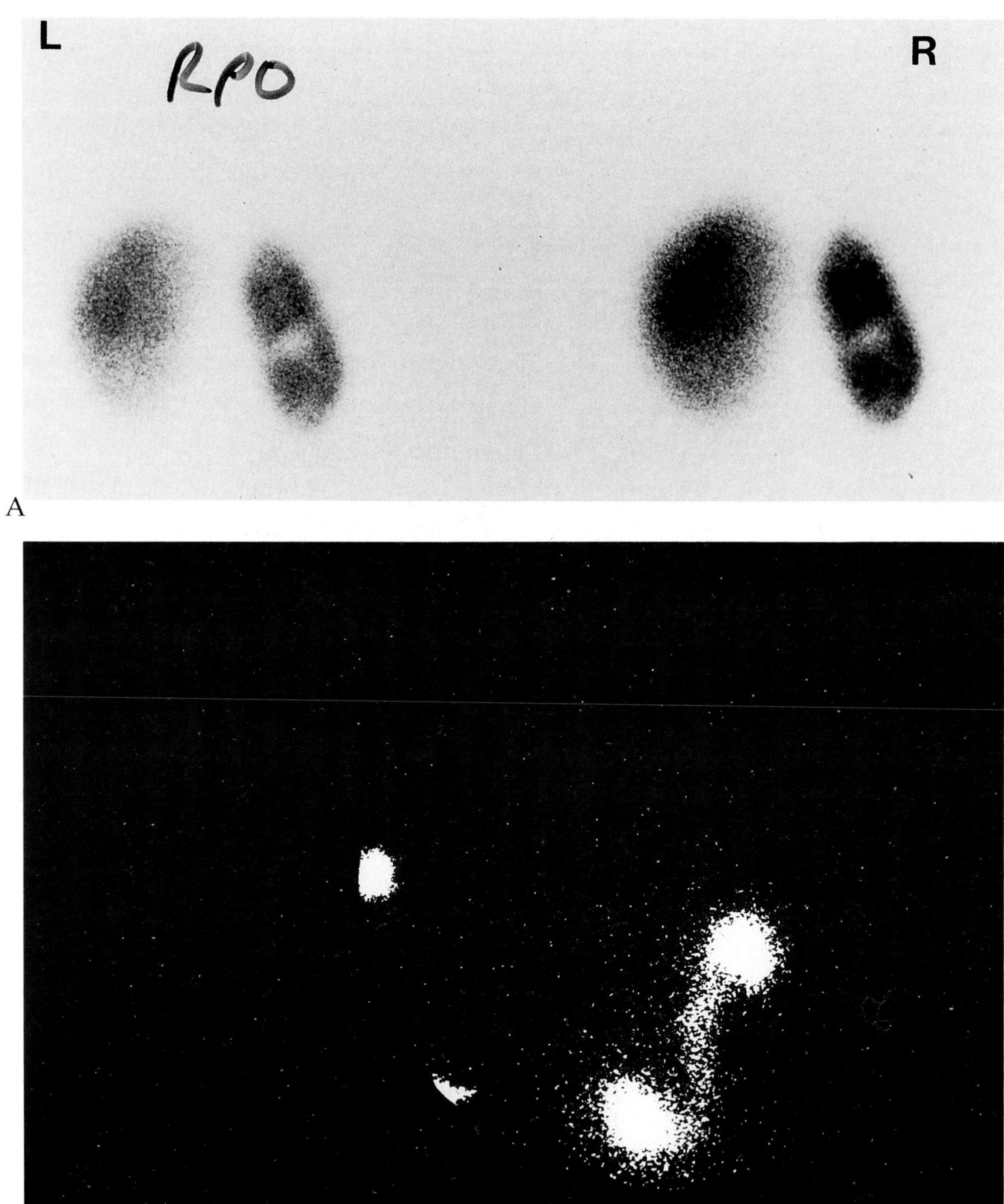

Figure 18.   This 5-year-old girl presented with recurrent episodes of pyelonephritis. Voiding cystourethrogram, IVU, and renal ultrasound scan were all within normal limits. (A, top) The DMSA renal scan demonstrates a photon-deficient area in the middle of the right kidney, consistent with acute pyelonephritis. (B, bottom) Isotope cystogram demonstrates reflux into the right kidney. Antireflux surgery was performed because of a failure to control infections with continuous chemoprophylaxis.

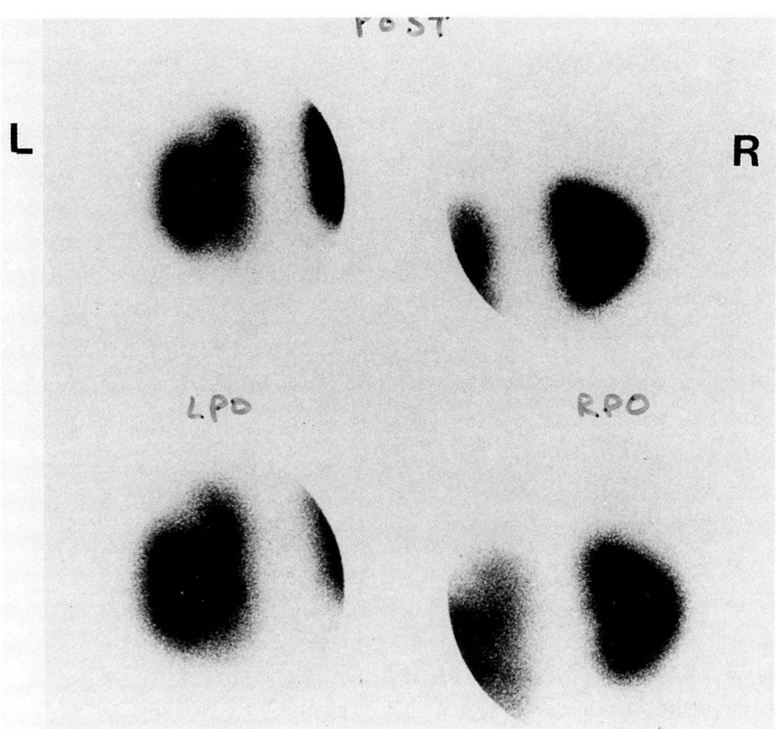

Figure 19A. Utility of isotope studies in reflux. The IVU and renal ultrasound scan were normal in this 3-year-old girl with a grade 3 left-sided reflux, but Tc-99m DMSA renal scan demonstrates significant left parenchymal scarring.

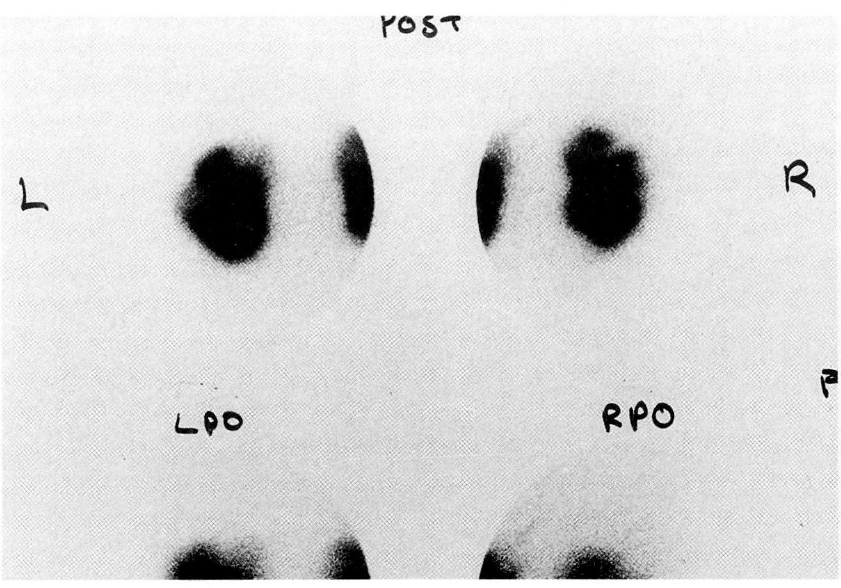

Figure 19B. A Tc-99m DMSA renal scan in a child with bilateral grade 4 vesicoureteral reflux demonstrates bilateral renal parenchymal scarring. Intravenous urogram demonstrated a mild hydronephrosis but no obvious renal parenchymal loss.

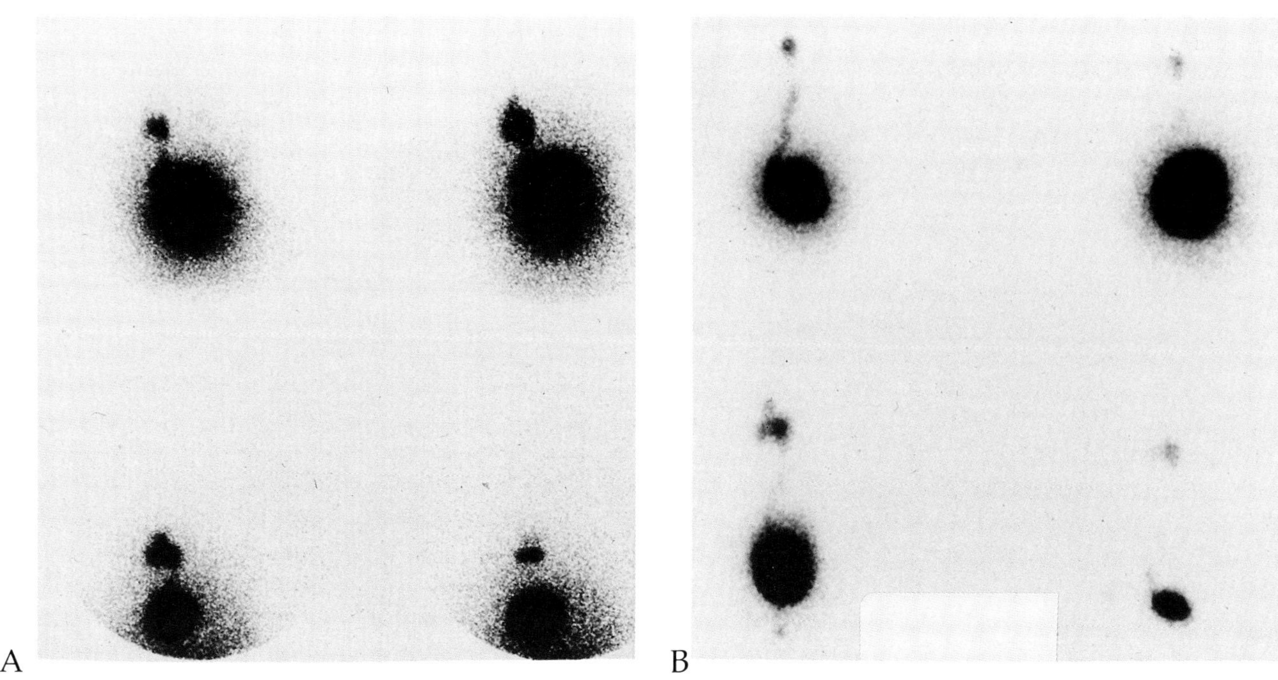

Figure 20.   Follow-up of reflux. (A, left) Left vesicoureteral reflux is demonstrated. Annual isotope cystography and renal ultrasonography are recommended. (B, right) Three years later, the reflux continues. The child remains infection free on continuous prophylaxis, and the renal ultrasound picture remains normal. Therefore, medical management is continued.

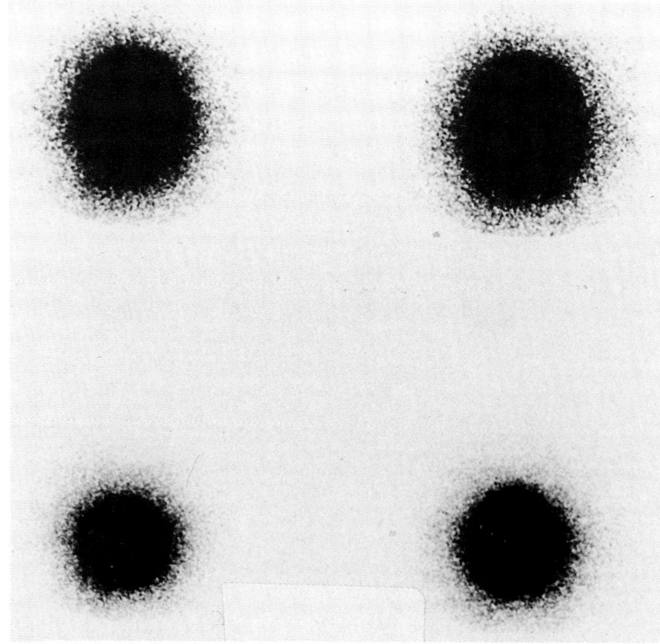

Figure 20C.   Nuclear cystogram demonstrates a complete resolution of the reflux after 4 years. Ultrasound scan was normal, and no further imaging studies were performed.

Imaging Protocol for Obstruction and Dilatation

Until recently, many urologists relied on the IVU to evaluate a child with hydronephrosis and made a decision for or against surgery according to their interpretation of the degree of enlargement of the collecting system. However, recent evidence[10] has demonstrated that much of this enlargement of the collecting system is not the result of an obstruction and that the degree of enlargement may not be an accurate indicator of obstruction (Figs. 21 and 22). In addition, the IVU is not a reliable measure of renal function; therefore, nuclear medicine imaging should be part of the evaluation of every child with significant urinary tract dilatation in order to measure renal function and to assess obstruction objectively (Fig. 23).

In all children with hydronephrosis, a VCUG should be routine to exclude infravesical obstruction or vesicoureteral reflux. In many instances, high-grade reflux will be identified in the absence of obstruction (Fig. 24). In this circumstance, the imaging algorithm and management protocol proceed as previously described in the section Integrated Imaging for Urinary Tract Infection. However, occasionally, reflux and obstruction coexist (Fig. 25), and it may be necessary to address both problems.

When hydronephrosis is identified by ultrasonography, a Tc-99m DTPA diuresis renal scan should follow (the IVU, although occasionally helpful, is not routine). However, it is important to remember that the results of diuretic renography are critically dependent on the technique employed. Unfortunately, the test is not performed in a standardized fashion in every institution, yet all authors refer to their studies as "diuresis renal scans." Without some understanding of the details of the study, it is difficult for the urologist to know whether the diuresis scan at a given institution will provide valid information.

The standard pediatric protocol[3] should include adequate prehydration and bladder catheterization whenever there is evidence of vesicoureteral reflux, a dilated ureter, an abnormally enlarged bladder, or infravesical obstruction (Fig. 26A). The diuretic should be adminis-

tered only after the dilated portion of the collecting system has completely filled with tracer. When the collecting system does not fill completely within 60 minutes after administration of the radiopharmaceutical, there may be insufficient renal function for a reliable study (Fig. 26B). A false-positive study may result when the child is not adequately hydrated, the bladder is not emptied, the diuretic is administered at the wrong time, or renal function is inadequate.

When the renal scan demonstrates that the hydronephrotic kidney has good function (at least 30% of the total renal function) and the T½ of washout of the radiotracer from the dilated collecting system is less than 15 minutes, the hydronephrosis is considered to be nonobstructive, and no surgery or pressure perfusion study is routinely performed (Fig. 27). A repeat diuresis renal scan is performed 6 months later and then annually. As long as the follow-up scans demonstrate that individual kidney function has not deteriorated and the T½ remains less than 15 minutes, no surgery is recommended.

The exact end-point for discontinuing follow-up testing has not been established, and, until the long-term prognosis of these children is known, it seems reasonably prudent to perform an annual diuresis renal scan in all children with significant persistent hydronephrosis. If at any time during follow-up, the scan demonstrates that the kidney in question has lost some of its function or a definite obstruction is identified scintigraphically, surgery is recommended.

In our experience, the majority of children (approximately 90%) with a T½ less than 15 minutes has maintained stable renal function and has not subsequently demonstrated an obstruction, with one very important exception—individuals with intermittent flank pain (Fig. 28). In these individuals, the diuretic scan may be normal unless the study is performed while they are having pain. Therefore, individuals with intermittent flank pain and a normal scan should have either an ultrasound scan or an IVU performed during the acute episode. If no increase in hydronephrosis is noted at that time, obstruction has been excluded, but if there is a significant increase in the degree of hydronephrosis, an obstruction is diagnosed.

When the T½ is greater than 15 minutes but

less than 20 minutes, the study is deemed indeterminate and is repeated 3 months later. As long as the renal function and the $T\frac{1}{2}$ remain stable or improve, these individuals are followed as if they were unobstructed. When the repeat study demonstrates a deterioration of renal function of a $T\frac{1}{2}$ greater than 20 minutes, an obstruction is diagnosed and surgery recommended. A pressure perfusion study is an option in this setting; however, when the function in the hydronephrotic kidney is good, we do not routinely perform a Whitaker test because of its invasive nature and the observation that it has been safe to follow these children. However, when the function is significantly reduced (less than 30% of the total renal function), a pressure perfusion study is frequently recommended.

When the diuresis renal scan demonstrates that the $T\frac{1}{2}$ of the hydronephrotic kidney is greater than 20 minutes, an obstruction is diagnosed and surgery recommended (Fig. 29). However, there are some very important exceptions. An obstruction should not be diagnosed when the $T\frac{1}{2}$ of the normal contralateral kidney exceeds 15 minutes, as this circumstance may reflect either the inability of the child's kidneys to respond to the diuretic or inadequate hydration (Fig. 30). Failure of the normal kidney to respond can occur at any age but is more common in neonates and in children who are not properly hydrated prior to the scan. In the older child, the scan should be repeated when the child has been adequately hydrated, and in the case of the neonate, it is usually repeated when the child is 3 months old. When the hydronephrotic kidney has less than 30% of the total renal function or the collecting system does not fill completely within 60 minutes after administration of the radiopharmaceutical, an obstruction cannot be diagnosed reliably on the basis of the diuretic renal scan alone. In this circumstance, placing a percutaneous nephrostomy tube can be very helpful. One can then perform a pressure perfusion study to determine whether an obstruction is present and an antegrade nephrostogram to demonstrate the anatomy of the upper collecting system, ureter, and the UVJ. When additional functional information is required, the nephrostomy tube may be left in place for 2 weeks and a Tc-99m DMSA scan then

performed to reassess renal function. When the pressure perfusion study demonstrates an obstruction and there has been a measurable improvement in renal function during drainage, reconstructive surgery is generally recommended. When the kidney in question has less than 20% of the total renal function, either nephrectomy or, occasionally, a temporary cutaneous diversion is a reasonable option, depending on the individual circumstances.

After reconstructive surgery, a repeat diuresis renal scan is usually performed at 6 to 10 weeks. At this time, the $T\frac{1}{2}$ will have improved significantly or normalized in the majority of kidneys (Fig. 31). However, when the $T\frac{1}{2}$ still exceeds 20 minutes, a satisfactory outcome can be expected as long as the differential renal function, as determined by nuclear scintigraphy, has either remained stable or improved (Fig. 32). On the other hand, when the renal function diminishes postoperatively, a persistent obstruction should be suspected and a pressure perfusion study performed. As long as renal function remains stable, a follow-up diuresis scan is usually obtained a year after surgery, at which time, the $T\frac{1}{2}$ should be less than 20 minutes. A prolonged $T\frac{1}{2}$ at this juncture suggests continued obstruction.

Renal sonography is an excellent means of following patients after reconstructive surgery. Typically, there is a marked reduction in the degree of hydronephrosis when the surgery has been successful (Fig. 33), although unchanging hydronephrosis does not necessarily indicate a poor result as long as the functional measures are improved.

Imaging Protocol for Congenital Neuropathic Bladder

The majority of children with congenital neuropathic bladder dysfunction has a normal urinary system at birth, and it is only with the passage of time that hydronephrosis, vesicoureteral reflux, renal parenchymal damage, and bladder diverticula develop (Figs. 34 and 35) as a consequence of a functional neurologic obstruction of the bladder outlet.[11] The severity of the obstructive uropathy and the rate at which it develops are related to the degree of the ure-throvesical obstruction. Therefore, the evaluation of children with neuropathic bladder dysfunction must have as its goal the early identification of urethrovesical obstruction and vesicoureteral reflux. All children should have a baseline renal and bladder ultrasound scan and VCUG at the time they are first evaluated. The IVU has limited usefulness in these children because bowel gas and stool often impair renal imaging. As long as the child's clinical circumstances remain unchanged, a nuclear cystogram and a renal ultrasound scan are usually repeated annually. When there is evidence of hydronephrosis or vesicoureteral reflux, cortical imaging studies (as previously outlined for vesicoureteral reflux) can provide significant clinical information (Fig. 36).[12]

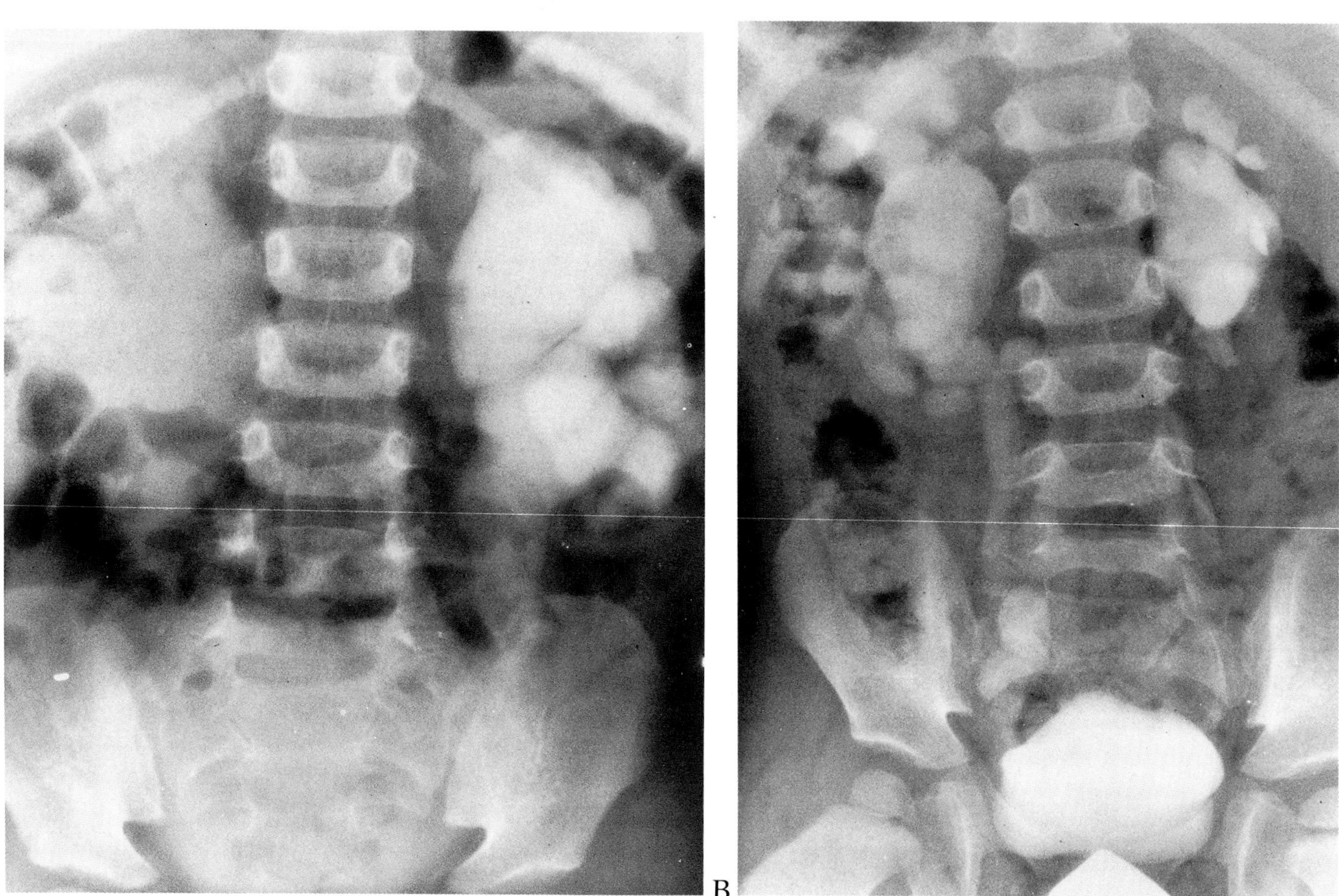

Figure 21.   These urograms (A, B, C) all demonstrate significant dilatation of the upper collecting systems. No evidence of mechanical obstruction was demonstrated on diuretic renography, and no surgery has been performed. The children remain asymptomatic with stable renal function.

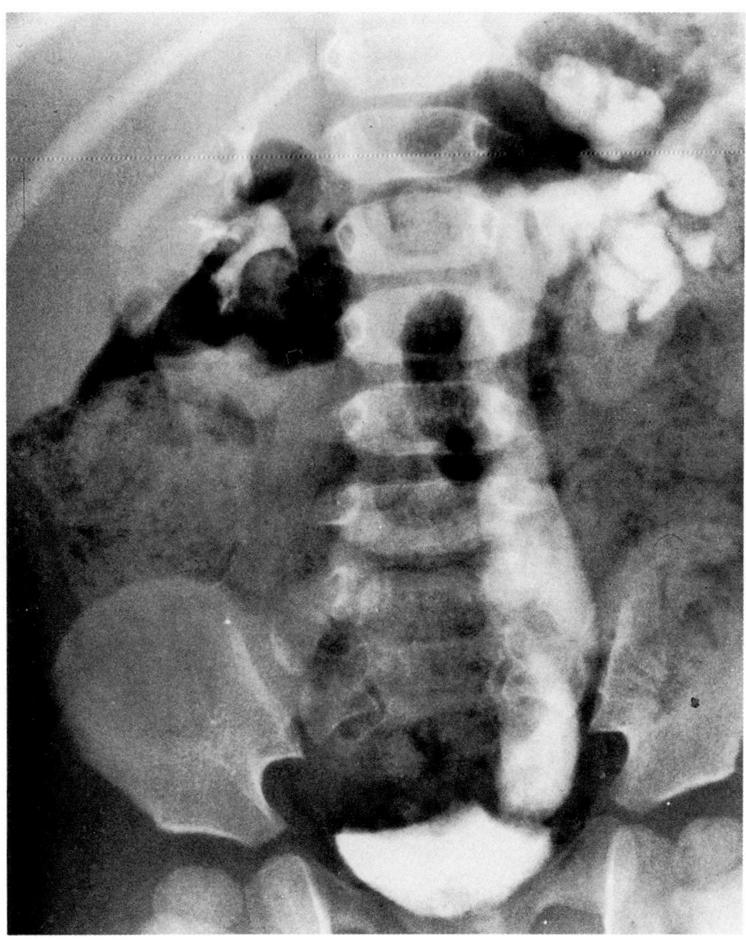

Figure 21C.

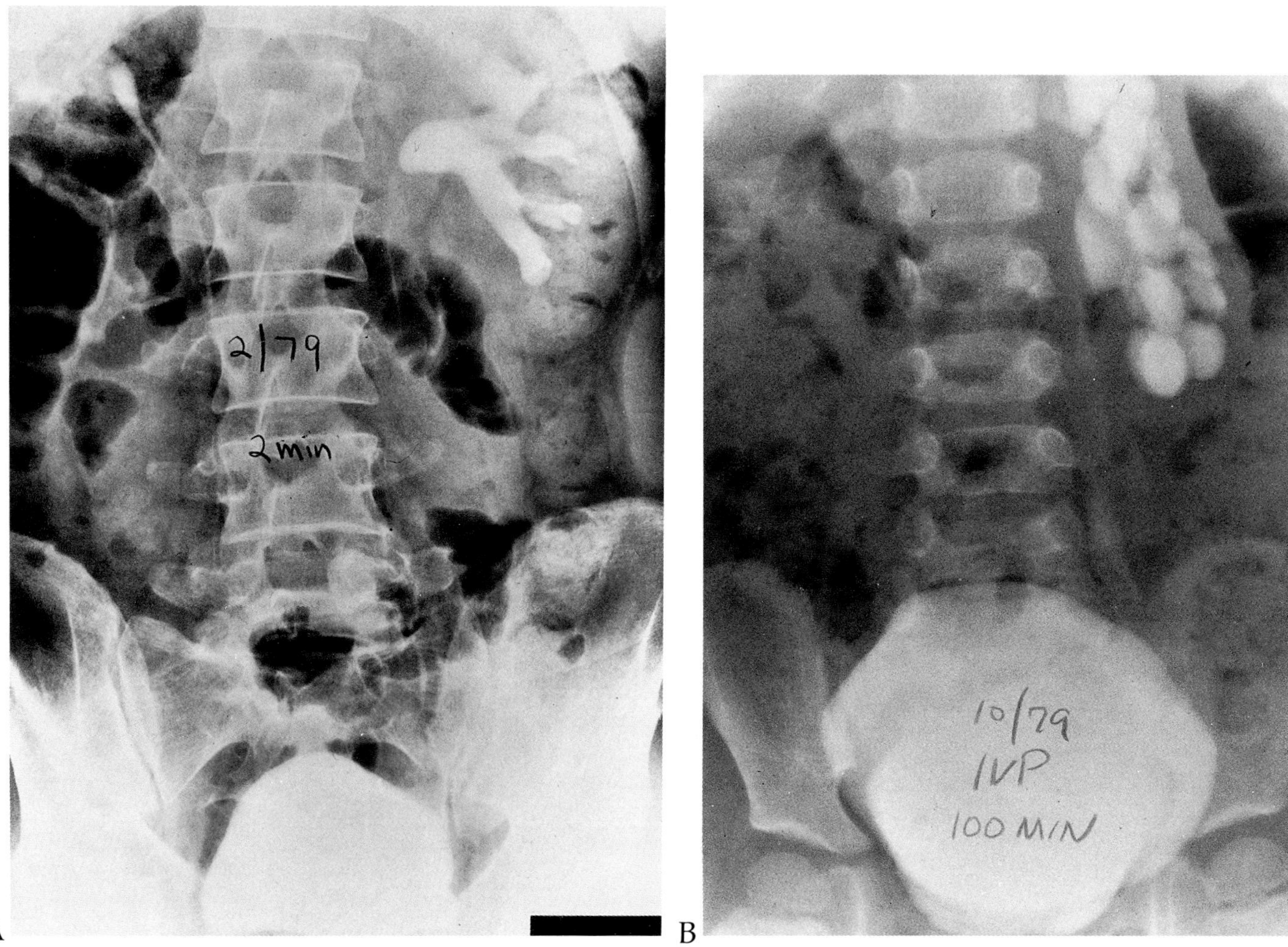

Figure 22.   These individuals (A, B, C) demonstrate degrees of enlargement of their collecting systems similar to those seen in Figure 21. Diuresis renogram showed mechanical obstruction, and surgery was performed.

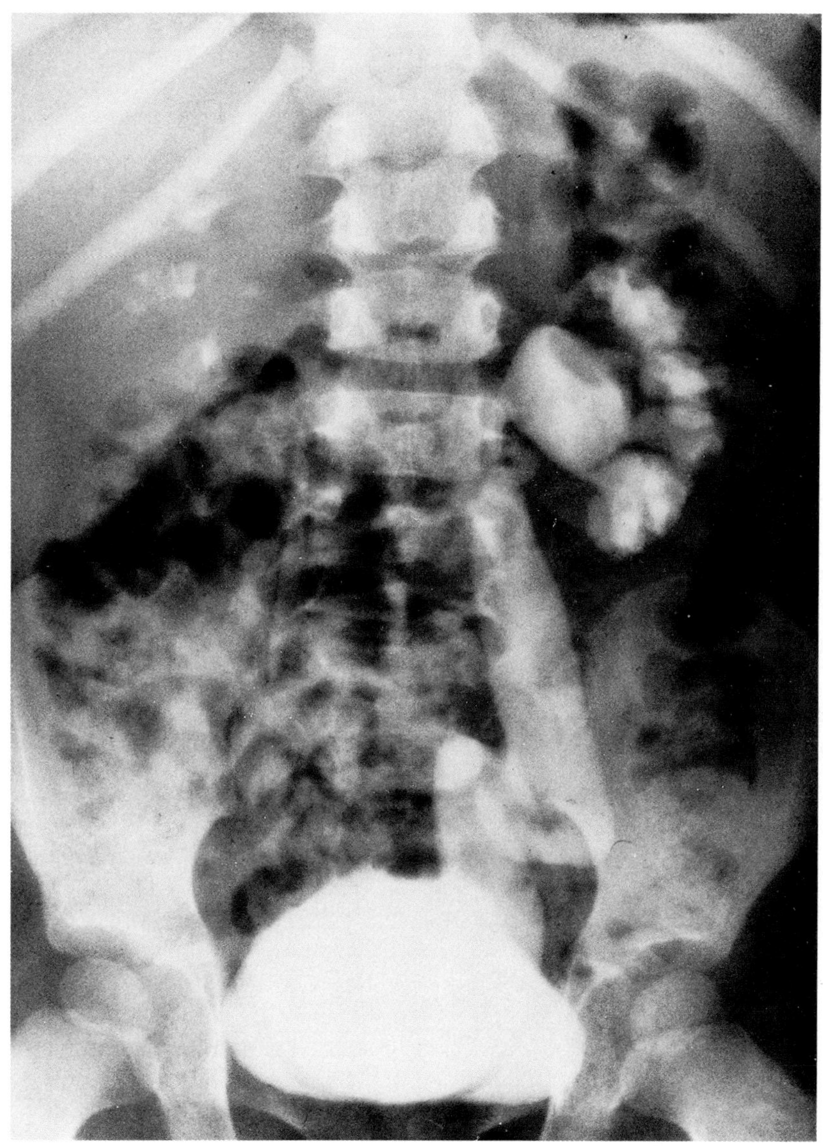

Figure 22C.

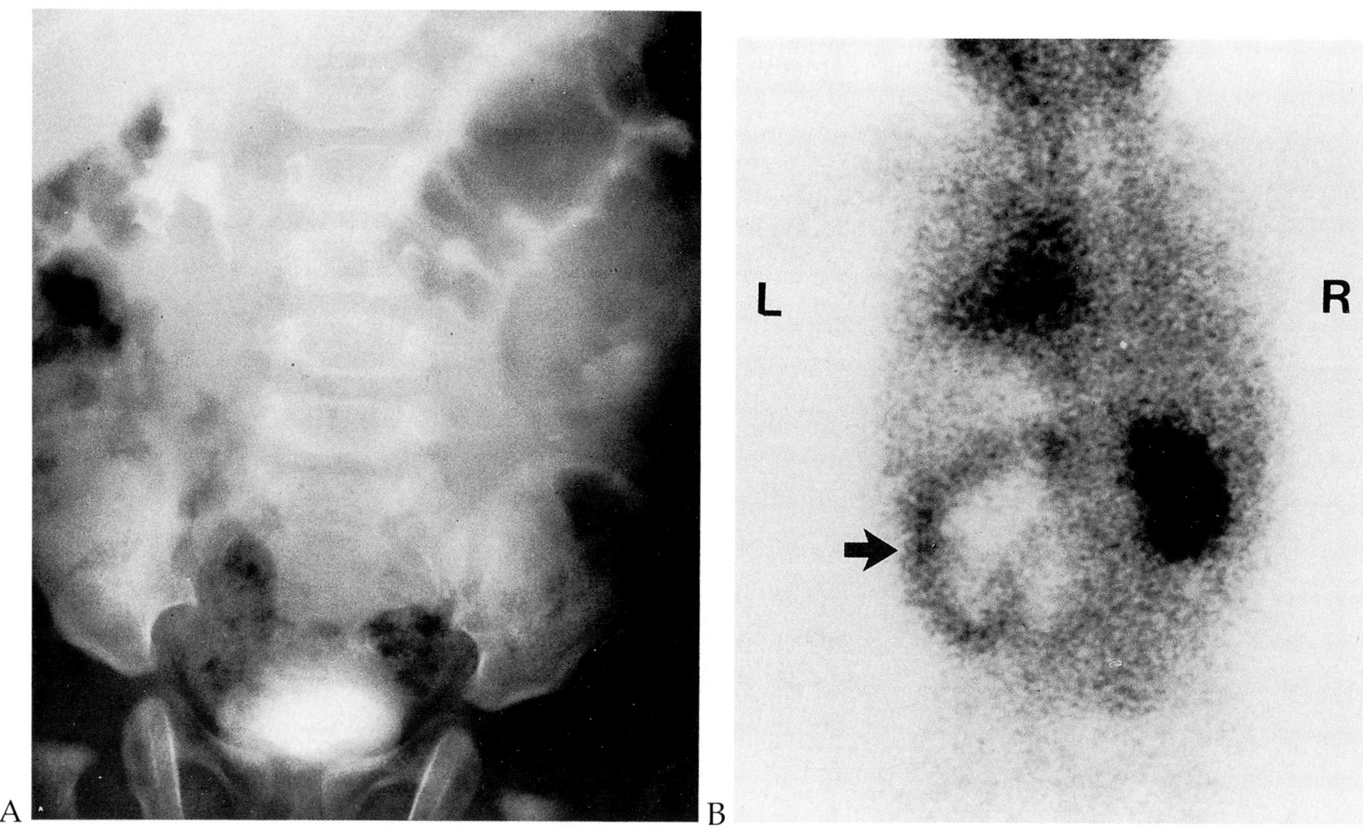

Figure 23.   A child with a possible left UPJ obstruction. (A, left) On IVU, the left kidney is not seen, but a large hydronephrotic kidney was seen on the renal ultrasound scan. (B, right) Renal scan in the same child demonstrates an enlarged and hydronephrotic left kidney with good rim of functioning parenchyma contributing more than 40% of total renal function (arrow). Half-time after diuretic stimulation was more than 20 minutes.

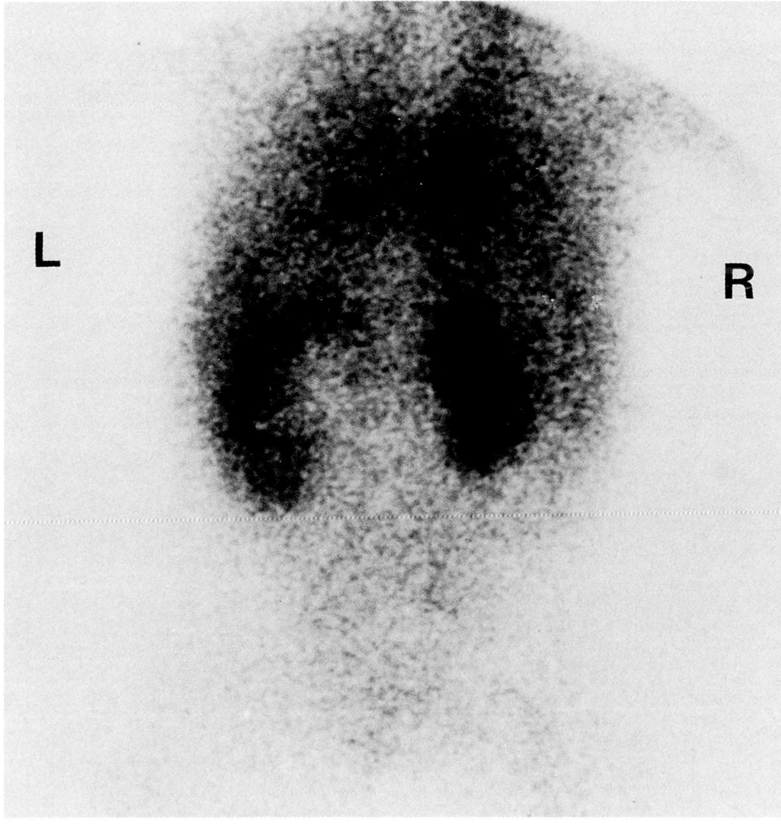

Figure 23C. After successful UPJ repair, nuclear study demonstrates a much more normal-appearing left kidney.

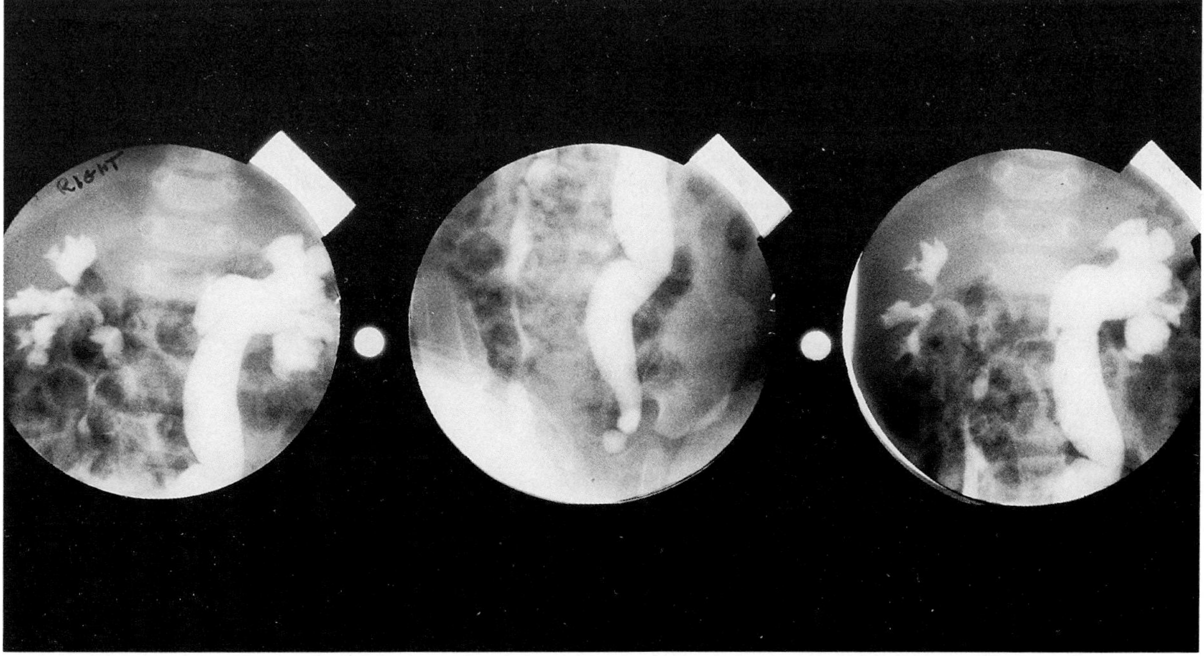

Figure 24. This child with prenatally detected hydronephrosis was found to have a bilateral vesicoureteral reflux. Subsequently, antireflux surgery was required because of breakthrough infections despite continuous chemoprophylaxis.

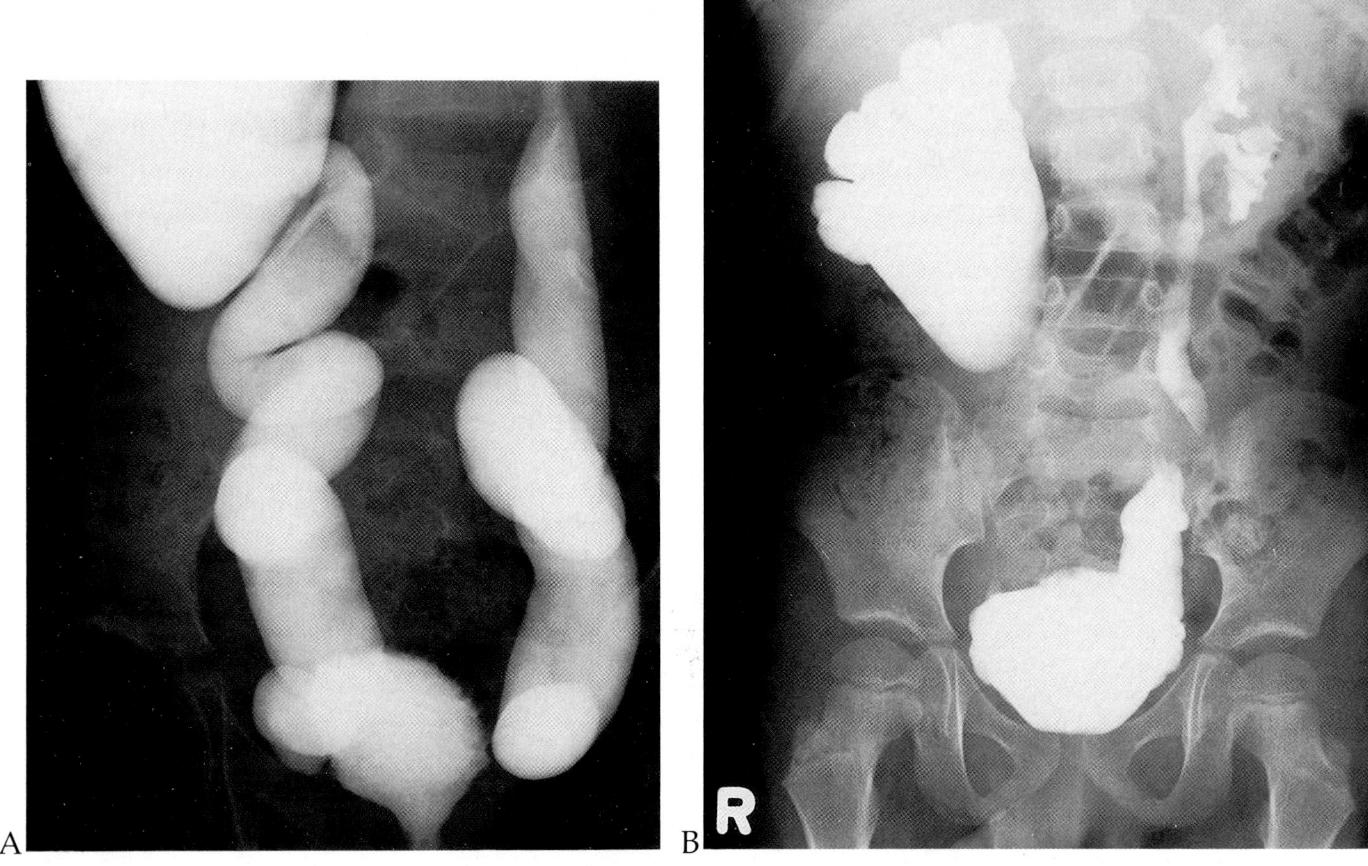

Figure 25.   Multiple problems. (A, left) Voiding cystourethrogram in a child with a possible right UPJ obstruction demonstrates significantly dilated ureters bilaterally. The bladder and urethra were normal. (B, right) Postvoiding film demonstrates residual contrast filling the dilated right collecting system, as well as a relatively normal left collecting system. Diuretic renal scan confirmed the presence of a right UPJ obstruction.

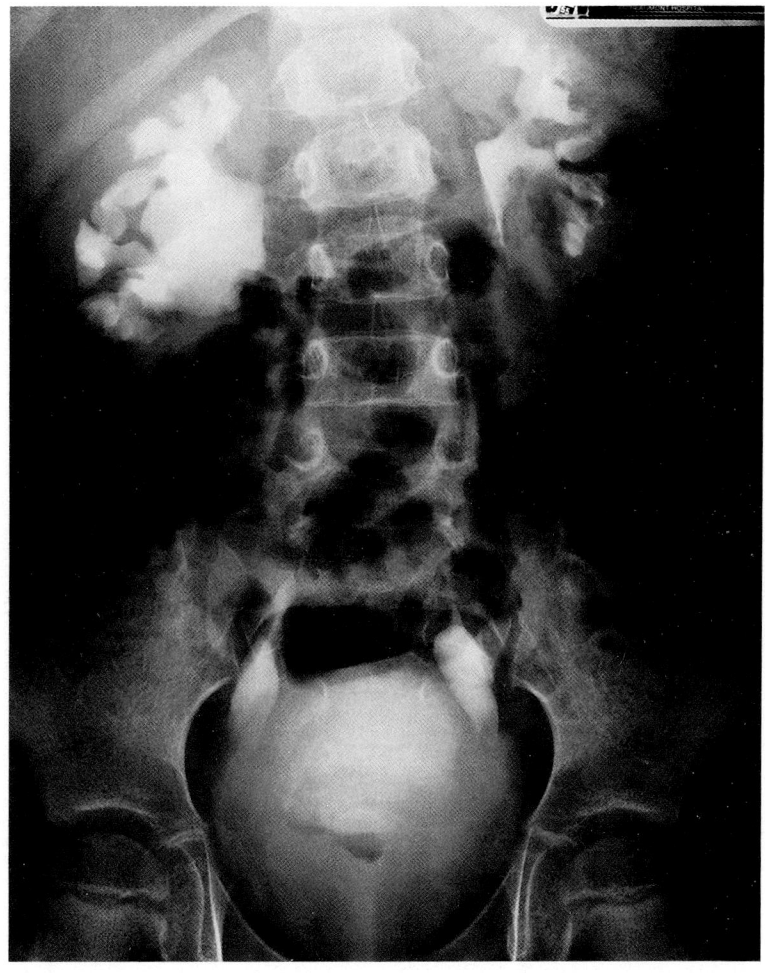

Figure 25C.   Excretory urogram after a right pyeloplasty and bilateral ureteral tapering and reimplantation. This child had a clinically significant reflux as well as a UPJ obstruction on the right side.

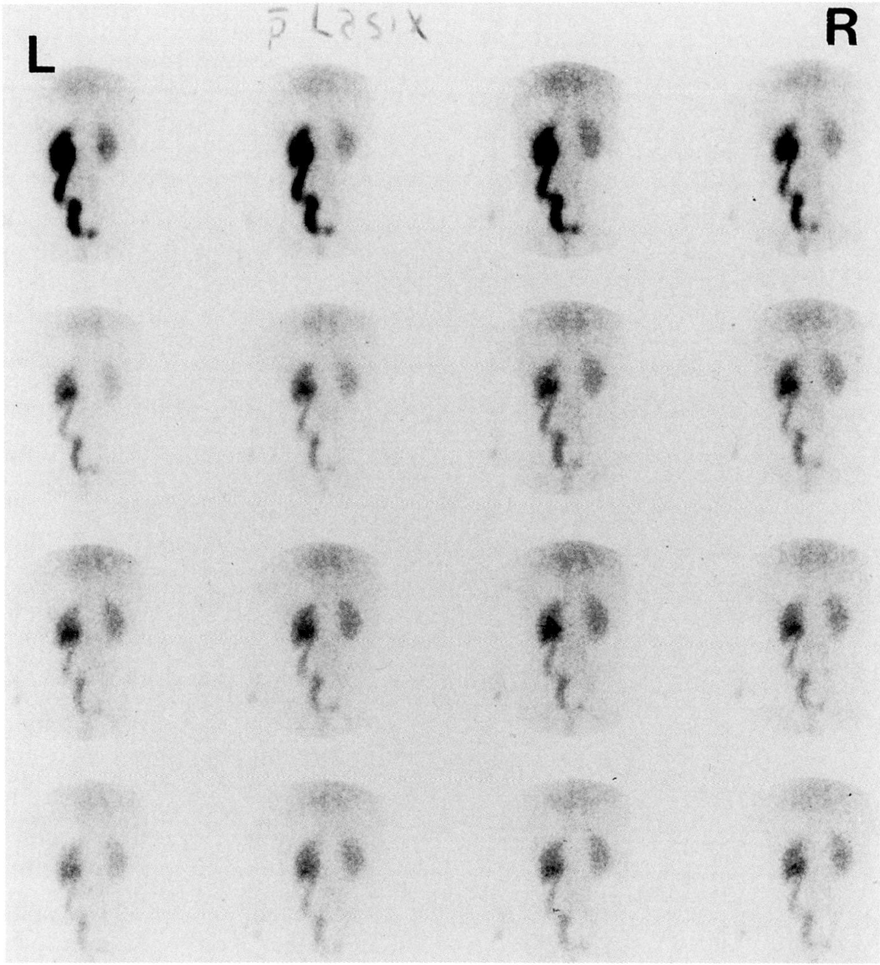

Figure 26A.   Proper technique of diuresis scanning. Scan demonstrating prompt drainage of the left collecting system after administration of diuretic. Drainage half-time was less than 10 minutes. Bladder catheterization ensures that accumulation of the radiopharmaceutical is not superimposed over the lower end of ureter, resulting in a false-positive study.

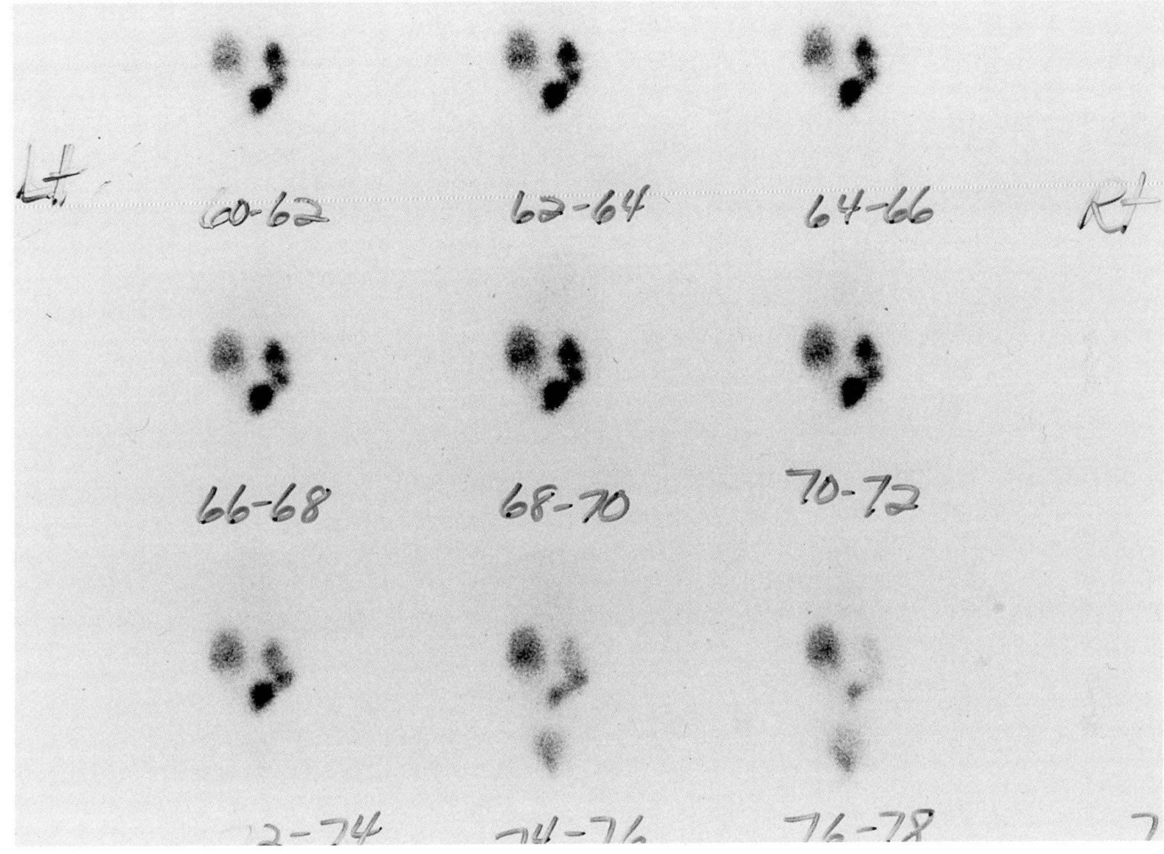

Figure 26B. Scan in a boy with significant bilateral hydroureteronephrosis. The right collecting system is filled completely by 60 minutes and responds nicely to the diuretic, thereby excluding a mechanical obstruction. The left collecting system does not fill adequately by 60 minutes, and therefore, a reliable diuresis renal scan cannot be obtained. Whitaker study demonstrated a significant mechanical obstruction on the left side. Left ureteral tapering and reimplantation was performed, and postoperatively, both collecting systems demonstrated significant reduction in the degree of hydronephrosis.

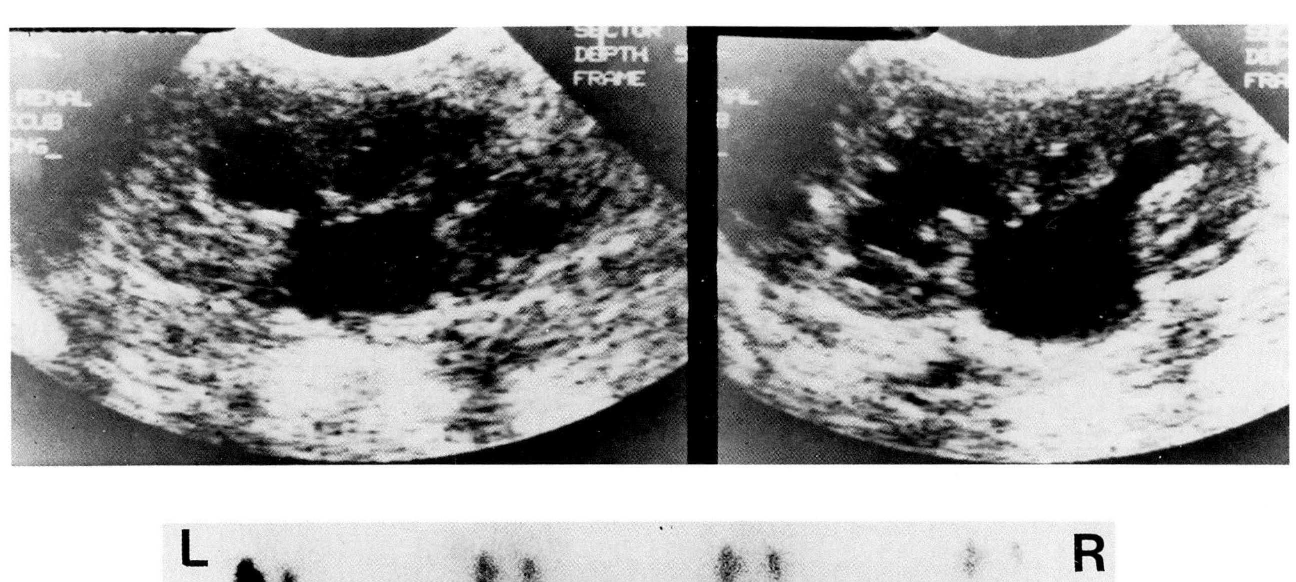

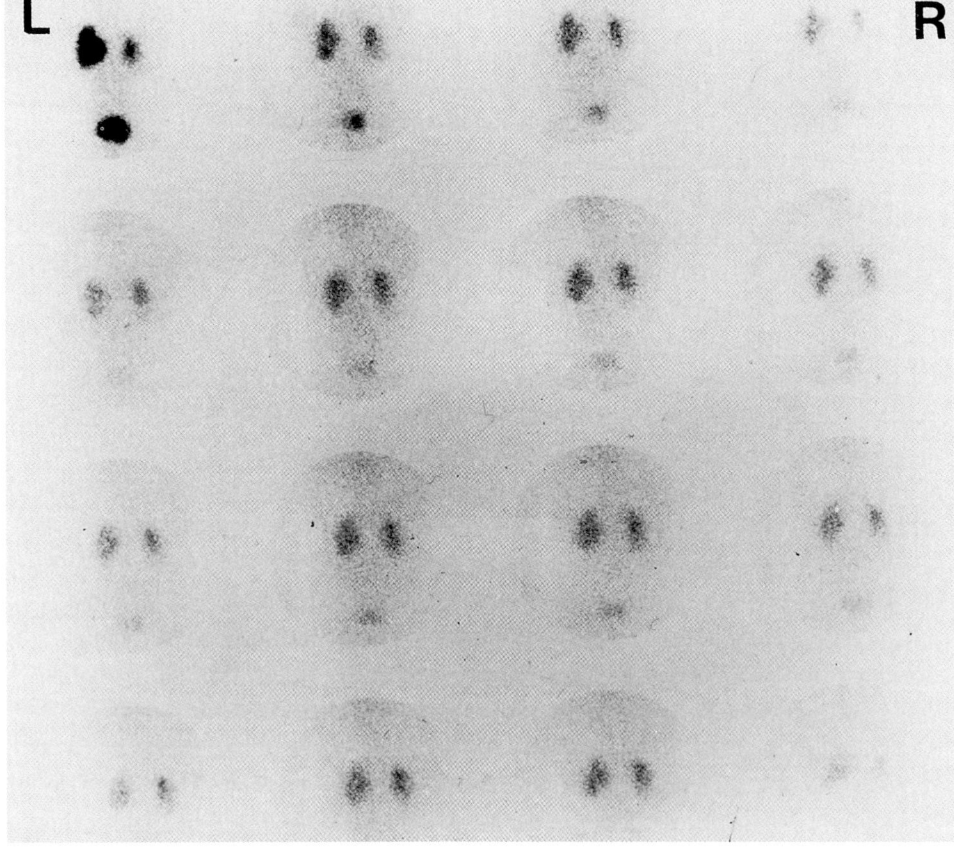

Figure 27. Scan results in cases of nonobstructive hydronephrosis. (A, top) Renal ultrasound in a child with prenatally detected hydronephrosis depicts enlargement of the renal pelvis and calices suggestive of a UPJ obstruction. (B, bottom) Diuresis renal scan demonstrates rapid washout of the radiopharmaceutical after the administration of the diuretic (T½ less than 10 minutes). No surgery has been performed. Renal function remains excellent, and the child is clinically well.

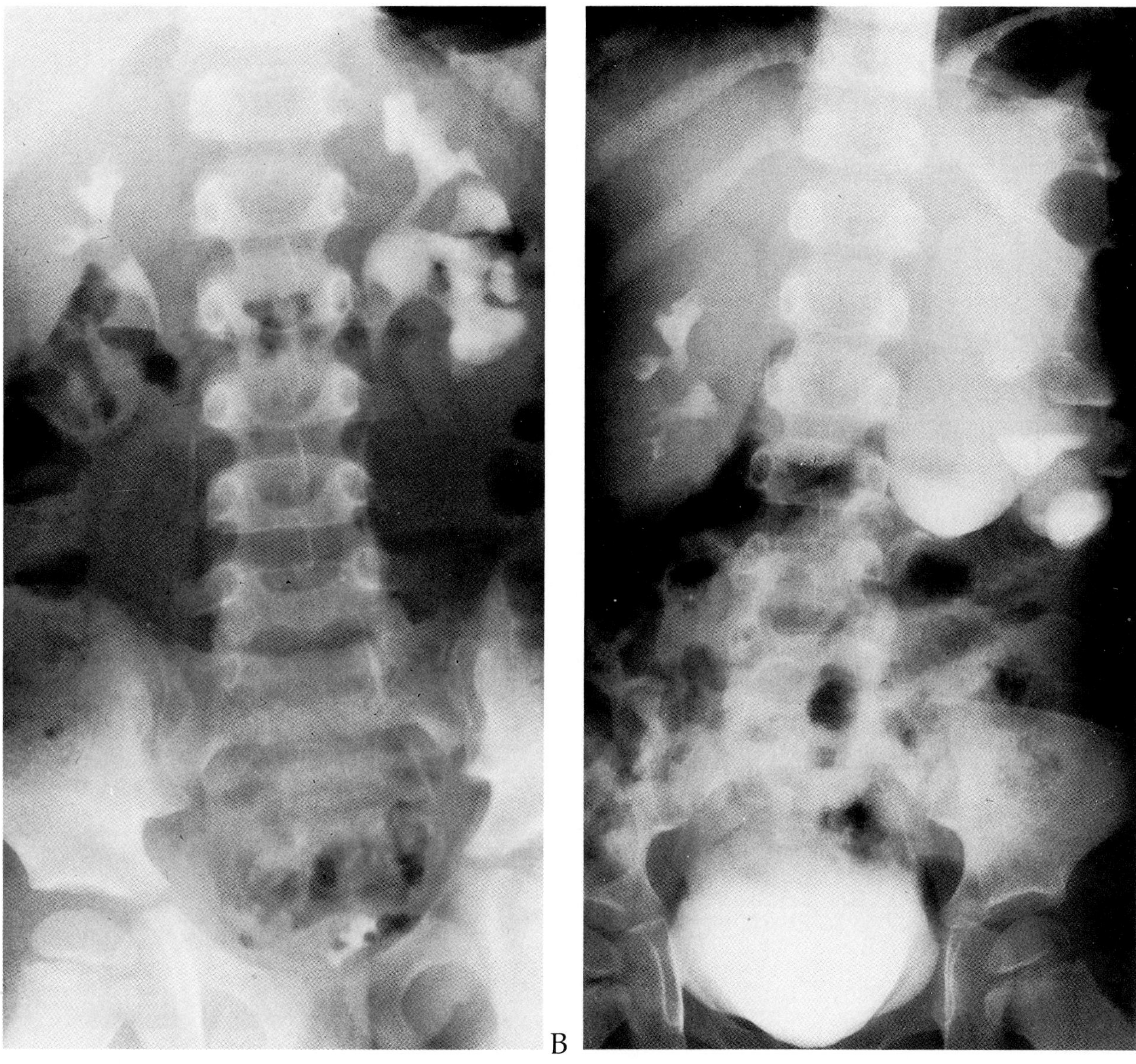

Figure 28.   Obstruction during flank pain. (A, left) IVU in a child with intermittent left flank pain. Diuresis renal scan demonstrated prompt and equal function bilaterally. The T½ for washout of the radiopharmaceutical was 12 minutes on the left side. (B, right) An IVU performed during an episode of pain demonstrates an obvious left UPJ obstruction. It is important to remember that in children with intermittent obstruction, diuresis renal scanning may not diagnose obstruction unless the child is having pain during performance of that study. In this circumstance, repeat ultrasound or IVU during an acute episode is often diagnostic.

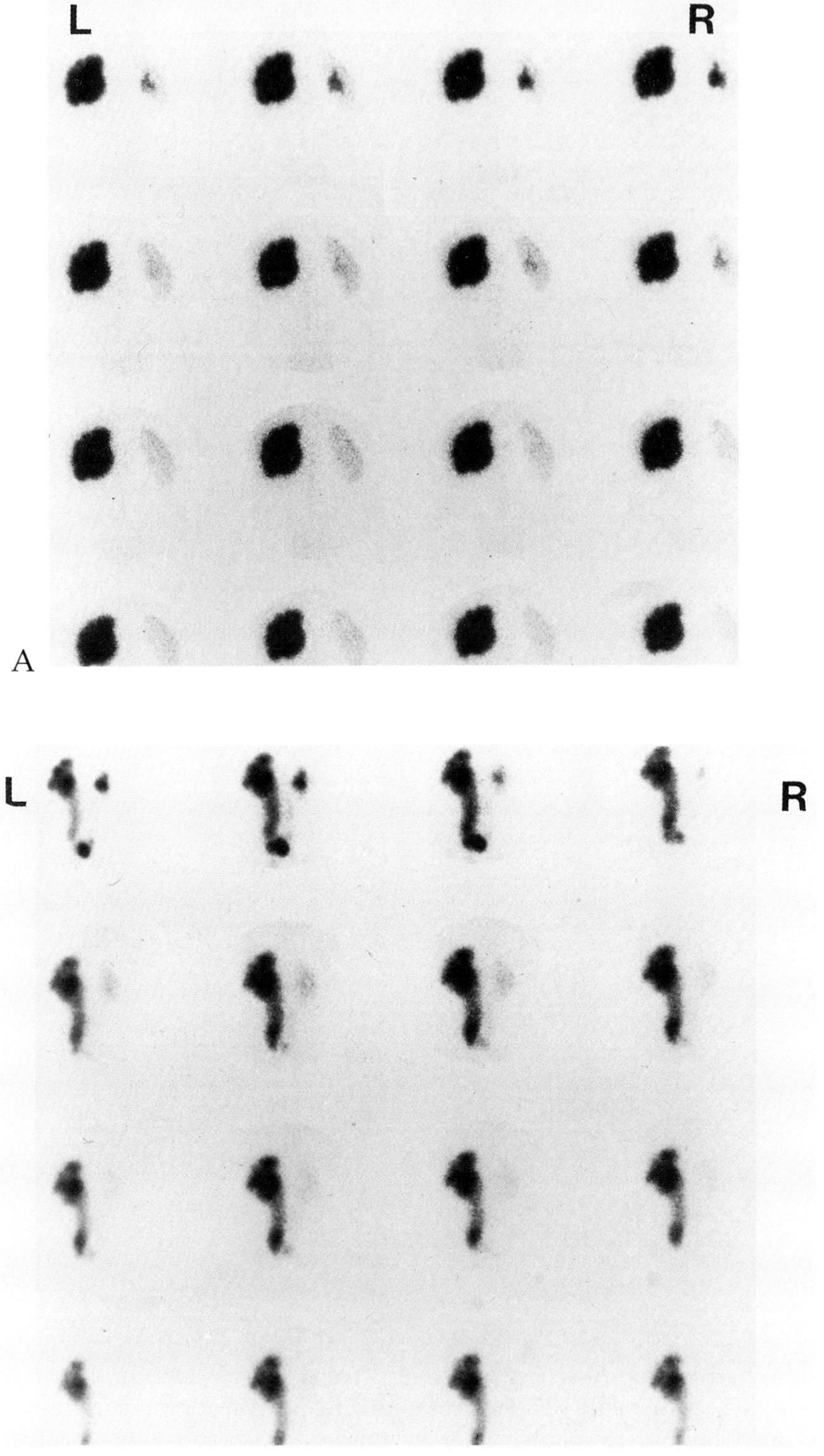

Figure 29.   Identification of an obstruction by diuresis renal scan. (A, top) Study in a child with a left UPJ obstruction. Note that after the administration of the diuretic, there is virtually no washout of tracer from the left collecting system. The T½ on that side was greater than 20 minutes. There is prompt washout from the right collecting system. A left pyeloplasty was performed. (B, bottom) This child has a left UVJ obstruction. The T½ for the left kidney was greater than 20 minutes. Note the prompt response to the diuretic from the right collecting system. A left ureteral tapering and reimplantation was performed.

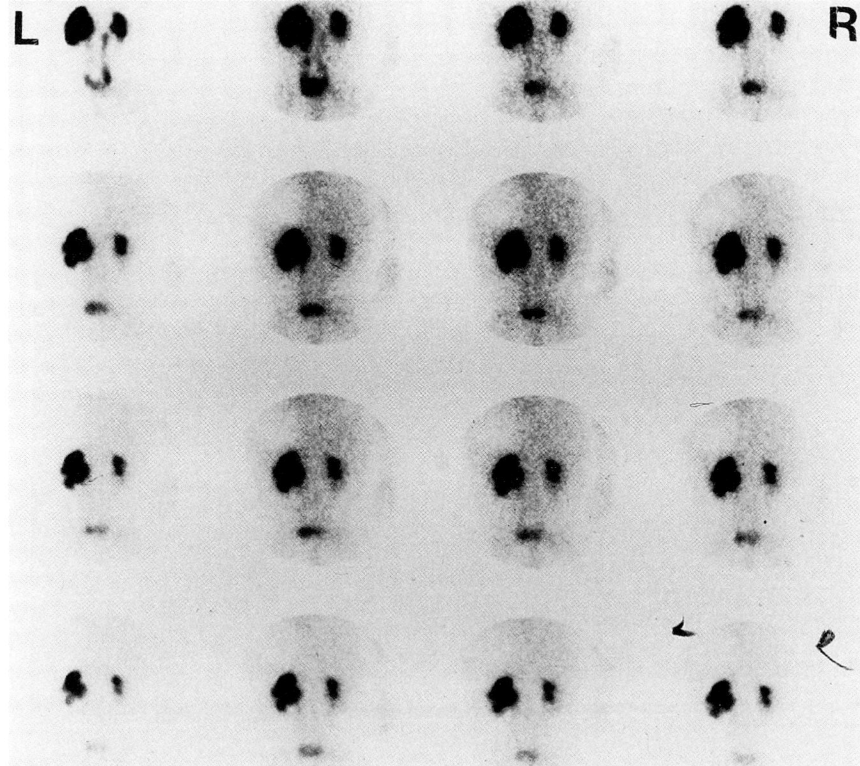

Figure 30.   This 1-month-old infant had prenatally detected left hydronephrosis suggestive of a UPJ obstruction. The right kidney was normal. After administration of the diuretic, there is sluggish washout of the radiopharmaceutical from the left kidney (T½: 22 minutes). However, note that there is also delayed washout from the normal right kidney. No obstruction should be diagnosed in this circumstance, because this study merely reflects an inability of the kidney to respond to the diuretic at this young age. Repeat study should be performed when the child is 3 months of age.

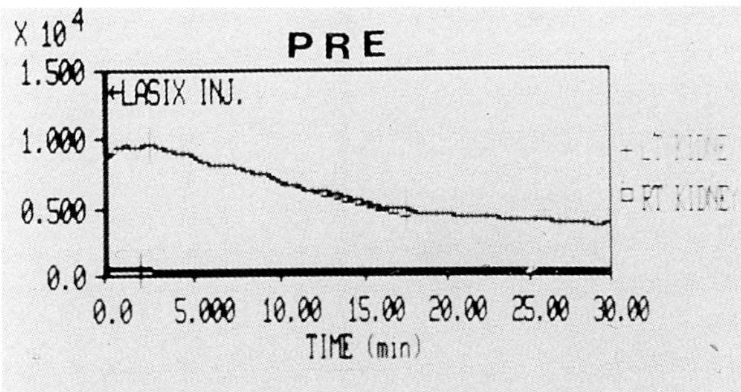

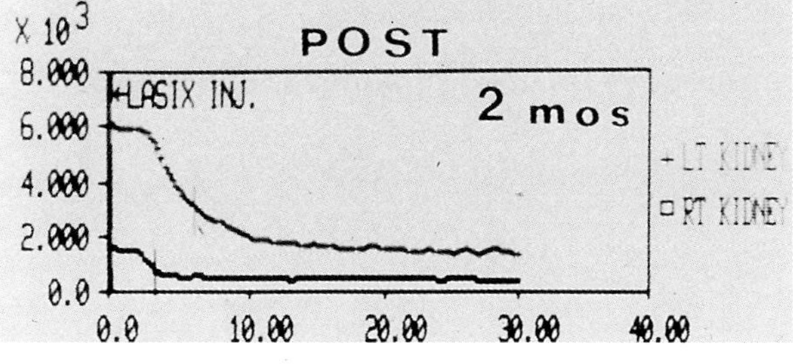

Figure 31.   Washout curves preoperatively and postoperatively in a child with a UPJ obstruction. Preoperative study demonstrated that T½ was greater than 20 minutes. Two months after surgery, T½ was less than 10 minutes, confirming a satisfactory surgical result.

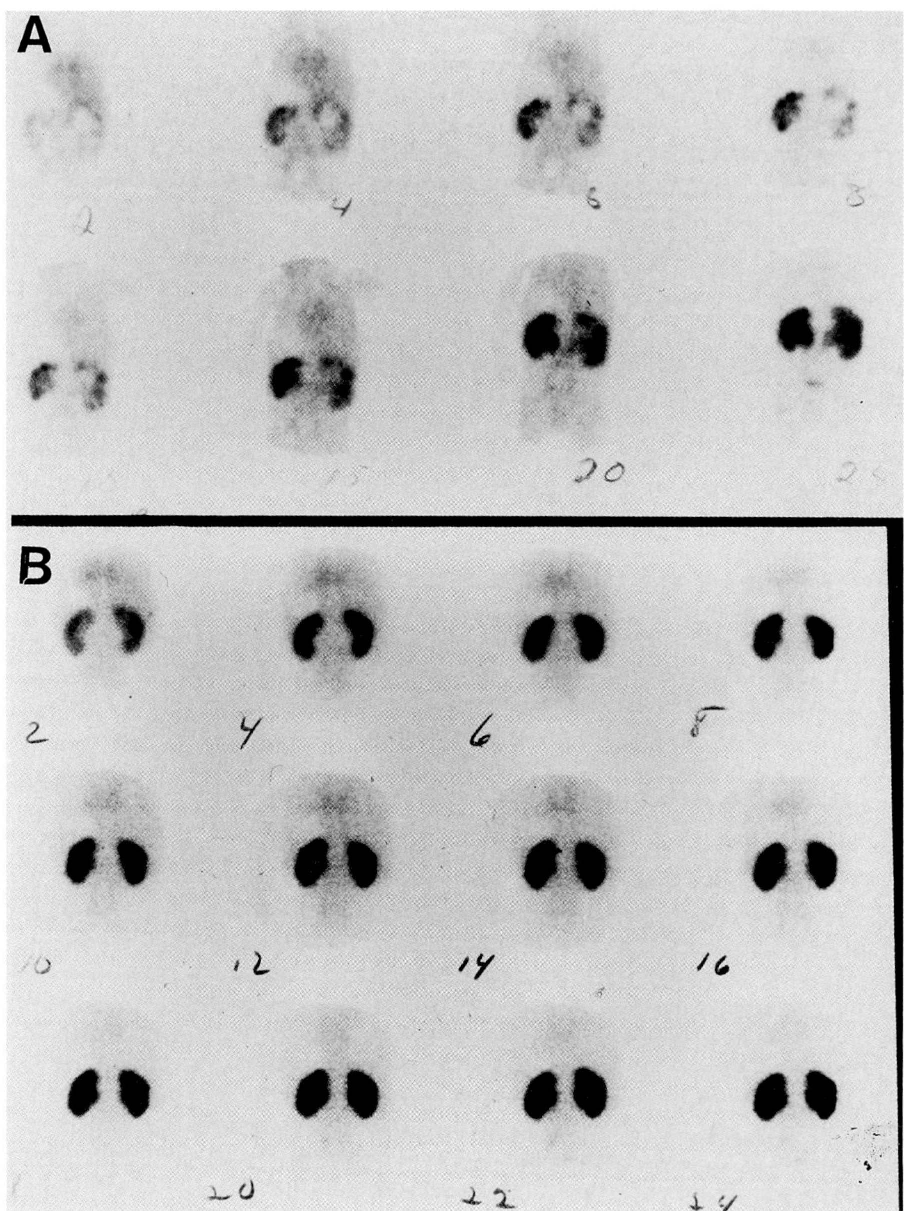

Figure 32. Assessment of surgical outcome with DTPA renal scanning. (A) A child with bilateral UPJ obstruction. Note bilateral decrease in the uptake of the radiopharmaceutical on early images. (B) After bilateral pyeloplasty, there is obvious functional improvement, although washout T ½ remained prolonged for 6 months.

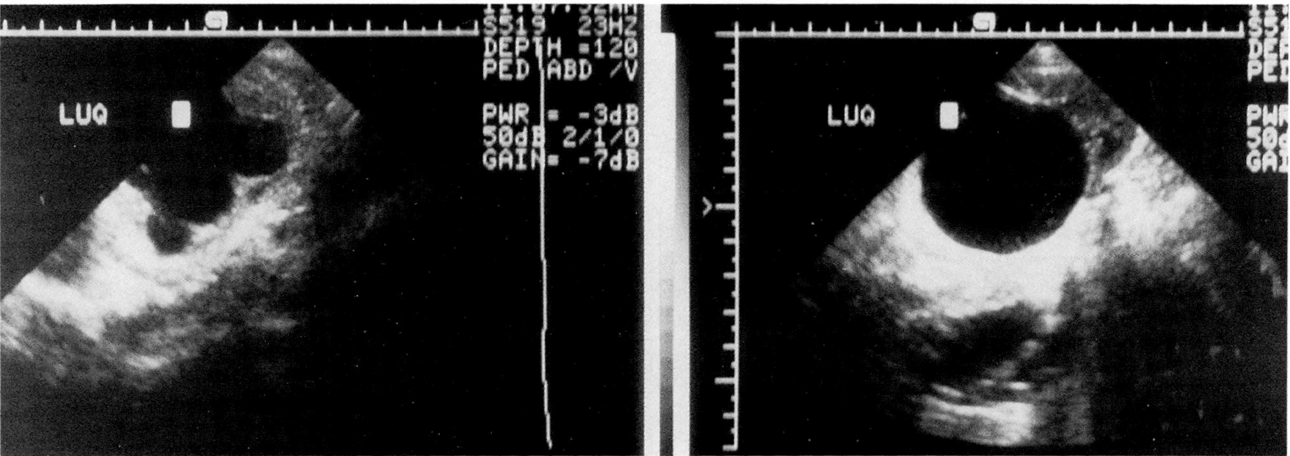

Figure 33A. Assessment of operative outcome with ultrasound. Preoperative renal scan a in child with a UPJ obstruction.

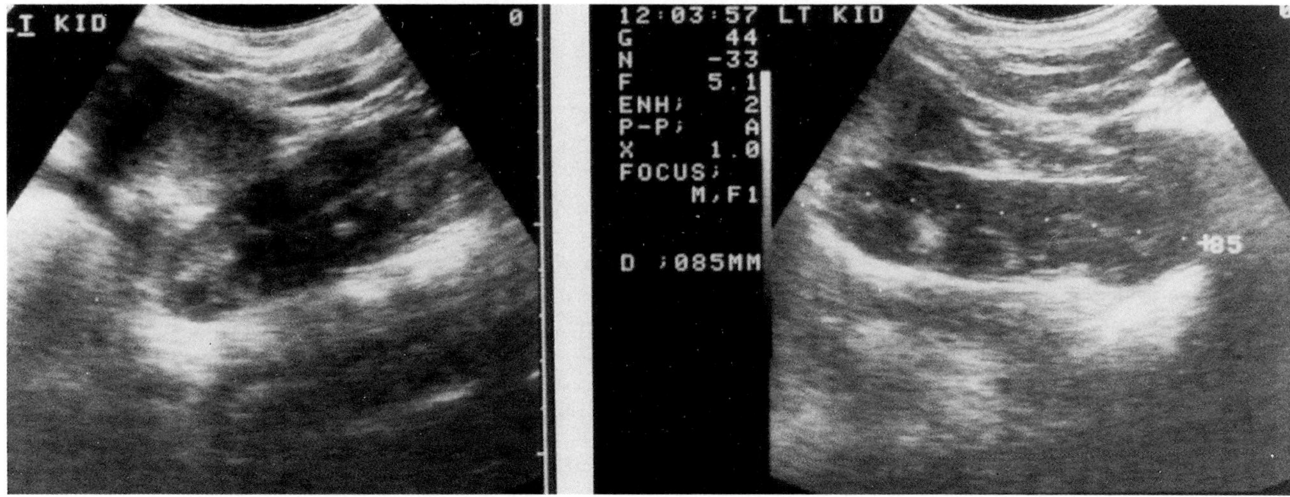

Figure 33B. Postoperative scan demonstrates satisfactory resolution of hydronephrosis.

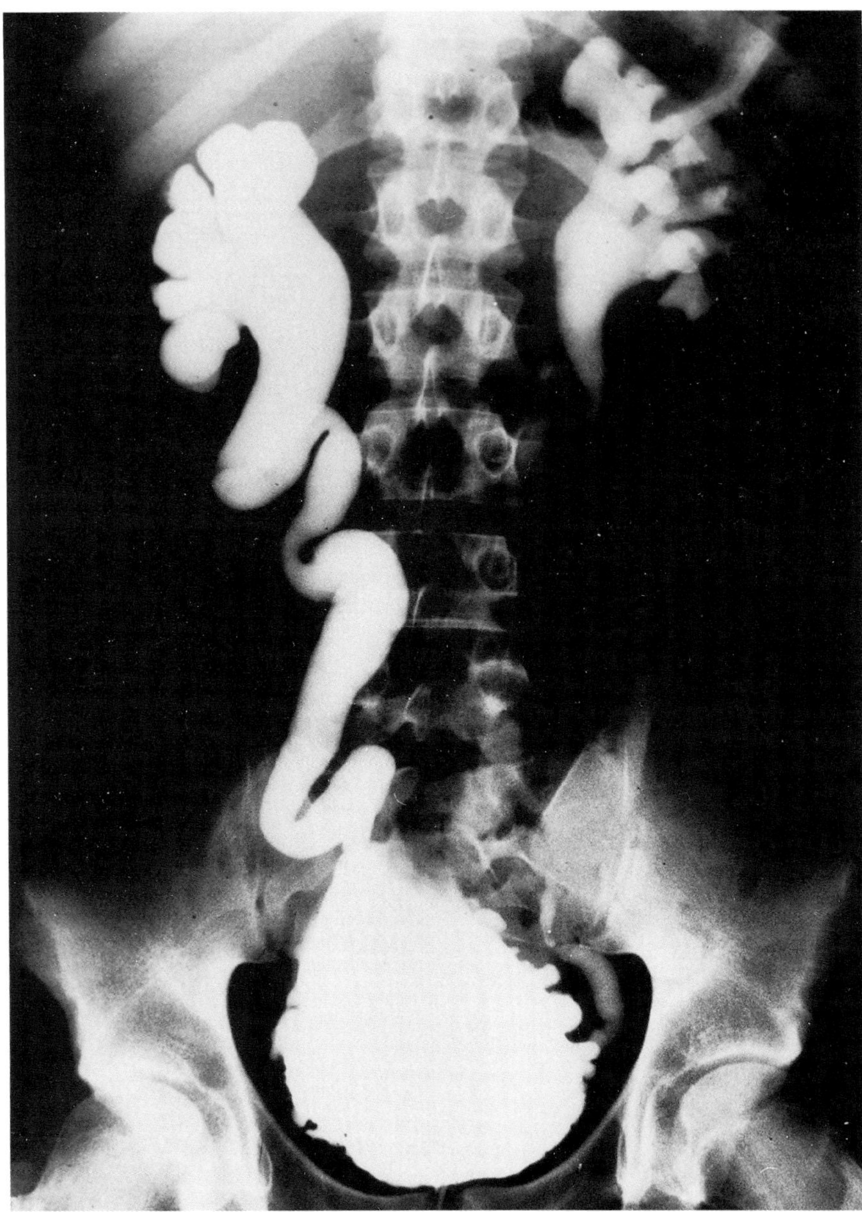

Figure 34.   This child has obvious bilateral vesicoureteral reflux and significant bladder diverticula formation. Similar studies performed during the first few years of life demonstrated normal upper tracts and absence of reflux. Both reflux and bladder changes are secondary to increased intravesical pressure.

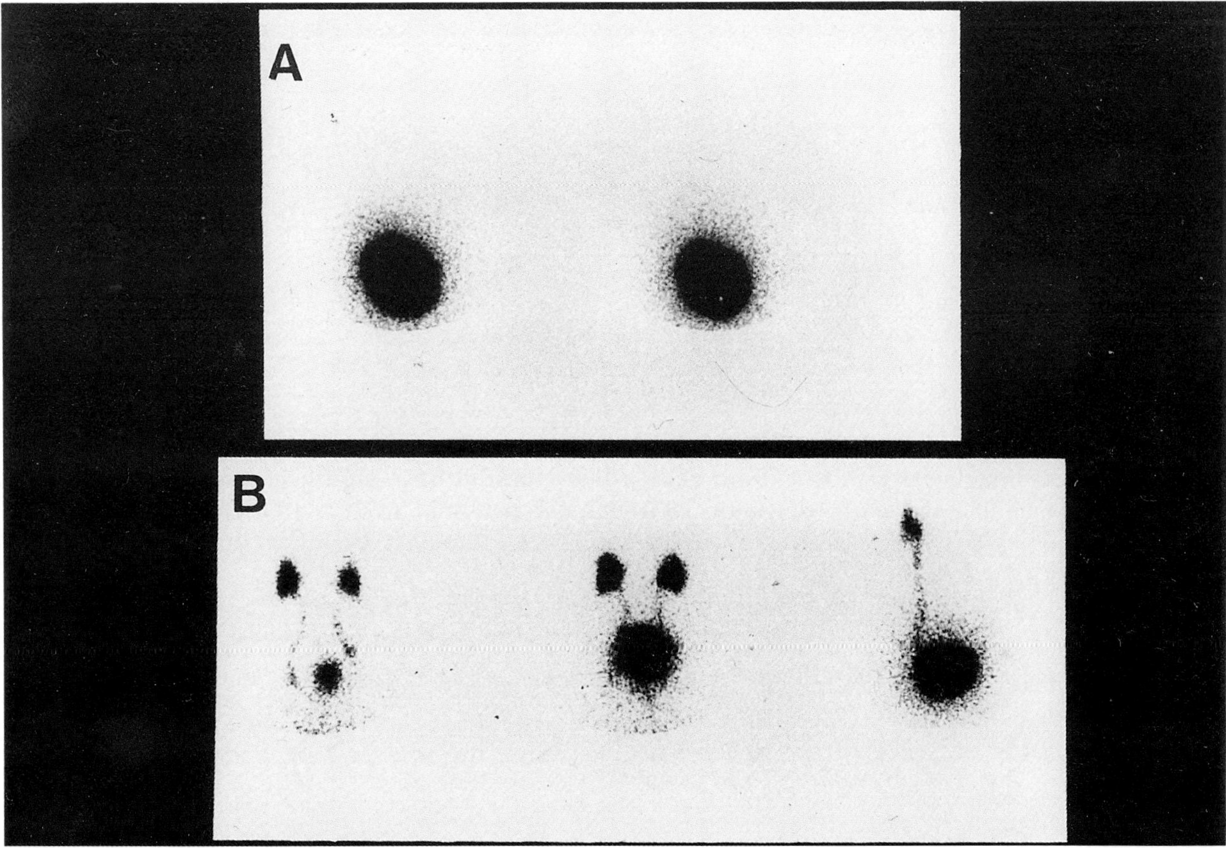

Figure 35.   Another child with vesicoureteral reflux that developed secondarily to bladder dysfunction. Nuclear cystograms are usually performed annually in children with spina bifida. Initially, no reflux was demonstrated; however, on subsequent studies, there is obvious bilateral vesicoureteral reflux. (A) Nuclear cystogram at 1 year of age does not demonstrate reflux. (B) At 3 years of age nuclear cystogram demonstrates a bilateral vesicoureteral reflux, which has developed as a result of abnormal bladder function.

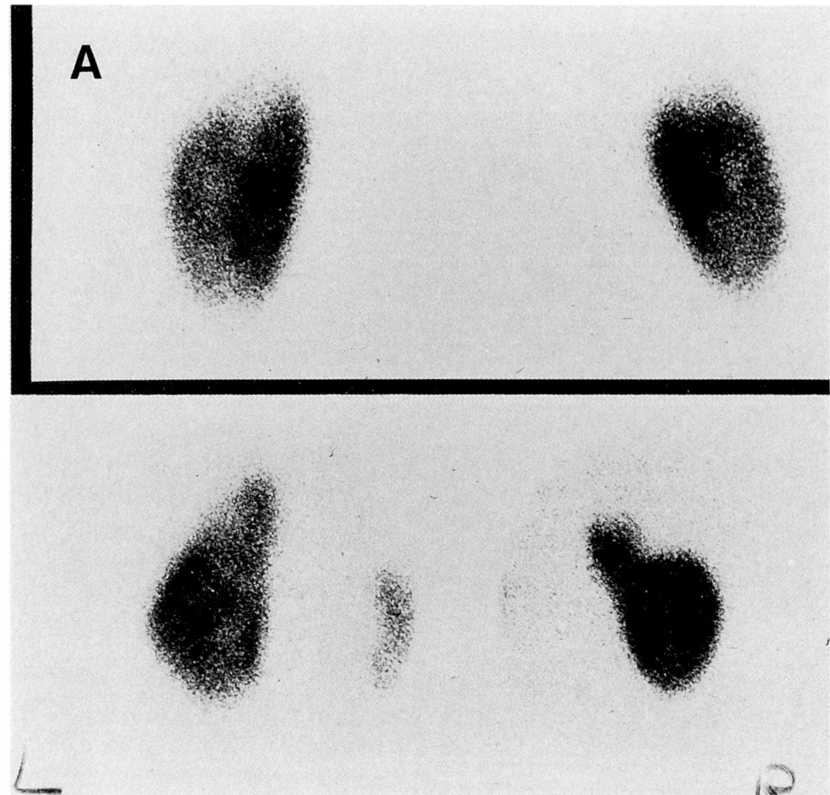

Figure 36A. Cortical imaging is performed annually when children have significant vesicoureteral reflux or hydronephrosis to facilitate the early detection of renal parenchymal injury. (A) This child has obvious right-sided scarring on a DMSA renal scan. Appearance of new scars in a child with reflux may be an indication for antireflux surgery.

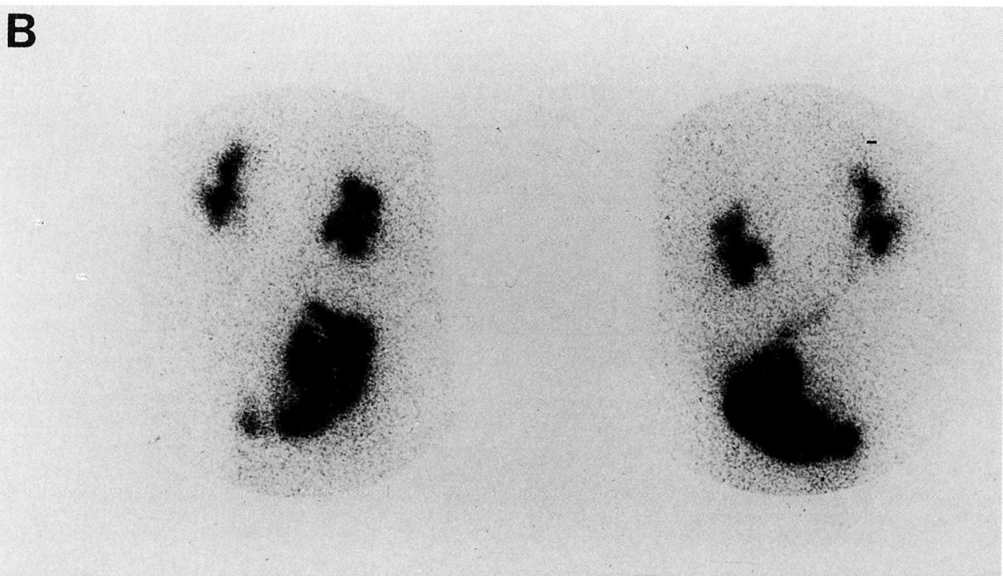

Figure 36B. This child had a urinary undiversion including right-to-left ureteroureterostomy and bladder augmentation. Glucoheptonate renal scan demonstrates a patent ureteral anastomosis without obstruction, as well as augmentation.

References

1. Cacciarelli AA, Kass EJ, Yang SS: Urachal remnants: sonographic demonstration in children. Radiology 1990; 174:473.
2. Russell CD, Bischoff PG, Kontzen F, et al: Measurement of glomerular filtration rate using 99m Tc-DTPA and the gamma camera: a comparison of methods. J Nucl Med 1985; 26:1243.
3. Kass EJ, Fink-Bennett D: Contemporary techniques for the radioisotopic evaluation of the dilated urinary tract. Urol Clin North Am 1990; 17:273.
4. Traisman ES, Conway JJ, Traisman JS, et al: The localization of urinary tract infection with Tc-99m glucoheptonate scintigraphy. Pediatr Radiol 1986; 16:403.
5. Majd M: Nuclear medicine. In Kelalis PP, King LR, Belman AB (eds): Clinical Pediatric Urology. Philadelphia: WB Saunders, 1985; p 140.
6. Al-Nahhas AA, Jafri RA, Britton KE, et al: Clinical experience with 99m Tc-MAG3, mercaptoacetyltriglycine, and a comparison with 99m Tc-DTPA. Eur J Nucl Med 1988; 14:453.
7. Kass EJ: Acute and recurrent urinary tract infections in children. Primary Care 1985; 12:607.
8. Kass EJ, Lebowitz RL, Reda EF, et al: Imaging modalities: their use in UTI. Dialogues Pediatr Urol 1986; 12:2.
9. Silver TM, Kass EJ, Thornbury JR, et al: The radiological spectrum of acute pyelonephritis in adults and adolescents. Radiology 1976; 118:65.
10. Kass EJ, Majd M, Belman AB: Comparison of the diuretic renogram and the pressure perfusion study in children. J Urol 1985; 134:92.
11. Kass EJ, Koff SA, Diokno AC: Fate of vesicoureteral reflux in children with neuropathic bladders managed by intermittent catheterization. J Urol 1981; 125:63.
12. Cohen RA, Rushton HG, Belman AB, et al: Renal scarring and vesicoureteral reflux in children with myelodysplasia: evaluation with technetium-99m DMSA renal scans. J Urol l990; 144:541.

Chapter 7

Renovascular Diseases of the Kidney

John F. Cardella, M.D.

Renovascular diseases of the kidney encompass a broad spectrum of clinical and radiologic entities, all of which have the common denominator of a pathologic process in either the arterial supply of or the venous drainage from the kidney. Because this spectrum of disorders shares basically the same two defects, the clinical presentations of many of the disorders are identical and fall into two categories. Arterial-side disorders present as insidiously rising blood pressure, diminishing renal function, and loss of renal parenchyma; the time course of these changes is variable and depends on the rapidity of onset and the rate of progression of the arterial pathology. Venous-side disorders generally present as hematuria and pain (secondary to edematous capsular stretching), with diminishing renal function generally occurring late; hypertension and parenchymal loss are uncommon manifestations of renal venous pathology and occur late if they do occur.[1]

The radiologic evaluation of renovascular disorders of the kidney has long played an important role in the diagnosis of this group of diseases, along with the history, physical examination, and laboratory studies.

Origin of Renovascular Hypertension

It is the intent of this discussion to present a logical and effective means to diagnose renovascular disease of the kidney using currently accepted imaging modalities.

By far the most renowned of the vascular diseases of the kidney is renovascular hypertension (RVH), in which compromise of the arterial supply to the kidney gives rise to systemic arterial hypertension. The arterial compromise has many possible etiologies, including atherosclerotic, fibromuscular dysplastic, arteritic, inflammatory, iatrogenic, post-traumatic, and thromboembolic. Despite its notoriety, the term "renovascular hypertension" implies more cause-and-effect relation than has actually been proven in the considerable literature dealing with the subject (reviewed in reference 2).

The mechanism by which a renal arterial stenosis causes hypertension is by way of the renin-angiotensin-aldosterone humoral system. Renin, an acid protease produced by the juxtaglomerular cells of the afferent arterioles, is secreted in response to hypoperfusion of the kidney by three identified control mechanisms: a vascular stretch-sensing baroreceptor in the afferent arteriole, a sodium-sensing chemoreceptor in the macula densa tubular mechanism, and a nonadrenergic secretory mechanism mediated by betareceptors. In addition, renin secretion is directly inhibited by circulating vasopressin and angiotensin II.

The renin secreted by the ischemic kidney(s) converts angiotensinogen, a tetradecapeptide produced in the liver, to angiotensin I, a decapeptide.

From *Imaging of Urologic Disorders* edited by Alexander S. Cass, MBBS, © 1992, Futura Publishing Inc., Mount Kisco, NY.

Angiotensin I is converted to the vasoactive octapeptide, angiotensin II by converting enzyme (ACE), a hydrolase found in the pulmonary vascular endothelium. In addition to its potent vasoconstrictor action, angiotensin II stimulates aldosterone secretion from the zona glomerulosa of the adrenal cortex, which causes sodium resorption from the distal tubules. A breakdown product of angiotensin II, known as angiotensin III, is also believed to be a moderately potent vasoconstrictor and stimulator of aldosterone secretion.

The renin-angiotensin-aldosterone system is very effective in raising blood pressure to serve its telelogic function of protecting renal blood flow. However, left to its own devices, the system can do more harm than good by increasing the blood pressure to harmful levels, leading to stroke, intracranial hemorrhage, myocardial hypertrophy, accelerated atherosclerosis, and hypertensive nephrosclerosis, in which hypertension begets more hypertension. The goal of diagnosis and treatment, then, is to interrupt this cycle before it spirals upward out of control.

Clinical, Laboratory, and Historical Evaluation

The exact incidence of RVH is unknown. Estimates exist that 10% to 15% of American adults have high blood pressure[3] and that 25% of persons age 50 to 70 have hypertension.[4] Of these persons with high blood pressure, it is estimated that 2% to 5% will subsequently be shown to have renovascular disorders,[5,6] although much higher incidences of RVH have been reported in subgroups of hypertensive patients.[7,8]

Early diagnosis of RVH is crucial. The primary defect in the disease is correctable, and early treatment avoids the morbidity and mortality risks of elevated blood pressure (myocardial infarction, thrombotic and hemorrhagic stroke, renal failure, congestive heart failure, and accelerated atherosclerosis).

A family history of hypertension is not a particularly sensitive or specific symptom of RVH, because primary "essential" hypertension is so common that many family members of a patient with RVH may have unrelated hypertension. Historical information regarding the duration of hypertension has similarly been shown to be relatively insensitive and nonspecific for RVH. The one historical feature that is helpful is a relatively young age at the time of presentation, particularly in women, in whom the renal artery stenosis is more likely to be secondary to fibromuscular dysplasia.

According to the Cooperative Study on Renovascular Hypertension,[6] nocturia and weakness or fatigue occur more often in patients with atheromatous renal artery stenosis than in those with fibromuscular dysplasia or essential hypertension. In addition, 20% of patients with atherosclerotic renal artery stenosis manifest arterial occlusive disease of the brain, heart, or extremities; this compares with only 10% of patients with essential hypertension or fibromuscular dysplasia manifesting these symptoms. Although a history of flank pain is not specific for RVH, its presence should raise the possibility of this etiology in a hypertensive patient, because in a small percentage of patients with RVH, renal cortical infarcts occur.

Physical findings in patients with RVH include obesity far less frequently than in patients with essential hypertension. Deep abdominal or flank bruits occur 8 to 20 times more frequently in patients with RVH than in those with essential hypertension. Retinal examination in the patient with RVH demonstrates focal arteriolar constrictions thought to be of spastic origin. These "angiospastic changes" are believed to be indicative of the severity of the hypertension and its rapidity of onset but cannot be considered specific for RVH since patients with essential hypertension also can have markedly elevated blood pressures of rapid onset.

The laboratory investigation of the RVH patient is relatively limited and is not helpful in differentiating RVH from essential hypertension. Peripheral vein renin measurements are advocated by some investigators but have been disregarded as insensitive and nonspecific by other investigators.

Imaging Evaluation

Intravenous urography (IVU), when properly performed, remains the most cost effective and informative screening examination for the patient with suspected RVH. The radiographic signs of discrepant renal size, unilaterally diminished nephrographic blush (both diminished in intensity and delayed), and decreased excretion of contrast into the intrarenal collecting system all reflect the physiologic changes of decreased renal blood flow and blood volume, ischemic atrophy, decreased glomerular filtration rate, and increased urinary transit time present in patients with RVH.

Proper intravenous urography should be performed without ureteral compression and with rapid-sequence films to demonstrate the discrepancy in contrast appearance time in the kidneys adequately. Ideally, nontomographic cone-down views of the kidneys are taken at 30 seconds, 1 minute, 2 minutes, and 3 minutes after injection of contrast material. Tomographic cuts, if desired, should then be performed 5 minutes after injection. An 8 minute film centered over the kidneys should be taken and renal size measured on this film, as tomograms may distort the renal size. Ten- and fifteen-minute, 14- × 17-inch films should then be taken to depict the ureters and bladder. Cone-down and oblique views of the bladder generally contribute little in the diagnostic evaluation of the patient with suspected RVH and should be avoided in the generally younger patient population to minimize radiation exposure to gonadal tissue.

Figure 1 demonstrates the radiographic signs seen on an intravenous urogram in a patient with proved RVH. Renal size discrepancy of greater than 1.5 cm pole to pole is generally felt to be significant, suggesting an ischemic process in the smaller kidney. A delay in the appearance of the nephrographic blush and in the appearance of contrast in the intrarenal collecting system are additional signs of unilateral renal ischemia and are best seen on the early-phase IVU films. Generally, the tighter the renal artery stenosis, the greater the discrepancy in appearance times, although this cannot be absolutely relied on, particularly if there are well-developed collaterals around the renal artery stenosis. Diminished contrast density and a diminished amount of contrast in the intrarenal collecting system are also radiographic signs of possible RVH and are related to the decreased renal blood flow and decreased

glomerular filtration, respectively, within the ischemic kidney. A rare, interesting sign of an ischemic kidney is the presence of ureteral notching in which enlarged retroperitoneal collaterals indent the ureter extrinsically.

According to the Cooperative Study on Renovascular Hypertension,[6] the most common abnormality, appearing in 59% of patients with renovascular disease and in only 2% of patients with essential hypertension, was delayed appearance of contrast material. Disparity in renal size was present in 38.6% of patients with renovascular disease and in only 5.6% of patients with essential hypertension. Renal size discrepancy of greater than 1.5 cm pole to pole occurred in approximately 60% of patients with severe renal artery stenosis, but discrepant renal size can also occur in patients with essential hypertension and concomitant unilateral renal artery atherosclerosis. Discrepant renal size occurs more frequently in essential hypertension than in the normal person.

Another excellent imaging modality for the evaluation of RVH is the isotope renogram. The IVU gives primarily anatomic information about the kidneys, whereas the isotope renogram provides information about the physiologic status of the kidney. The isotope method most popular in the evaluation of RVH is the technetium-99m diethylenetriamine penta-acetic acid (Tc-99m DTPA) flow study, either alone or in combination with a captopril challenge.

On the DTPA flow study, images are obtained at 2-second intervals for 30 seconds (15 images), with additional images at 1 and 5 minutes. These latter images are taken to evaluate the amount of activity in the intrarenal collecting system, ureters, and bladder. Computer software packages are available in most nuclear medicine facilities to analyze the rapidity of appearance of activity in the renal cortex and also to measure the accumulation of activity within the intrarenal collecting system using operator-determined regions of interest. The activity intensity curve in the aorta is them compared with that in the renal cortex; these curves should be nearly parallel with a slight (less than 1-second) interval between the appearance times of activity in the aorta and renal cortex. Side-to-side discrepancies in the activity appearance time suggest renal arterial compromise on the delayed side and correspond to the excretory urographic finding of a delayed nephrographic blush (Fig. 2).

Although not routinely used at our institution, The Milton S. Hershey Medical Center, captopril challenge has utility in some cases. With the administration of this ACE inhibitor, the relative ischemia of the involved kidney worsens, and this change accentuates the discrepancy in the appearance time of activity in the involved kidney. The standard DTPA renogram and the captopril challenge renogram must be performed 48 hours apart to allow clearing of the technetium-99m activity from the first examination.

The second portion of the isotope renogram is designed to assess renal excretory function by acquiring images out to 60 minutes at 5-minute intervals. By selecting regions of interest over the renal pelves and bladder, the excretion of activity into the pelvis and subsequent drainage of activity into the bladder can be followed. In a normal functioning kidney, activity should accumulate promptly in the renal pelves if excretory function is normal and it should also drain promptly from the renal pelves into the urinary bladder if there is no ureteral obstruction. Decreased excretory function on the renogram is less specific for renovascular disease and generally indicates significant loss of glomerular filtration of whatever cause. Such decrease in excretion is seen only in moderately to far advanced RVH. Isotope renography is a very useful tool for qualitatively following both the progression of RVH and improvements after revascularization. The technique is noninvasive and can be repeated at frequent intervals.

When the IVU and isotope renogram are used in combination, 91% to 96% of patients with one or both positive studies will show improvement in their hypertension after revascularization of the kidney.[9,10] Additionally, in a patient with an abdominal bruit, abnormal IVU, and abnormal isotope renogram, the chance of finding a renal artery stenosis of greater than 50% is 95%[11]

Ultrasonography provides a noninvasive way to access renal size and renal cortical thickness. When decreased, the features may be late findings of RVH, but they are nonspecific. In fact, decreased renal size and decreased cortical thickness occur with advancing age, so these findings become less helpful in elderly patients. Also, patients with longstanding essential hypertension may demonstrate these ultrasound findings secondary to small-vessel nephrosclerosis. A unilateral decrease in renal size and cortical thickness is more useful in diagnosing RVH, especially in younger patients. The additional information available from ultrasound examination of the kidneys from an imaging standpoint is insufficient to warrant the additional cost.

Duplex ultrasound evaluation of the renal arteries is a newer noninvasive modality that adds specificity and sensitivity to the conventional ultrasound study by providing hemodynamic information about the renal artery. Generally, stenosis of 50% luminal diameter reduction (75% reduction in cross-sectional area) are sufficient to create turbulent flow and high-velocity jets of blood, both of which can be detected by duplex scanning of the renal arteries. The technique gives good hemodynamic information about flow in the renal arteries but does require a skillful scanning technologist and a well-prepared abdomen (as gas free as possible in the small bowel). The renal arteries can be imaged in a high percentage of well-prepared patients, and areas of the artery can be interrogated using the Doppler mode of the duplex scanner. Hemodynamically significant stenoses create distal turbulent flow, which causes the sound wave to be dephased into multiple frequencies in the echo wave (that sound returning to the transducer); this phenomenon is seen as spectral broadening on the waveform analysis. Hemodynamically significant stenoses also cause "jet streaming" of blood right at the stenosis, and this creates a high-frequency shift in the returning sound signal, which is seen as a high spike on the spectral waveform analysis (Fig. 3).

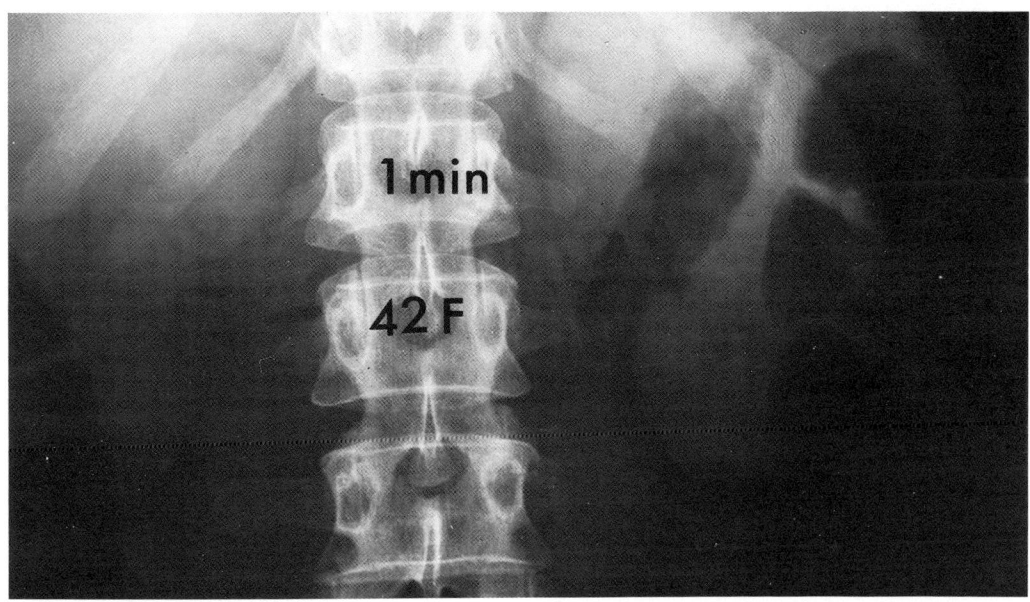

Figure 1A.   Intravenous urography picture of RVH. The one-minute film from rapid-sequence IVU in a 42-year-old woman shows a discrepant degree of nephrographic blush, with definite decrease on the right side.

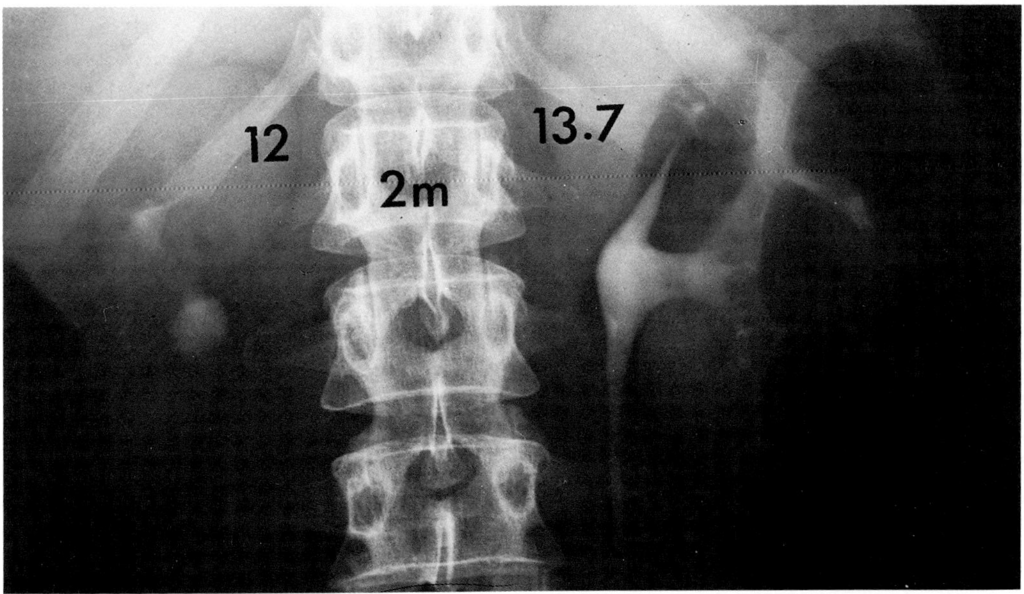

Figure 1B.   Two-minute film from the same sequence demonstrates a significant amount of contrast in the left collecting system and proximal ureter with only early appearance of contrast in the right intrarenal collecting system. Discrepant renal size is also appreciated, with a 12-cm right kidney and a 13.7-cm left kidney.

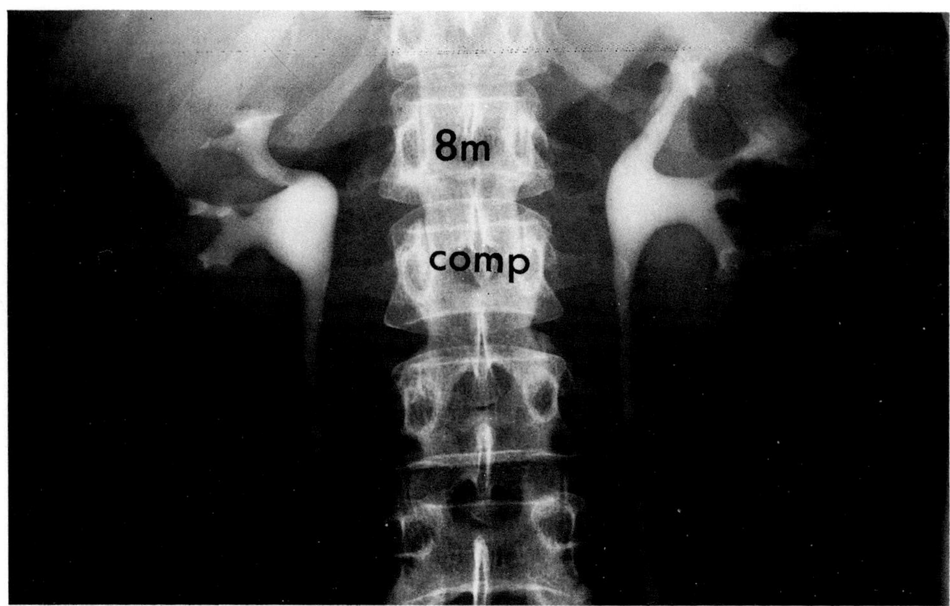

Figure 1C.   Eight-minute film demonstrates little discrepancy in nephrographic blush or in the amount of contrast material in the intrarenal collecting systems. This image emphasizes the fact that IVUs performed with only 5- and 8-minute films frequently miss subtle discrepancies in appearance time of contrast material in the collecting system.

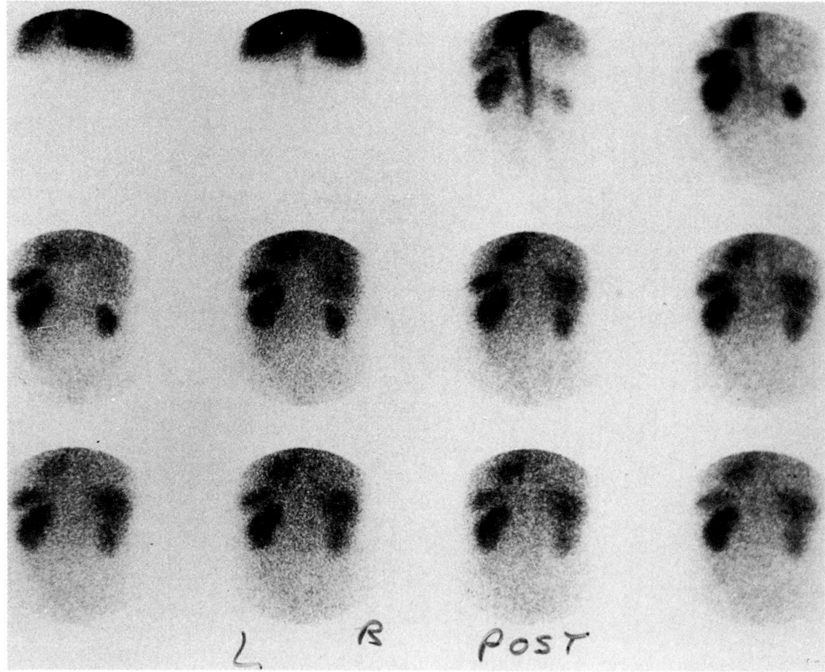

Figure 2.   Early images from technetium-99m DTPA renogram scanned posteriorly. Upper four scans demonstrate appearance of activity in the left kidney nearly simultaneously with its appearance in the aorta. Note significant decrease in activity in the right kidney, as well as significantly decreased size of that kidney. Nephrogram intensity in the left kidney increases and is always greater than activity level in the right kidney. This scan demonstrates the classic findings of renal artery stenosis on the right side. A 90% right renal artery stenosis was confirmed angiographically.

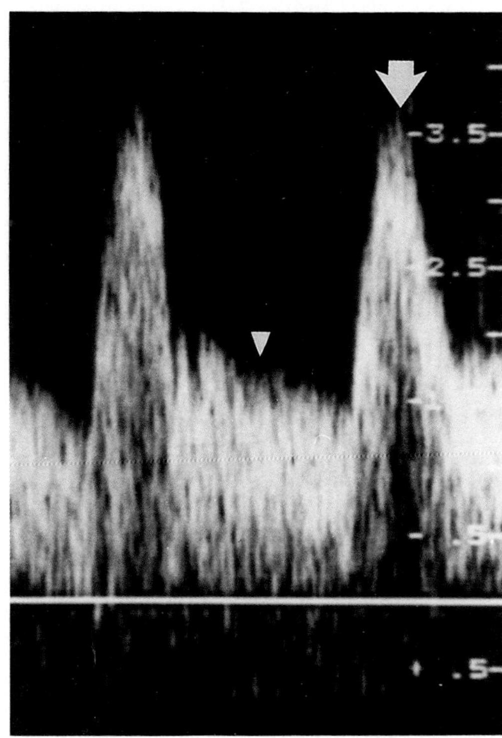

Figure 3A.   Duplex ultrasound evaluation of a 43-year-old woman with hypertension. Normal examination of the left renal artery. Note frequency shift to only 3.5 kHz (arrow) with relatively homogeneous diastolic flow pattern (arrowhead).

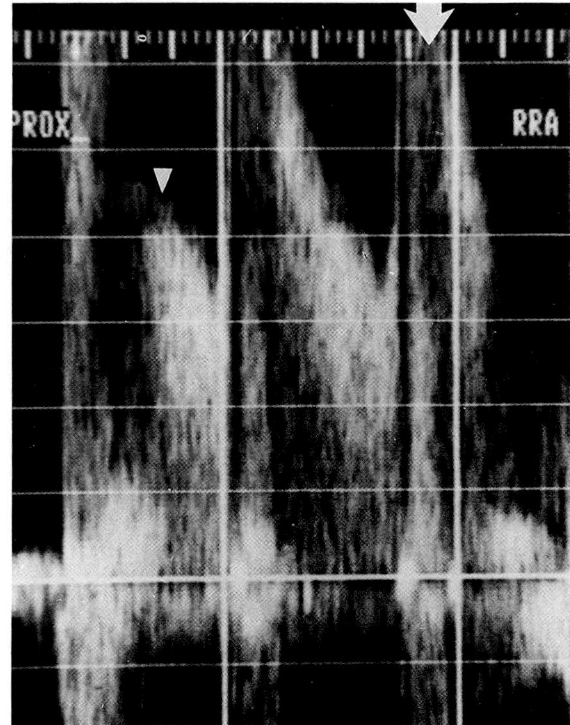

Figure 3B.   Scan of an abnormal right renal artery demonstrates high peak systolic velocities with frequency shifts above 6 kHz (arrow) indicating high-velocity blood flow secondary to jet-stream phenomenon. Also seen is nonhomogeneous chaotic diastolic pattern (arrowhead) consistent with significant degree of turbulent blood flow.

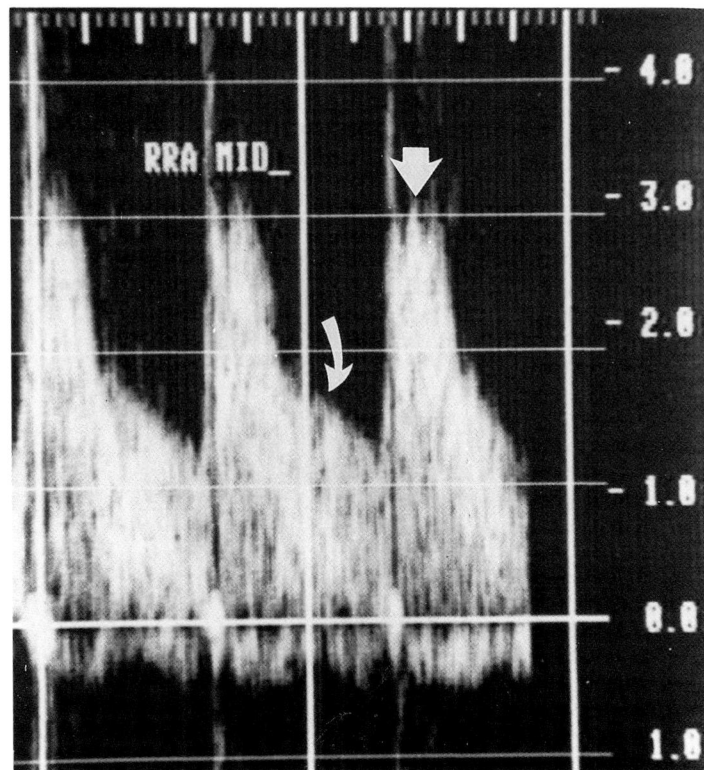

Figure 3C. Examination of the right renal artery after percutaneous transluminal angioplasty demonstrates frequency shifts returning to 3-kHz range (arrow) and return of a more homogeneous pattern in diastole (curved arrow) consistent with more laminar-type flow. Duplex spectral pattern now closely approximates normal tracing from the left renal artery.

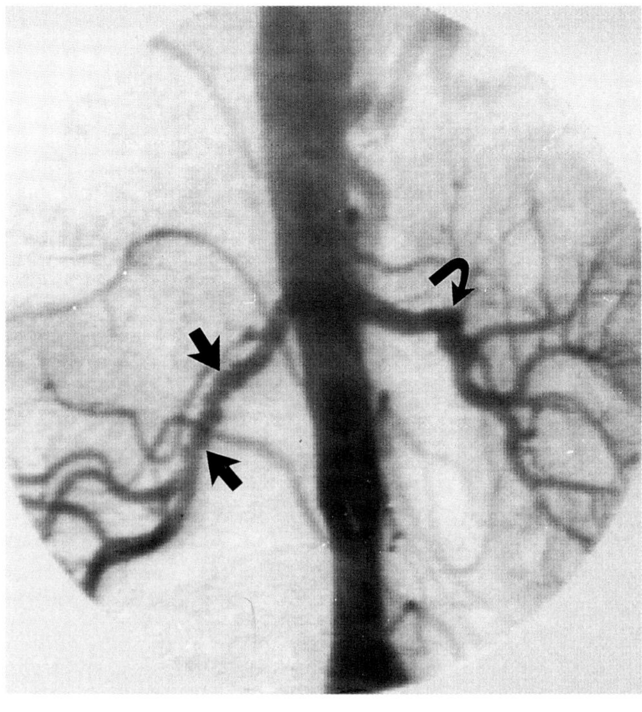

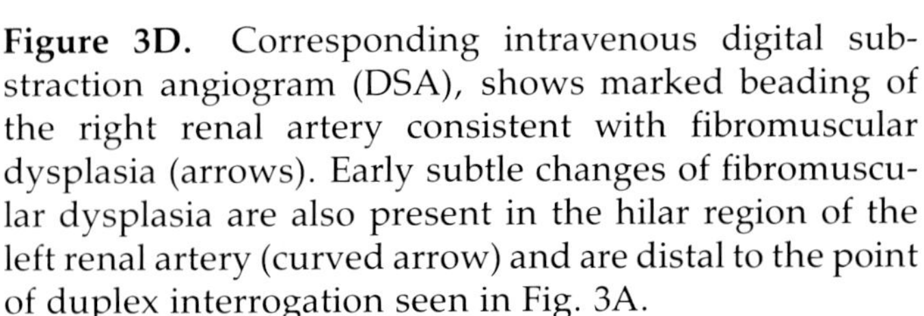

Figure 3D. Corresponding intravenous digital subtraction angiogram (DSA), shows marked beading of the right renal artery consistent with fibromuscular dysplasia (arrows). Early subtle changes of fibromuscular dysplasia are also present in the hilar region of the left renal artery (curved arrow) and are distal to the point of duplex interrogation seen in Fig. 3A.

Invasive Imaging Evaluation

The standard examination for evaluation of RVH, against which all other modalities must be judged, is aortorenal arteriography with selective renal arteriography if indicated. At our institution, RVH arteriography is performed with a single-plane anteroposterior cut-film run of the aortorenal area using a high-volume flush abdominal aortic injection. Filming is carried out for 12 seconds to ensure an adequate nephrogram phase. The 14- × 14-inch field of view is large enough to include both renal outlines, both renal arteries, and the aorta in a single injection. This study can usually be performed with 40 to 50 ml of contrast material, depending on the size of the patient and the velocity of flow in the aorta as judged by fluoroscopic test injections.

If unilateral or bilateral renal artery stenoses are demonstrated, these lesions are not crossed selectively unless angioplasty during the initial session has been arranged. If renal artery stenoses are suspected from the flush aortogram but are not well seen on the study, we add oblique DSA (digital subtraction angiography) of the involved side. In the majority of patients, because of the slightly posterolateral course of the renal artery from the aorta, the right renal artery is best studied by a right anterior oblique DSA, while the left renal artery is best studied with a left anterior oblique DSA. These oblique subtraction angiograms are obtained using the pigtail catheter in the aorta. Atherosclerotic involvement of the renal arteries is generally in the proximal portion, and, as mentioned above, when such lesions are encountered, selective renal artery injections are not performed unless the patient has been scheduled for a concomitant renal artery angioplasty or unless pressure gradient data have been requested.

If, however, the patient demonstrates the more peripherally located lesions of fibromuscular dysplasia or stenoses of first- and second-order renal artery branches, selective injection of the involved renal artery is performed with magnification cut-film angiography centered over the involved kidney. These magnification views can also be performed on DSA. In this way, less contrast material can be injected for the study, which may be particularly important in patients with early renal failure as a result of their renal artery stenosis. However, those centers utilizing small field-of-view DSA equipment should be aware that although they can perform each individual angiogram with smaller volumes of contrast, they will have to administer multiple injections to include the aorta, renal artery origins, and renal parenchyma itself. In our experience, the performance of a three-view DSA study of the renal arteries and kidneys utilizes more contrast material than a single anteroposterior cut-film run on 14- × 14-inch film. Figure 4 demonstrates a typical intraarterial DSA study of bilateral renal artery stenoses caused by atherosclerosis. Figure 5 presents a comparison of DSA and cut-film aortorenal angiograms in a patient who has had successful angioplasty for right renal artery fibromuscular dysplasia.

Although shortly after the introduction of DSA, it was predicted that intravenous study intravenous digital subtraction angiography (IVDSA) would become the gold standard screening test for renal artery stenosis, this prediction has not come true. In our experience, IVDSA does not depict the renal arteries as effectively as direct intra-arterial studies on either cut-film or DSA, and it requires far more contrast material. In our experience, patients whose IVDSA studies suggested renal artery stenosis ultimately required an intra-arterial study prior to any contemplated angioplasty or surgical correction of the renal artery stenosis.

The IVDSA concept was popular initially because it enabled concomitant renal vein renin sampling utilizing the same femoral vein puncture site. With the recent trend toward performing renal artery angioplasty for renal function preservation, our clinicians have relied less on the renal vein renin results. We currently evaluate the patient with suspected renal artery stenosis using a cut-film angiogram initially, and renal vein renin sampling is considered only if moderate stenotic disease is present bilaterally. Renal vein renin measurements are being obtained in only 10% to 15% of all patients with renal artery stenosis. Our approach represents a trend away from the classic evaluation of RVH, in which renal vein renin samples were always obtained initially followed by aortorenal arteriography.

The current lack of consensus about how, when, and if to obtain renal vein renin data is nicely addressed in the recent literature,[1] which should be consulted by those interested in the debate. We have relied more heavily on the appearance of the renal artery stenosis and its pressure gradient than on renal vein renin measurements in our recent practice. Unilateral moderate to high-grade renal artery stenoses are being corrected with angioplasty without renal vein renin measurements. Unsuccessful unilateral angioplasties or lesions unsuitable for angioplasty are corrected surgically, also without renin determinations.

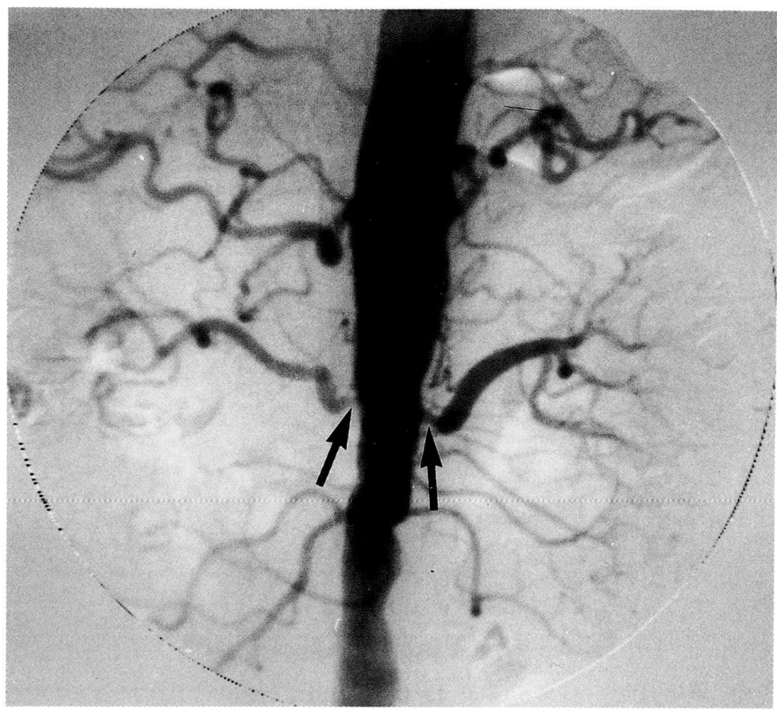

Figure 4A. Typical intra-arterial DSA study for atherosclerotic renal artery stenosis. Nonmagnification anteroposterior aortorenal angiogram demonstrates bilateral proximal renal artery stenoses secondary to atherosclerosis (arrows). Note that even with 11-inch field of view, much of the renal parenchyma is excluded from image.

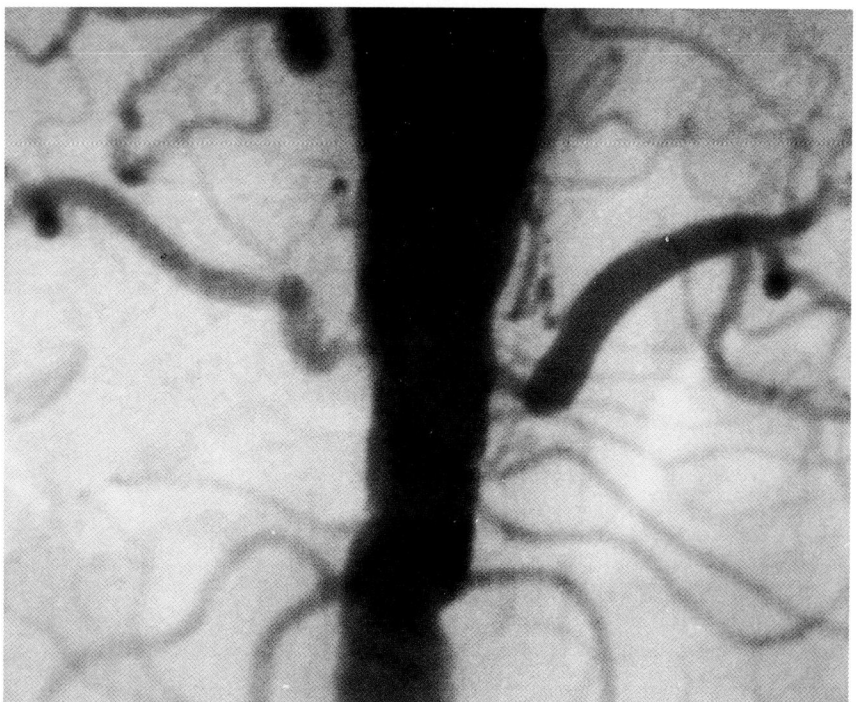

Figure 4B. Magnification cone-down view of anteroposterior aortorenal angiogram shows bilateral renal artery stenoses clearly. Magnification technique further reduces available field of view. First- and second-order renal artery branches are excluded from the field of study in the magnification mode.

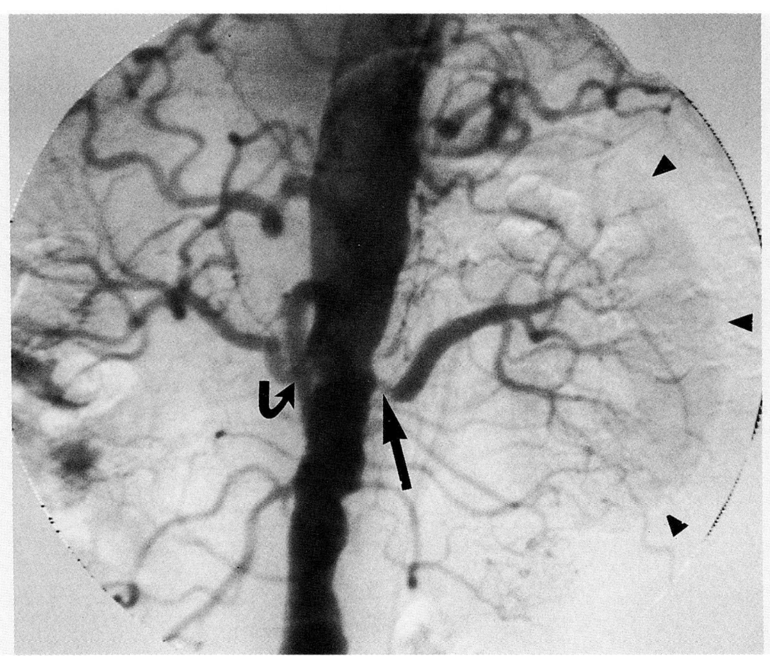

Figure 4C.   Left anterior oblique aortorenal injection performed in nonmagnification mode to profile proximal left renal artery stenosis more extensively (arrow). Although this oblique view shows the left renal artery origin to better advantage, it causes significant foreshortening of the right renal artery origin and superimposes the superior mesenteric artery over the right renal artery origin (curved arrow). In the oblique projection, nephrogram of the left kidney is totally included (arrowheads). Moderate diffuse infrarenal atherosclerosis is also appreciated in the distal abdominal aorta. The patient was referred for study for a blood pressure of 220/120 mm Hg poorly controlled with antihypertensives.

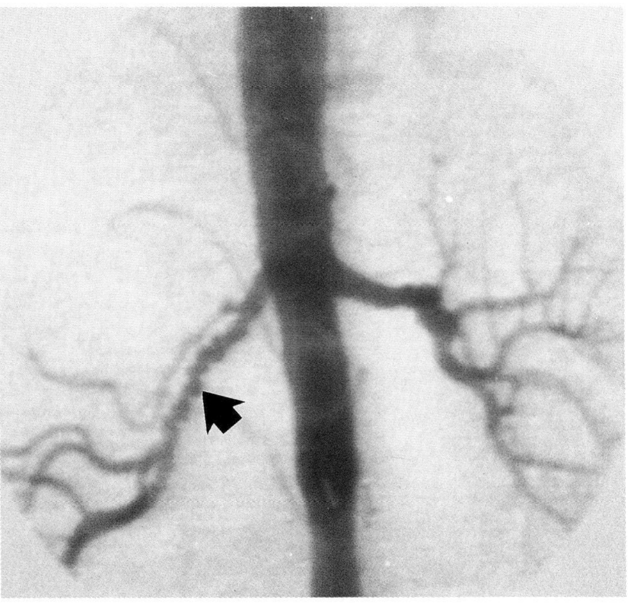

Figure 5A.   Intravenous DSA study in an ideally prepared (gasless abdomen) 42-year-old woman with excellent cardiac output and hypertension. The study reveals extensive fibromuscular dysplasia in the right renal artery (arrow). Although not all of the renal parenchyma is included because of limited field of view, study is diagnostic. (Same patient as in Figure 3).

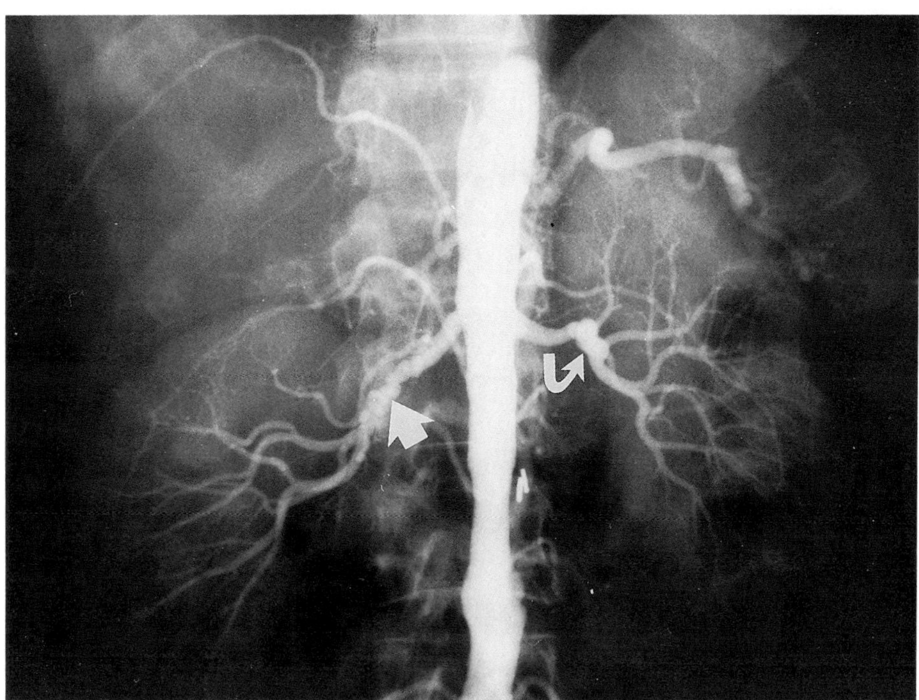

Figure 5B. Cut-film aortorenal angiogram performed the same day shows improved visualization of the right renal arterial fibromuscular dysplasia (arrow). Subtle early changes of fibromuscular dysplasia in the left renal hilar region (curved arrow) are shown to better advantage than on IVDSA study. Excellent nephrogram phase represents significant advantage over DSA study. The IVDSA study was performed using 40 ml of contrast material; cut-film aortorenal angiogram also performed with 40 ml of contrast material.

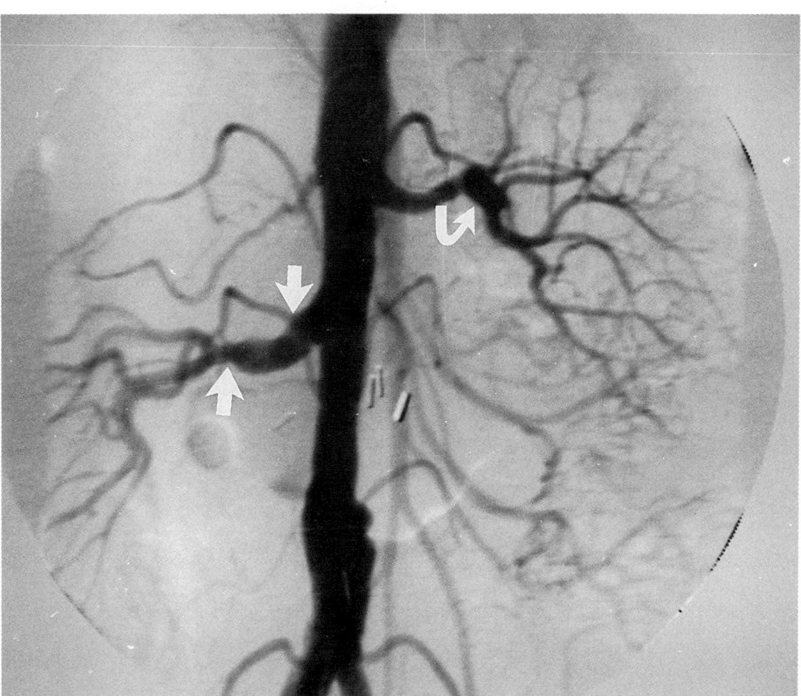

Figure 5C. Intra-arterial DSA study (right anterior oblique projection) performed 18 months after a successful percutaneous transluminal angioplasty of right-sided fibromuscular dysplasia. Angioplasty site is readily apparent throughout the proximal and mid right renal artery (arrows). Fibromuscular dysplasia in the left renal artery has shown little progression (curved arrow).

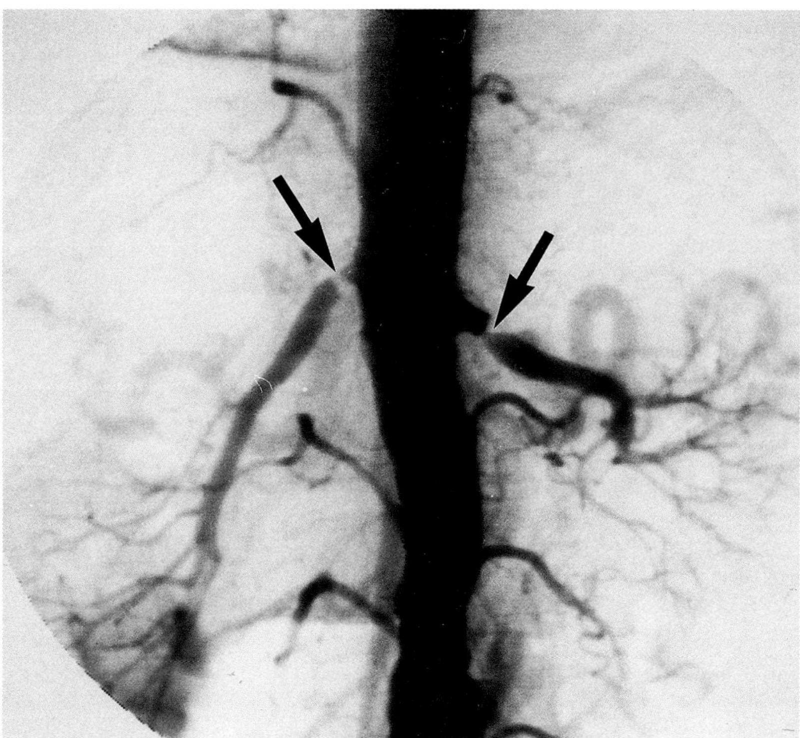

Figure 6A.   Intra-arterial DSA aortorenal angiogram showing bilateral atherosclerotic renal artery stenoses; both ideal lesions for percutaneous transluminal angioplasty (arrows). This left anterior oblique view profiles the 95% of left renal artery stenosis while foreshortening right-sided stenosis.

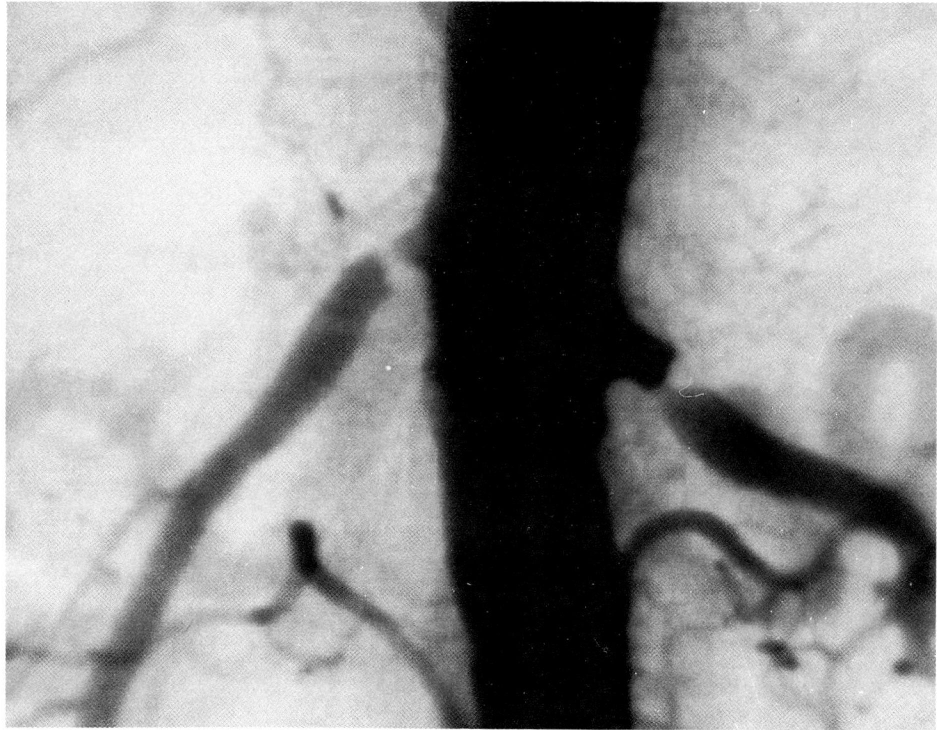

Figure 6B.   Cone-down magnification view of bilateral renal artery stenoses. Left anterior oblique projection (post-processing magnification of image in A).

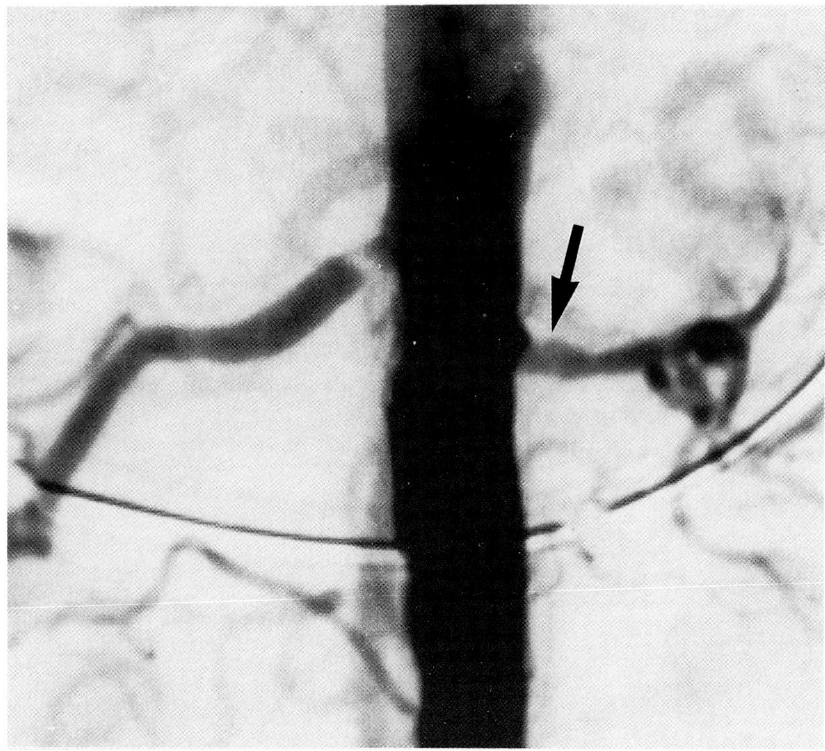

Figure 6C. The patient presented with a blood pressure of 240/140 mg Hg without medication, and, because of the bilaterality of disease, renal vein renin measurements were obtained. Convincing lateralization of renin values prompted left renal angioplasty to be performed first. Magnification left anterior oblique post-angioplasty angiogram shows excellent reduction in degree of stenosis with, at most, a residual 20% lesion (arrow). Bulbous appearance of the proximal left renal artery is evidence of successful dilatation.

Acknowledgments: The author wishes to thank Christine Lear for secretarial assistance in the preparation of this manuscript.

References

1. Pollack HM (ed): Clinical Urography: an Atlas and Textbook of Urological Imaging. Philadelphia: WB Saunders, 1990, p 2119.
2. Emmett JL, Myers GH, Witten DM, Utz DC: Emmett's Clinical Urography: Clinical Urography: An Atlas and Textbook of Roentgenologic Diagnosis, ed 4. Philadelphia: WB Saunders, 1977, p 1979.
3. Wilber JA, Barrow JG: Hypertension: a community problem. Am J Med 1972; 52:653.
4. Hodges CV: Hypertension of renal vascular origin. J Michigan Med Soc 1962; 61:1236.
5. Smith HW: Unilateral nephrectomy in hypertensive disease. J Urol 1956; 76:685.
6. Maxwell MH: Demographic analysis of the cooperative study of renovascular hypertension. JAMA 1972; 220:1195.
7. Poutasse EF, Dustan H, Page IH: Surgical treatment of hypertension due to renal vascular lesions. Med Clin North Am 1961; 45:479.
8. Burbank MK, Hunt JC, Tauze WN, et al: Radioisotopic renography: diagnosis of renal artery disease in hypertensive patients. Circulation 1963; 27:328.
9. Juncos LI, Strong CG, Hunt JC: Prediction of results of surgery for renal and renovascular hypertension. Arch Intern Med 1974; 134:655.
10. Strong CG, Hunt JC, Sheps SG, et al: Renal venous renin activity: enhancement of sensitivity of lateralization by sodium depletion. Am J Cardiol 1971; 27:602.
11. Bookstein JJ, Abrams HL, Buenger RE, et al: Radiologic aspects of renovascular hypertension 2: the role of urography in unilateral renovascular disease. JAMA 1972; 220:1225.

Chapter 8

Cystic Diseases of the Kidneys

John F. Cardella, M.D.

Renal cystic disease (RCD) includes many congenital, developmental, inflammatory, infectious, neoplastic, obstructive, and iatrogenic processes. An excellent discussion and classification of these entities is included in the recently released textbook, *Clinical Urography*.[1] Regardless of the particular etiology, the imaging evaluation always has at its center the differentiation of benign from malignant processes, which will be the emphasis of this discussion. The discussion of RCD evaluation will be general in approach, rather than an encyclopedic cataloging of the specific finer diagnostic features of specific cystic entities.

No single imaging modality has done more to advance the diagnosis of RCD than ultrasonography. Computed tomography (CT) has added considerably to the evaluation but has the disadvantage, in children, of involving ionizing radiation. Fine-needle cyst puncture for fluid sampling and renal cystography is an excellent adjunct for definitive tissue cytology diagnosis.

Detection

Patients with RCD generally come to clinical attention because of pain in the back or costovertebral angle and, occasionally, hematuria or because of a palpable mass. Others are discovered incidentally during imaging studies, including intravenous urography (IVU), CT, or ultra-

sonography. Indeed, with the widespread use of ultrasound and CT scanning, the number of incidentally discovered, asymptomatic renal cysts has increased dramatically in recent years.

Once cysts have been found, the clinician and radiologist are confronted with a problem of choosing further diagnostic procedures. The following sections discuss the imaging options.

Imaging Evaluation

Intravenous Urography

Intravenous urography has historically been the imaging examination most commonly responsible for the detection of RCD, whether performed specifically for this purpose or for some other reason. The cystic mass produces a number of findings: (1) a spherical (round) area of relative decrease or absence of nephrographic blush, either within the renal parenchyma or at the margin of the kidney, causing the well-known "drop-out" of the renal margin; (2) splaying or distortion of the contrast-filled intrarenal collecting system; (3) enlargement of the kidney outline; and (4) distortion of renal or ureteral location (in the case of very large cysts). In this study, RCD is best detected if the lesion is near the renal margin, abuts and distorts the intrarenal collecting system, or is very large (Fig.

From *Imaging of Urologic Disorders* edited by Alexander S. Cass, MBBS, © 1992, Futura Publishing Inc., Mount Kisco, NY.

1). The IVU is not a good study for detecting small intraparenchymal cystic lesions. This study also lacks the ability to differentiate among soft-tissue densities of whatever nature and therefore cannot distinguish serous fluid (simple cyst) from blood or pus (hematoma or abscess) or from solid soft tissue (necrotic nonfunctioning tumor) (Figs. 1 and 2). Because of these limitations, the IVU generally only detects a mass of some type, and the differentiation of solid from cystic must be done by other means.

Ultrasonography

Ultrasonography has proved to be the least invasive, least expensive modality for the reliable differentiation of solid masses from cystic ones and has rapidly become the next or first step in the evaluation of RCD. Figure 3 demonstrates the classic ultrasonographic findings in simple cysts, which include enhanced through-transmission of sound, crisp signal interfaces at both the front and back walls of the cyst without tissue nubbins along the walls, and absence of internal echoes and fluid-fluid interfaces within the cyst.[2]. Cystic masses demonstrating all the classic criteria of a cyst can, with a high degree of certainty (98% to 100%), be diagnosed accurately as simple cysts.[2-4] This degree of accuracy requires state-of-the-art equipment and a high level of expertise of the ultrasonographer.

Solid renal masses, on the other hand, demonstrate the following ultrasonographic characteristics: (1) absence of enhanced through-transmission of sound; in fact, they may have decreased through-transmission depending on the acoustic impedance of the tissue; (2) absence of crisp walls; (3) internal echoes, either hyperechoic or hypoechoic relative to normal renal parenchyma; and (4) possible fluid-fluid or fluid-solid interfaces within the mass. Several of these findings are apparent in Figure 4.[3,4]

In the proper clinical setting, when ultrasonography confirms the lesion as a benign simple cyst, frequently, that is sufficient to stop the evaluation. In the cases in which ultrasonography indicates other than a simple cyst, further study is warranted, especially in the clinical setting of hematuria, weight loss, fever

and chills, decreasing renal function, or abnormal urinalysis. The ultrasound findings of complex fluid (moderate-level echoes within the central or dependent portions of a predominantly cystic mass, floating debris, fluid-fluid interfaces) within a cystic mass point away from simple cyst and toward acute or chronic hematoma, abscess, hemorrhagic cyst, or necrotic liquified tumor. Ultrasound findings of solid mass (hyperechogenicity or hypoechogenicity in a mass contiguous with renal parenchyma without a wall, decreased through-transmission of sound, and mixed solid and cystic [solid predominant] components) suggest hematoma, renal cell carcinoma, tuberculoma, or angiomyolipoma. Additional evaluation of these latter categories of ultrasonographic findings includes CT scanning of the kidneys, angiography, and magnetic resonance imaging (MRI). Cyst puncture and cystography also play a role in the evaluation of difficult RCD problems.

Computed Tomography

On CT, simple renal cysts have sharply marginated edges, with an imperceptibly thin wall, CT numbers in the range of -10 to $+10$ HU (Houndsfield units), and no enhancement after intravenous contrast administration. Strict adherence to these criteria results in accuracy approaching 100% (Fig. 5).[5-7] Generally, at our institution, The Milton S. Hershey Medical Center, patients with masses that meet the classic criteria of a simple cyst by both ultrasound and CT scanning are not worked up further.

Pus, blood, and other complex fluids within cystic masses give higher HU numbers than simple serous fluid or urine. Typically, pus will produce values in the $+20$ to $+40$ HU range, and the internal quality of the fluid takes on a more irregular appearance, with more inhomogeneity and alternating high- and low-density areas. Well walled-off abscesses of the kidney develop a thick, ragged wall, which enhances variably with intravenous contrast administration (Fig.5).

Hemorrhage into the kidney, whether it be into a cyst or a tumor or the result of trauma or bleeding diathesis, presents a similar CT scan appearance, depending on the age at which the blood collection is scanned. Acute bleeding appears as a hyperdense area (relative to renal parenchyma) on unenhanced scans, which becomes hypodense (relative to renal parenchyma) on enhanced scans (Fig.5). This is known as the "flip-flop" phenomenon. Typical densities for acute hemorrhage are in the +40 to +70 HU range. These types of hemorrhages rarely have thick surrounding walls or curvilinear calcifications. *Chronic* hemorrhage into the kidney (or, more correctly, chronic hematoma) demonstrates curvilinear wall calcifications and inhomogeneous texture of the fluid as the blood is liquefied. The wall calcifications are very easily seen on CT scans (Fig. 5). As the hematoma becomes organized, the "flip-flop" phenomenon disappears and is replaced by an area of low attenuation within the kidney.

Magnetic resonance imaging has not been shown to be of benefit in simple renal cysts but is useful in differentiating hemorrhagic from simple cysts. The MRI appearance of hemorrhagic cysts varies with the age of the blood; fresh blood produces high-intensity signals at all pulse sequences. The MRI scan cannot, unfortunately, differentiate hemorrhagic cyst from hemorrhagic neoplasm.[8–10]

Angiography

Angiography plays little role in the general modern-day evaluation of RCD and is only used to clarify complex cases. The angiographic findings of RCD are marked draping of the normal renal vessels around the mass, an avascular area corresponding to the cystic mass, and no wall enhancement surrounding the mass. These findings are moderately specific (see Fig. 1).

There are two noteworthy angiographic findings in RCD. The first is rim enhancement, which is an angiographic blush seen around walled-off abscesses or chronic hematomas. The blush represents hyperemia in the lining wall, and *diffuse* neovascularity may be seen because of the granulation tissue that forms the walls of these two entities. This type of neovascularity must be distinguished from the focal neovascularity, the second significant angiographic find-

ing in RCD, which may indicate a neoplastic nubbin in the wall of what otherwise appears to be a simple cyst. The angiographic findings in solid tumor masses of the kidney, including dense tangles of neovascularity throughout the mass, puddling of contrast material, and complete derangement of the normal arborized pattern of branching of the intrarenal vessels, are readily distinguishable from the findings in RCD (see Fig. 2).

In kidneys with multiple cysts, the angiographic findings are less specific than in those with solitary cystic lesions, as the kidneys generally enlarge, and the draping of vessels is less apparent because intrarenal vessels are pushed in multiple directions at once. Frequently, the only angiographic signs are renal enlargement, mild splaying of vessels, or the impression that there are too few intrarenal branches (because the same number of vessels has been separated throughout the larger multiple cysts in the kidney).

Renal Cyst Puncture

With the high sensitivity and specificity of ultrasonography and CT scanning, the use of cyst puncture has decreased sharply in recent years. At this time, the technique is reserved for problematic cases and for those situations in which cyst puncture is performed for therapy.

The technique is best performed under ultrasound guidance with the patient in a prone position on the procedure table. Using a 22-gauge Chiba needle, the kidney can be punctured safely in everyone with normal coagulation, using local anesthesia only. Cyst fluid is taken for Gram stain and culture and sensitivity in the case of suspected abscess or for cytology study in the case of suspected carcinoma, or for both in cases of confusing clinical presentations. The fluid can be submitted to virtually any biochemical, hematologic, or immunologic test available given the proper clinical setting and provided the specimen is procured and processed in the appropriate manner.

Following removal of as much of the fluid as aspirates freely, contrast material is injected into the cyst under fluoroscopic monitoring to avoid extravasation. If extravasation is encountered, the injection should be stopped immediately; overdistention of the cyst should also be avoided, as this causes discomfort, may cause transient bacteremia, and increases the chance of extravasation into the retroperitoneum. The patient is then positioned in multiple degrees of obliquity, attempting to cover the full 360° of patient rotation to position contrast material along all the interior margins of the cyst.

A variation of cystography is the "double-contrast" cystogram in which a small amount of gas (ideally, carbon dioxide to avoid air embolism to the lungs) is injected after the contrast material. This technique gives exquisite images of the inside lining of the cyst (akin to air-contrast colon examinations) and is the best way to document small mural nodules, which may represent carcinoma developing within the cyst.

The value of cyst puncture in RCD is equivocal, particularly for the evaluation of carcinoma arising in a simple cyst. Positive cytology from a cyst puncture will lead to surgical nephrectomy. Unfortunately, false-negative cytology findings occur and, therefore, open biopsy is required which, when positive, leads to nephrectomy.[11]

Multicystic Disease

Much of the above discussion has dealt with the appearances of solitary cystic and solid renal masses. There is a large component of RCD in which the cysts are multiple. The findings in multicystic disease are qualitatively the same as those in solitary cystic disease but differ quantitatively. A detailed discussion of the differential points of multicystic disease is beyond the scope of this work, and the interested reader is referred to the excellent treatise on the subject in reference.[1]

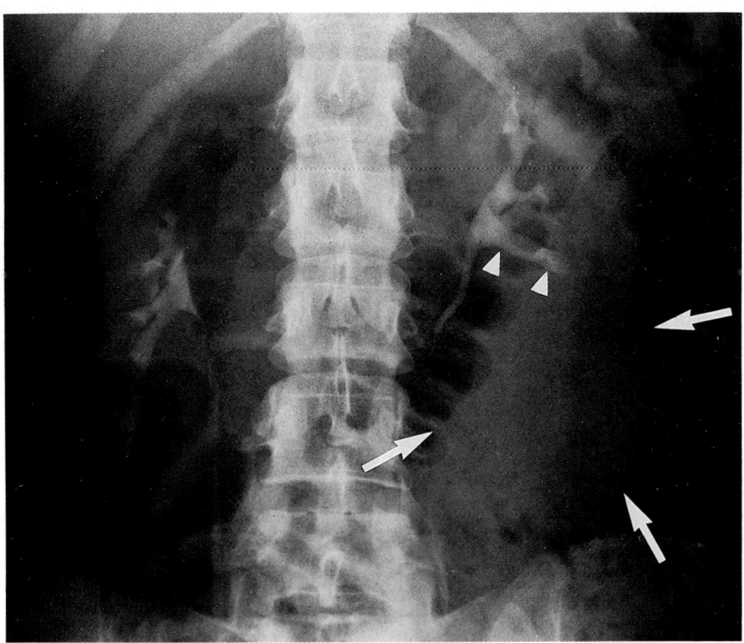

Figure 1A. Detection of cystic disease by IVU. Fifteen-minute film demonstrates medial deviation of the left ureter, absent nephrogram blush in the lower pole of the left kidney, a large second soft-tissue density projecting off the inferior aspect of the left kidney (arrows), and some superior distortion of the lower-pole calices (arrowheads).

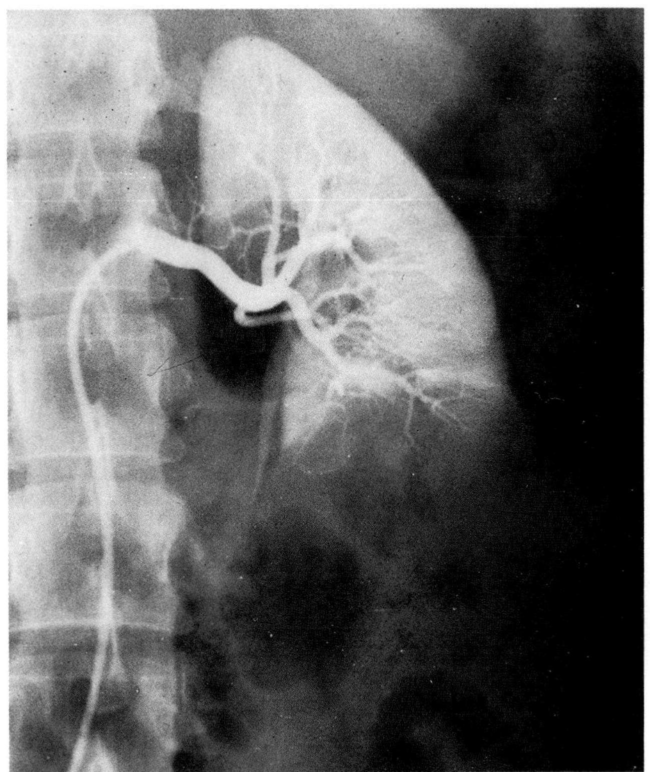

Figure 1B. Arteriography was performed on this patient because the IVU was obtained in the preultrasound era. Midarterial phase of selective renal arteriogram demonstrates absent nephrographic blush in the lower pole of the left kidney with no appreciable vascularity of the large left lower-pole mass. Margins of the large mass are obscured by bowel contents. No neovascularity is identified.

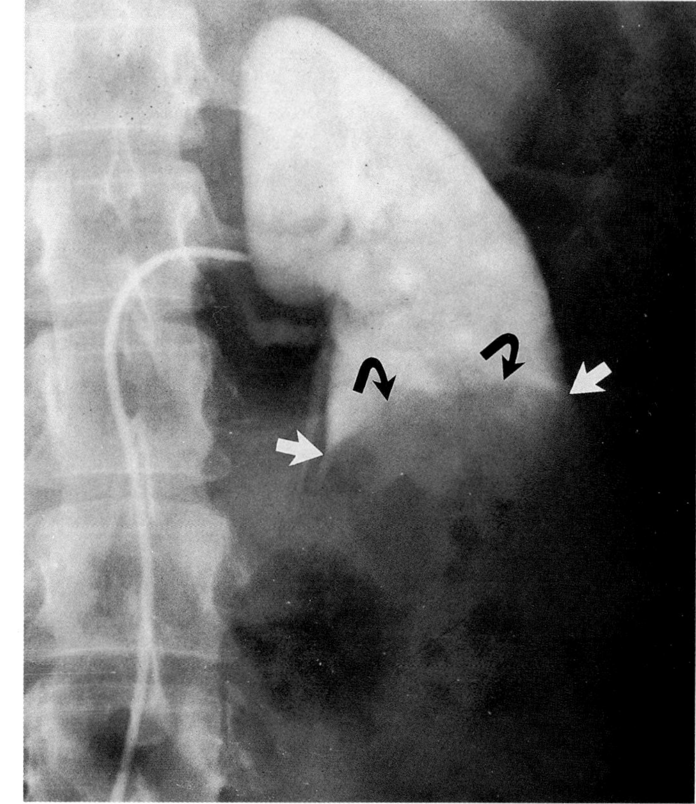

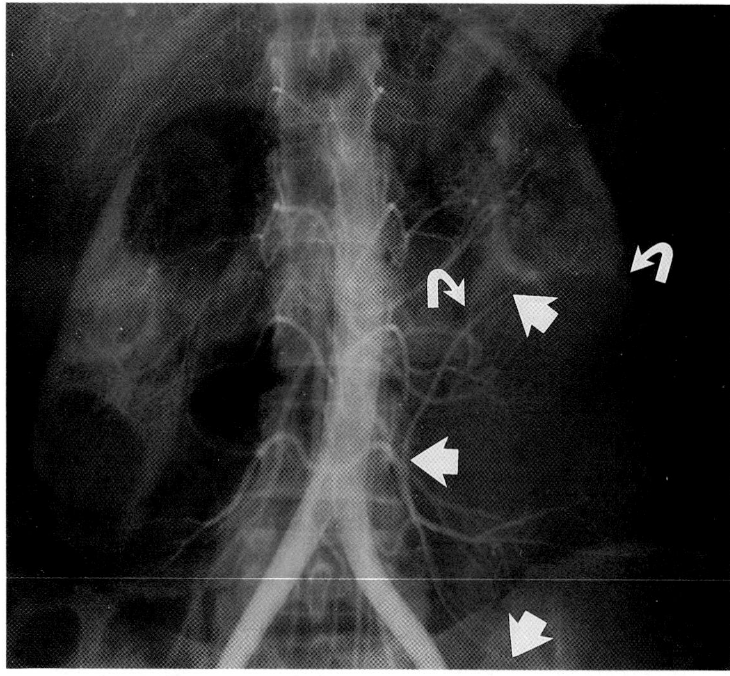

Figures 1C,D. (C, top) Nephrographic blush phase of arteriogram, demonstrating acute angulations of the normal renal parenchyma with cyst margin (arrows). Margin on the cyst is more apparent on this film (curved arrows). (D, bottom) Flush aortic injection performed as part of the arteriogram shows marked draping of the retroperitoneal and lumbar branches (arrows), giving greater appreciation of the true size of the left lower-pole cyst. Acute angles of the junction between the normal renal parenchyma and the cyst are again apparent (curved arrows).

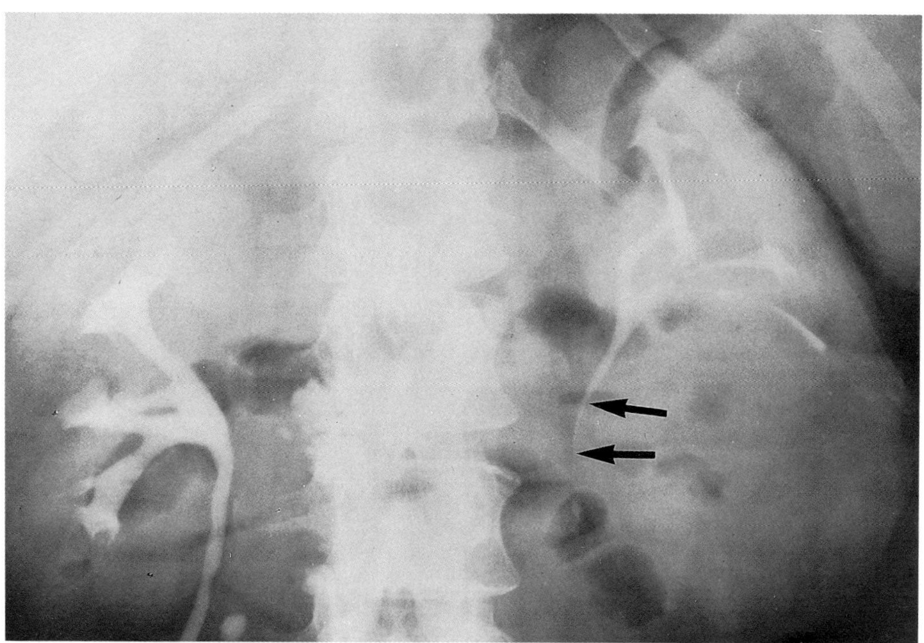

Figure 2A. Drawbacks of IVU in evaluating a renal mass. Eight-minute film showing marked distortion of the lower-pole collecting system of the left kidney with medial deviation of the proximal left ureter (arrows). Appearance is similar to IVU in Figure 1. Note, however, that there is a nephrographic blush in the renal mass.

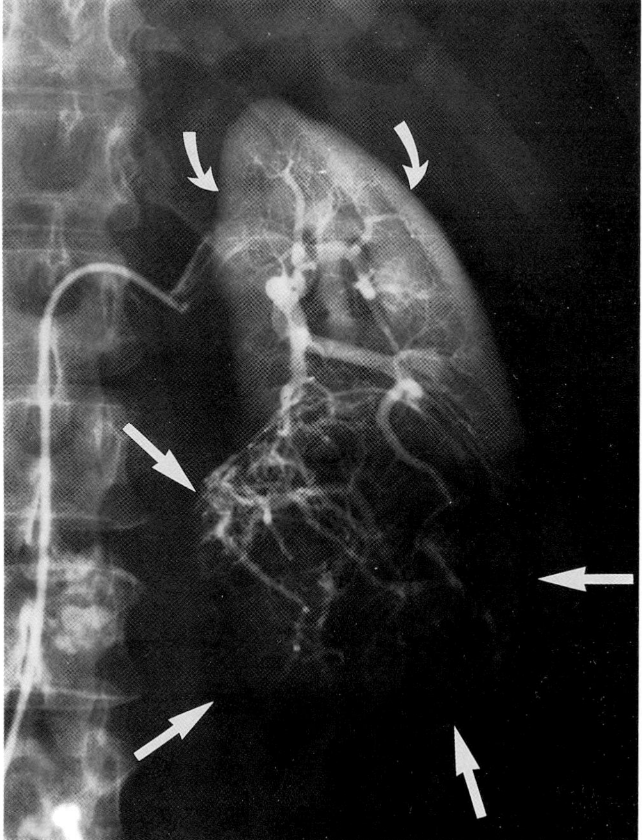

Figure 2B. Late arterial phase of the left selective renal arteriogram demonstrates tumor neovascularity in the mass (arrows) with disruption and destruction of normal arborization of the renal vessels seen in uninvolved upper pole (curved arrows).

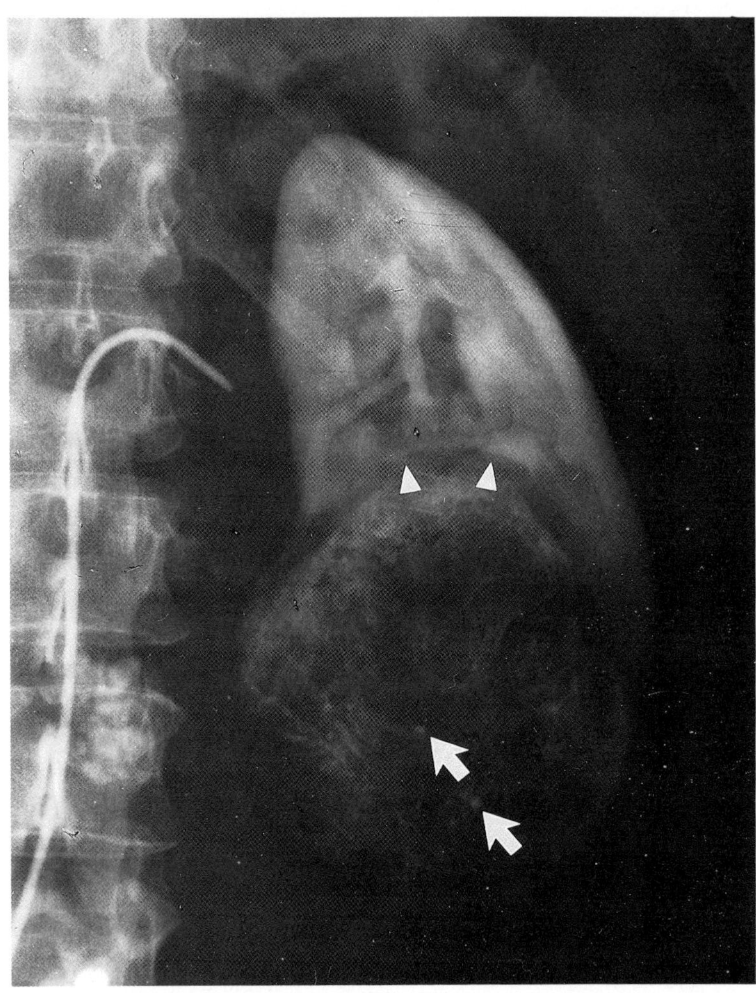

Figure 2C. Nephrographic phase of the left renal arteriogram demonstrates persistent chaotic tumor neovascularity with some puddling of contrast (arrows), as well as distortion of the lower-pole calices (arrowheads). Pathologically proved lower-pole renal cell carcinoma.

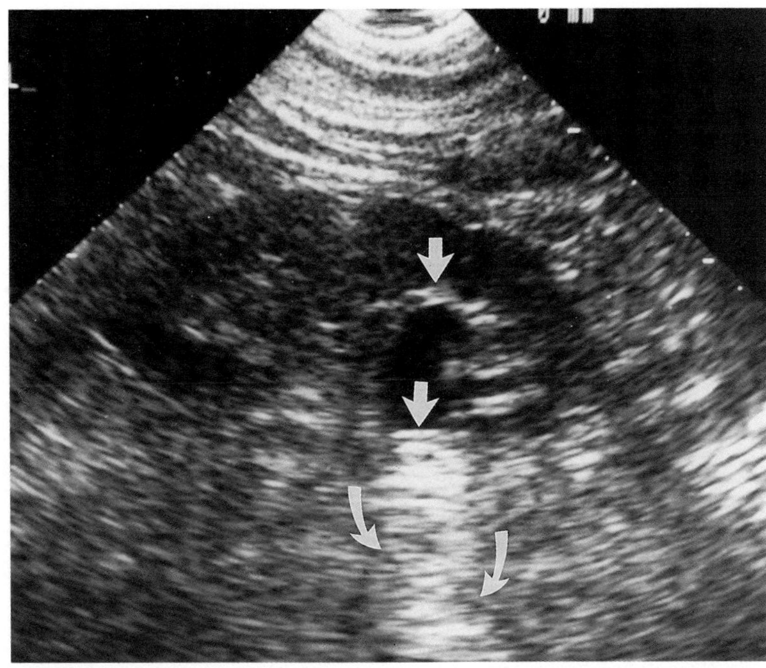

Figure 3A.   Longitudinal ultrasound study of the left kidney demonstrating classic findings of a simple renal cyst, in this case located in parapelvic region of mid-lower pole of the left kidney. Crisp echoes are present at the anterior and posterior wall interfaces of cyst (arrows). Cyst itself is free of internal echoes and fluid-fluid interfaces. Excellent example of enhanced through-transmission of sound (curved arrows).

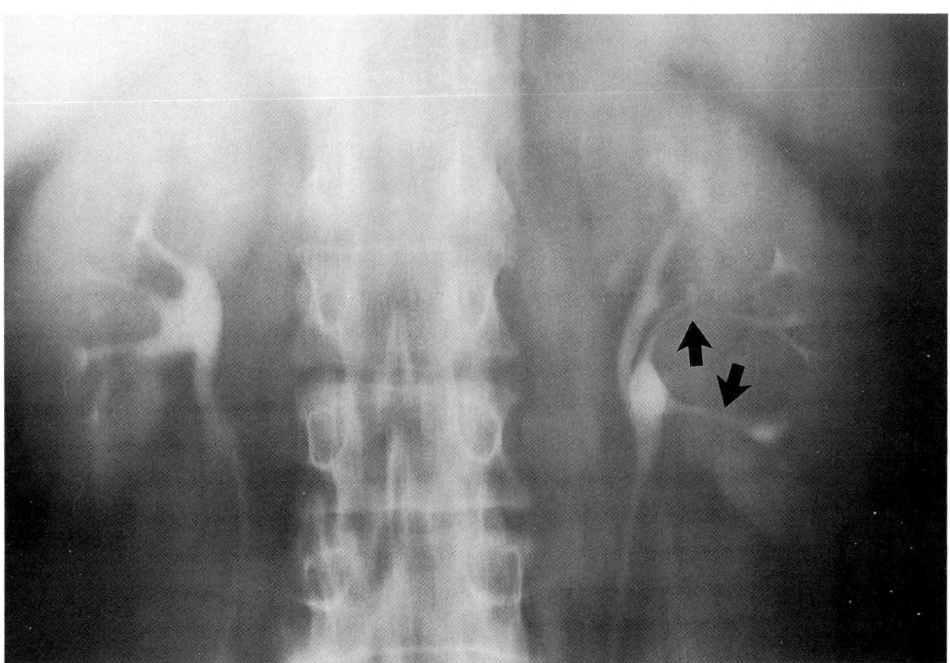

Figure 3B.   Corresponding IVU confirms the presence of an oblong mass causing distortion of middle- and lower-pole caliceal infundibula (arrows). Although generally spherical, it is not unusual for parapelvic cysts to be somewhat oblong.

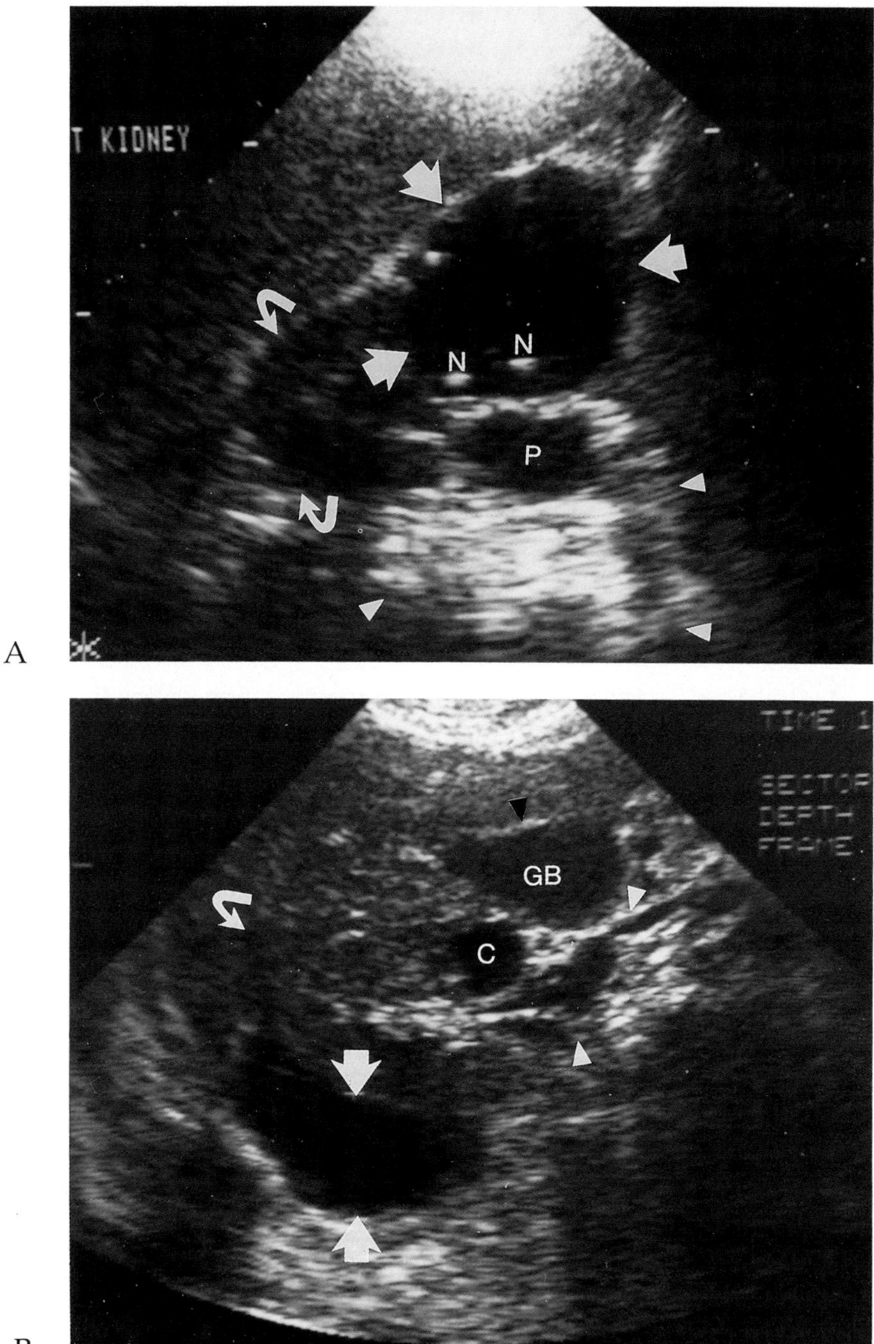

Figures 4A,B.   (A, top) Transverse axial scan of the right kidney demonstrates a large complex cystic mass projecting from the anteromedial aspect (arrows). Cystic mass contains mural high-level echoes consistent with nodules (N). Normal renal tissue is identified by curved arrows. Because the mass is predominately cystic, there is enhanced through-transmission deep to the large mass (arrowheads). Moderate hydronephrosis of the renal pelvis (P) and intrarenal collecting system is identified. Hemorrhagic cyst with mural calcifications. (B, bottom) Transverse axial sonogram of the right kidney showing irregular perirenal cystic mass posterolateral to the right kidney (arrows). Normal renal parenchyma indicated by a curved arrow. Renal hilar structures located anteriorly and to the mid-line (white arrowheads). Ill-defined and shaggy-appearing front and back wall make it unlikely that this is a simple renal cyst, but enhanced through-transmission of sound indicates a significant fluid component. Patient had undergone a renal biopsy 2 days prior to the scan, causing a medium-size perirenal hematoma. C = renal cyst. GB = gallbladder with strong acoustical interface of the anterior wall (black arrowhead).

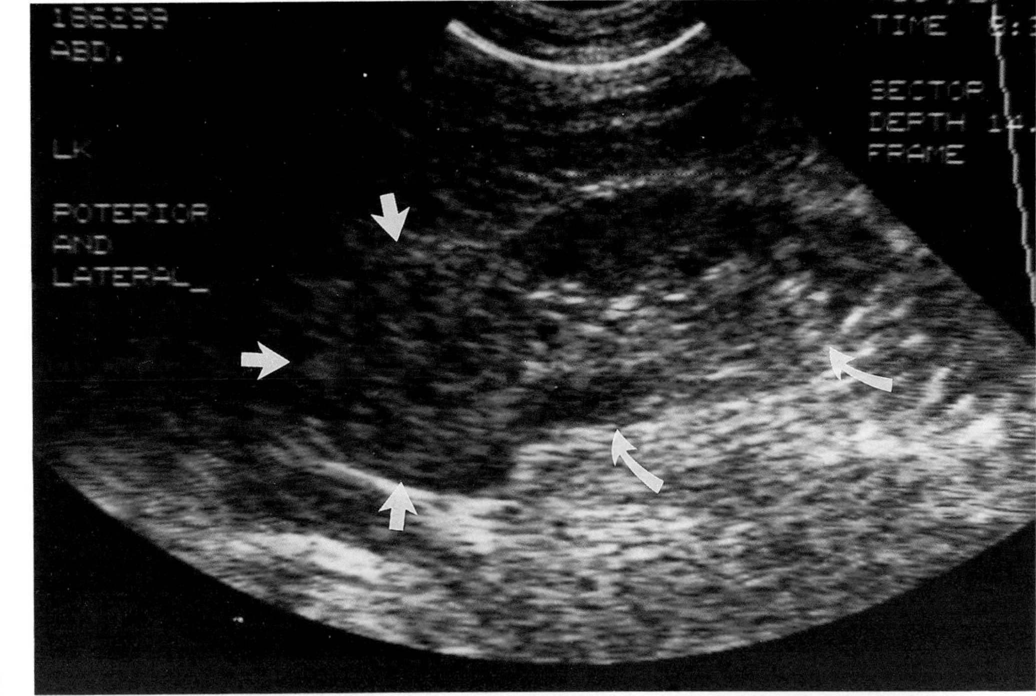

C

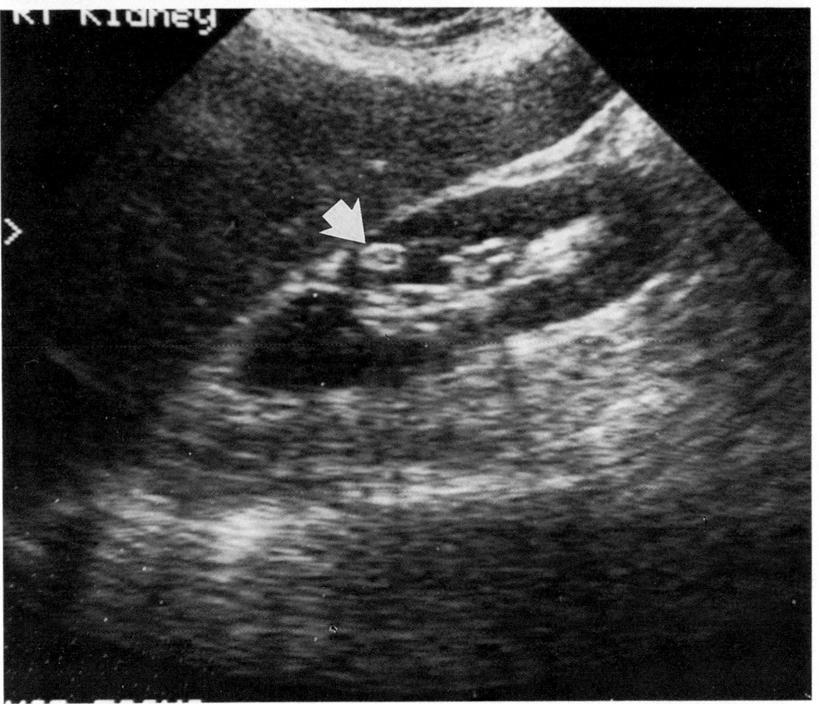

D

Figures 4C,D. (C, top) Longitudinal sonogram of the left kidney demonstrates a highly echogenic mass projecting from the posterior and lateral aspect of the superior pole. Mass (arrows) is nearly isoechoic with normal renal parenchyma (curved arrows). Absent anterior and posterior wall echoes, extensive internal echoing, absent enhanced through-transmission, and slightly inhomogeneous central portion of the mass all indicate a solid renal tumor with slight central necrosis. Pathologically proved superior-pole renal cell carcinoma. (D, bottom) Longitudinal sonogram of the right kidney demonstrates a very echogenic small mass in the anterolateral aspect (arrow). Remainder of the right kidney is within normal limits. High-level echogenicity with "bull's-eye" appearance is characteristic of an angiomyolipoma of the kidney. High-intensity echo is a result of chaotic internal architecture and multiple acoustical interfaces within an angiomyolipomas.

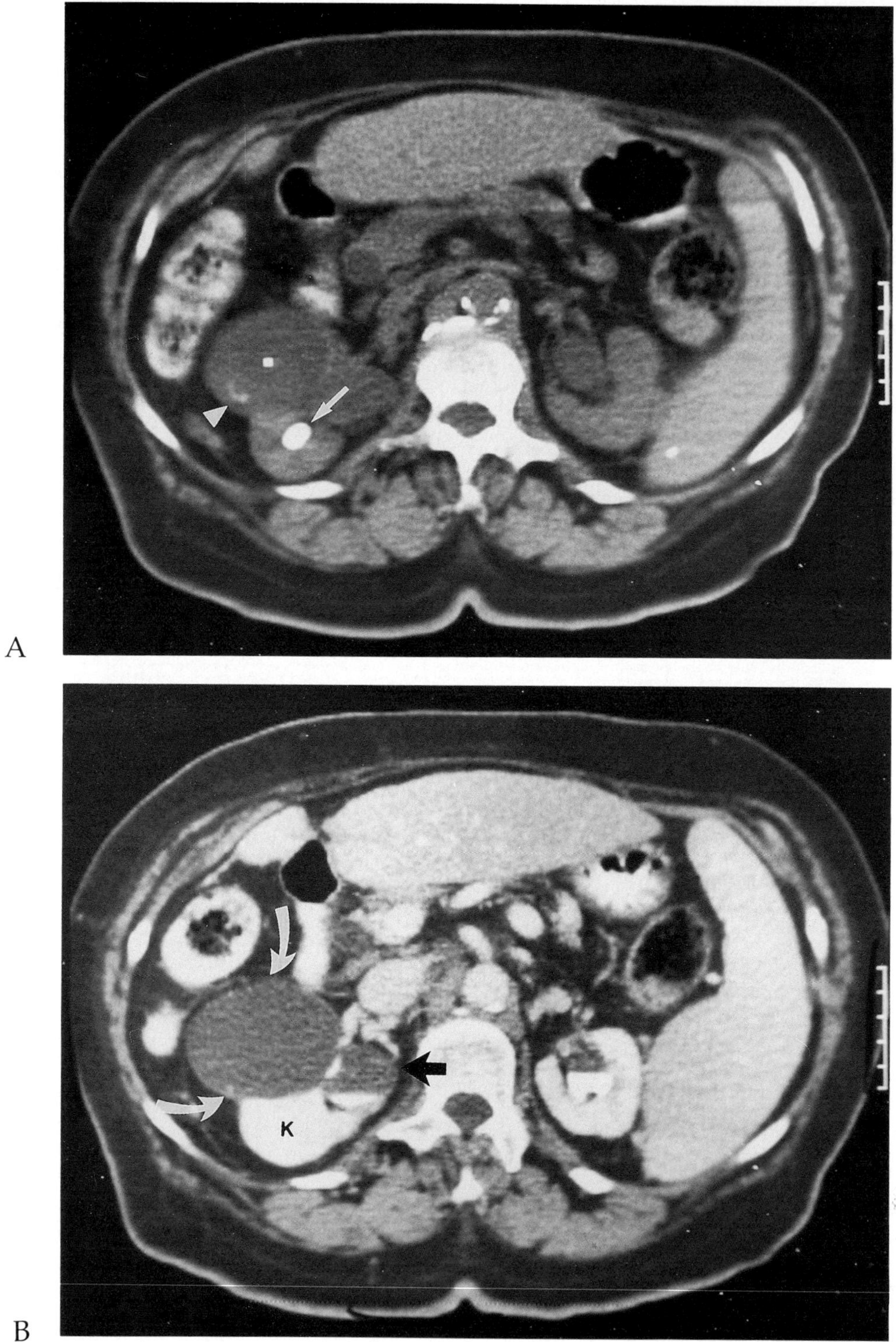

Figures 5A,B.   CT scans showing the same patients as in Figure 4. (A, top) Unenhanced CT scan demonstrates a stone in the right kidney (arrow) as well as some curvilinear calcification in the posterolateral aspect of the cyst (arrowhead). Mean Hounsfield number of cursor within the cyst (square box) is 4. This is consistent with water-density material and supports the diagnosis of chronic liquified and calcified hematoma. (B, bottom) Corresponding enhanced CT scan, confirming contrast accumulation in a moderately dilated renal pelvis (arrow), normally functioning renal parenchyma (K), and an unenhanced cystic mass in the anterolateral aspect of the kidney (curved arrows).

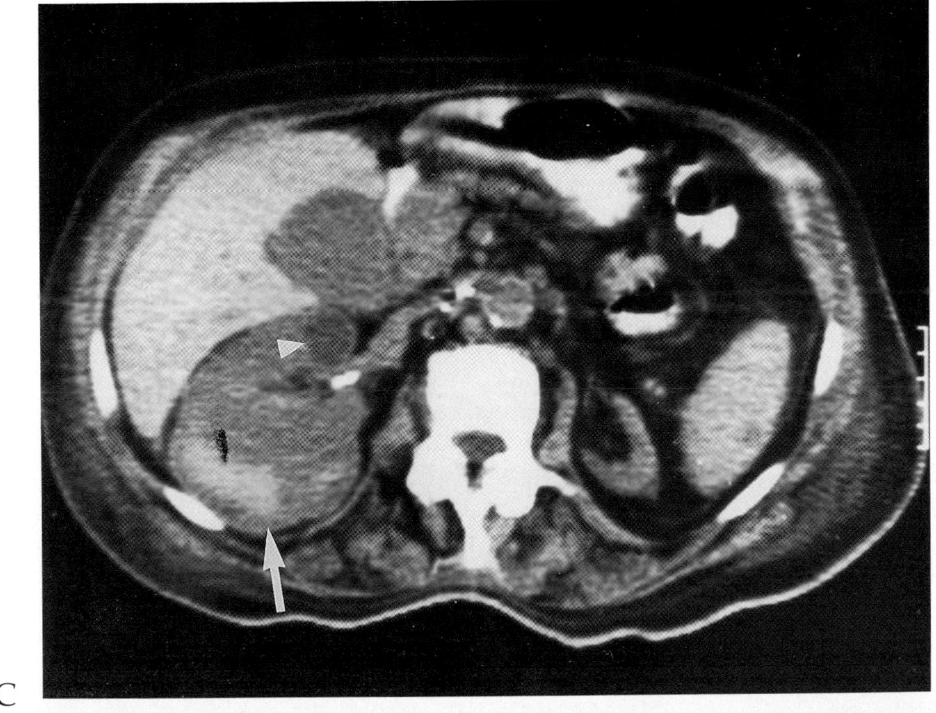

C

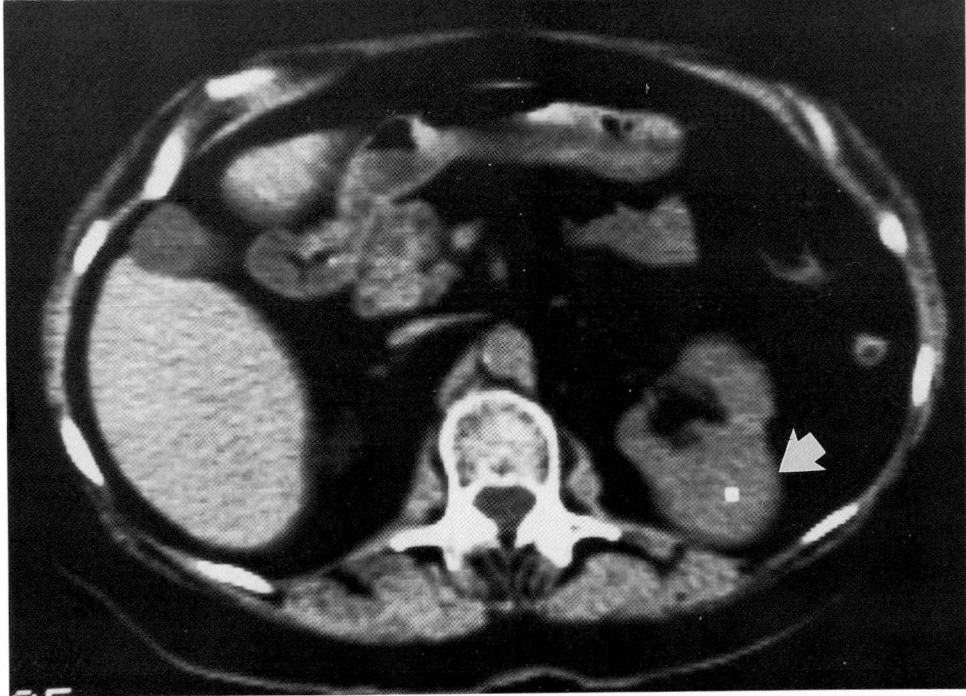

D

Figures 5C,D. (C, top) Unenhanced CT scan demonstrates high-attenuation material in the posterior right perirenal space consistent with an acute hematoma. Excellent correlation with the sonogram of Figure 4B. The CT finding of an acute perirenal hemorrhage is increased attenuation compared with renal parenchyma (arrow). Densely calcified right renal artery accounts for central calcification in the renal hilar region. Benign cyst demonstrated on ultrasound is also evident in the anterior portion of the right kidney (arrowhead). (D, bottom) Unenhanced CT scan of the left kidney demonstrates a solid-appearing mass projecting from the posterolateral aspect of the superior pole of the left kidney (arrow) with mean HU value of 40 (square box). Same patient as Figure 4C, with renal cell carcinoma diagnosed at nephrectomy. The CT density of tumor mass is nearly identical to that of renal parenchyma. Exophytic mass projected more superiorly above the left kidney on higher scans.

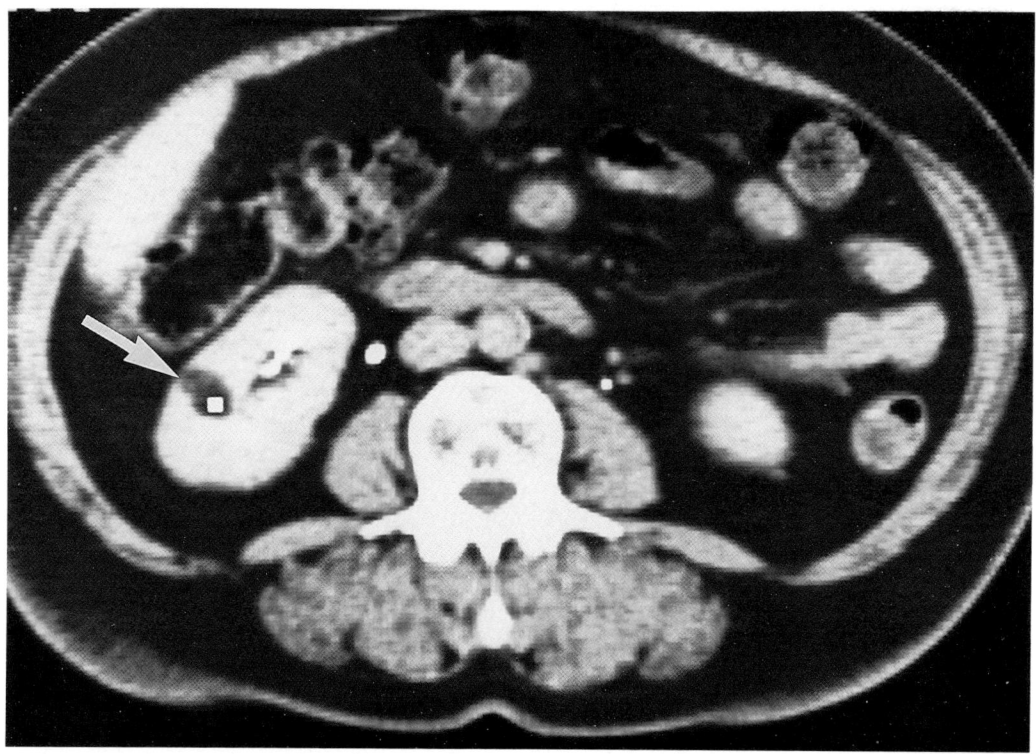

Figure 5E.   Enhanced CT examination demonstrates small, homogeneous low-attenuation area in the lateral aspect of the right kidney (arrow). Mean of −58 HU (square box) is consistent with a high proportion of fatty material in the lesion. In conjunction with the sonogram of Figure 4D, this finding is diagnostic of angiomyolipoma.

Acknowledgments: The author wishes to thank Drs. Brian Thiele, Gary Thieme, and Marsha Neumeyer for supplying case material for this manuscript. Also, special thanks to Christine Lear for assistance in manuscript preparation.

References

1. Pollak HM (ed): Overview of renal cystic disease. In Clinical Urography. Philadelphia: WB Saunders, 1990, p 1059.
2. Lingard DA, Lawson TL: Accuracy of ultrasound in predicting the nature of renal masses. J Urol 1979; 122:724.
3. Chan SL, Cooperberg P, McLoughin MG, et al: Grey-scale ultrasonography: a refined tool for differentiating renal mass lesions. Can Med Assoc 1980; 102:321.
4. Pollak HM, Banner MP, Arger PH, et al: The accuracy of grey-scale ultrasonography in differentiating cystic neoplasms from benign cysts. Radiology 1982; 143:741.
5. Mayer DP, Baron RL, Pollack HM: Increase in CT attenuation values of parapelvic cysts after retrograde pyelography. AJR 1982; 139:991.
6. McClellan BL, Stanely RJ, Melson GL, et al: CT of the renal cyst: is cyst aspiration necessary? AJR 1979; 133:671.
7. Shanser JD, Hedgcock MW, Korobkin M: Transit of contrast material into renal cysts following urography or arteriography. AJR 1978; 130:584.
8. Hricak H, Williams RD, Moon KL, et al: Magnetic resonance imaging of the kidney: renal masses. Radiology 1983; 147:765.
9. LiPuma JP: Magnetic resonance imaging of the kidney. Radiol Clin North Am 1984; 22:925.
10. Newhouse JH, Markisz JA, Kazam E: Magnetic imaging of the kidney. CardioVasc Intervent Radiol 1986; 8:351.
11. Marshall FF: The role of selective exploration in ambiguous renal cystic lesions. Urol Clin North Am 1980; 7:689.

Chapter 9

Imaging in Female Urology

Jay Hollander, M.D., Jalil Farah, M.D., and Michael Farah, M.D.

This chapter will focus on a number of gynecologic problems related to the urinary tract. We will also discuss the problems encountered with imaging of the urinary tract during pregnancy. The majority of the information presented in this text can apply to patients of either sex. Such is the case with most primary problems of the upper urinary tract. The lower urinary tract, however, is subject to several processes that are specifically female owing to the uniqueness of the anatomy and reproductive physiology.

The chapter will begin by briefly discussing the various imaging modalities useful for evaluating the female pelvis. An introduction to normal anatomy as it is pertinent to the urologist is all we hope to achieve. We will then discuss specific gynecologic conditions that can affect the urinary tract and the various imaging modalities useful in their diagnosis.

Normal Anatomy and Imaging Techniques

The intravenous urogram (IVU) has been the mainstay of urologic diagnosis for the last half century and remains of significant importance in urology. However, newer imaging modalities are becoming more important in gynecologic diagnosis, and IVU itself has limited usefulness to the gynecologist. Pelvic ultra-sound, computed tomography (CT), and magnetic resonance imaging (MRI) are clearly more useful in the workup of female pelvic processes. The urologist must be familiar with the appearance of normal female pelvic anatomy as imaged by these various modalities, as urologic involvement in pathologic processes is not frequent.

Plain Film and Intravenous Urogram

The IVU in the normal female patient differs from that in the male only in the distinct soft-tissue impressions made by either the uterus or the prostate, and the absence of male external genital signs.

Certain gynecologic conditions may result in pelvic calcifications that can be recognized by their appearance on the plain film. Calcified leiomyomas appear as round structures with a mottled appearance near the midline occupying a uterine or parauterine position within the pelvis (Fig. 1). Ovarian calcifications may represent benign or malignant changes. Calcifications resembling teeth can be formed in mature cystic teratomas. Ovarian fibroadenomas and carcinomas can also contain calcifications. Dermoid tumors of the ovary can contain fat and may be seen as radiolucent masses requiring ultrasound or CT confirmation (Fig. 2). In general, however, the IVU has a limited role in ruling out gyneco-

From *Imaging of Urologic Disorders* edited by Alexander S. Cass, MBBS, © 1992, Futura Publishing Inc., Mount Kisco, NY.

logic pathology, being useful only in ruling out urologic involvement by gynecologic processes. It can also be useful in looking for features associated with gynecologic conditions, such as renal agenesis, which may be associated with uterine anomalies.

Ultrasound

The essential anatomy of the female pelvis becomes simple when a systematic approach is utilized (Fig. 3). The urinary bladder is identified as an anechoic fluid-filled structure in the midline in both the sagittal and the transverse plane. The uterus is seen directly posterior to the bladder as a pear-shaped structure with a linear echogenic band on sagittal scans and as an oval structure with a central echogenic focus on transverse scans. The echogenic band represents the endometrial cavity. By following the posterior wall of the bladder inferiorly on sagittal scans, one can see an echogenic line parallel to the bladder wall that represents the vagina.

The ovaries are best seen in premenopausal females. They are oval homogeneous structures measuring approximately 3 to 4 cm with multiple small cysts that represent follicles (Fig. 4). The location of the ovaries is quite variable but usually is lateral to the uterus.

Computed Tomography

The interpretation of CT anatomy is greatly facilitated when oral, rectal, and intravenous contrast is administered (Fig. 5). The urinary bladder is easily identified as an anterior structure filled with intravenous contrast. The rectum is seen as a barium-filled structure anterior to the sacrum. The uterus lies between the rectum and bladder, appearing as an enhancing soft-tissue mass. Enhancement is the result of the vascularity of the myometrium. One can usually see a central area of low density within the uterus representing the endometrium. The cervix and vagina are not clearly seen as separate structures. However, by following the uterus inferiorly on serial scans, the region of the cervix and vagina can be identified. The ovaries are more difficult to identify on CT than with ultrasound. They are usually seen as small oval soft-tissue densities with small cysts (follicles). Differentiating the ureters from enhancing vessels is best done by following them over serial images either to the kidney and bladder or to the aorta or inferior vena cava.

Magnetic Resonance Imaging

Various parameters are set on the MRI scanner in order to produce a T1-weighted or T2-weighted image. The appearances of the pelvic structures are variable in signal intensity depending on whether the image is T1- or T2-weighted. MRI has the advantage of imaging in multiple planes including the axial, sagittal, and coronal.

On T2-weighted sagittal images (Fig. 6), the bladder is seen as a triangular area of increased signal intensity (opaque) posterior to the pubis, which is oval and has decreased signal intensity (dark). The uterus is identified as a pear-shaped structure with a linear band of increased signal intensity (endometrium) superior or posterior to the bladder, depending on how much the bladder is distended.

As with ultrasound, the vagina can be seen parallel to the posterior wall of the bladder. Also, like the uterus, the signal characteristics of the vagina change with the menstrual phase and hormonal stimulation. The ovaries are difficult to visualize on MRI because of surrounding bowel. The rectum is seen posterior to the uterus and anterior to the sacrum with areas of signal void (black) from gas.

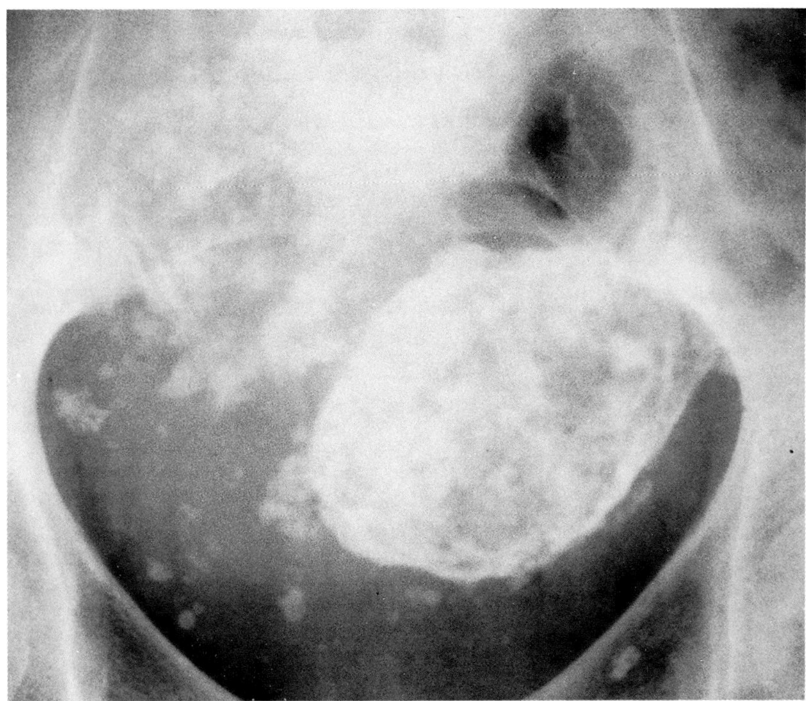

Figure 1. Leiomyoma of the uterus with diffuse calcification of the tumor mass in the pelvis.

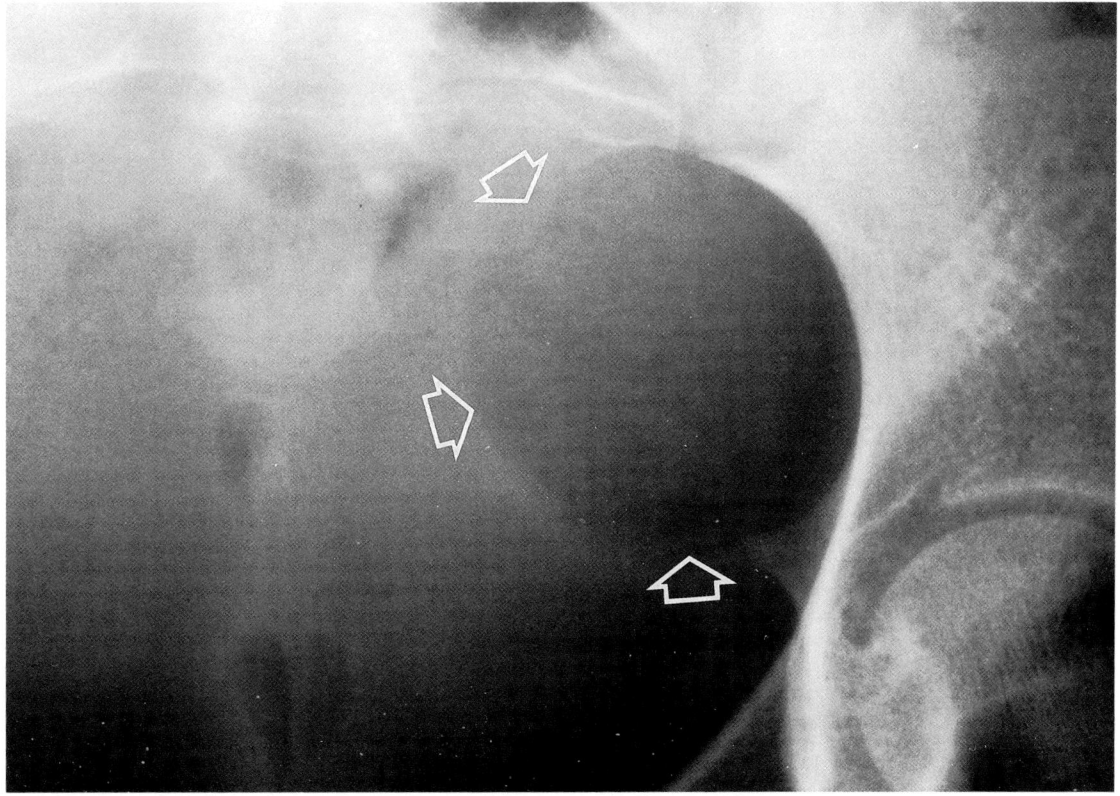

Figure 2. Dermoid tumor with a round area of decreased density representing fat (arrow).

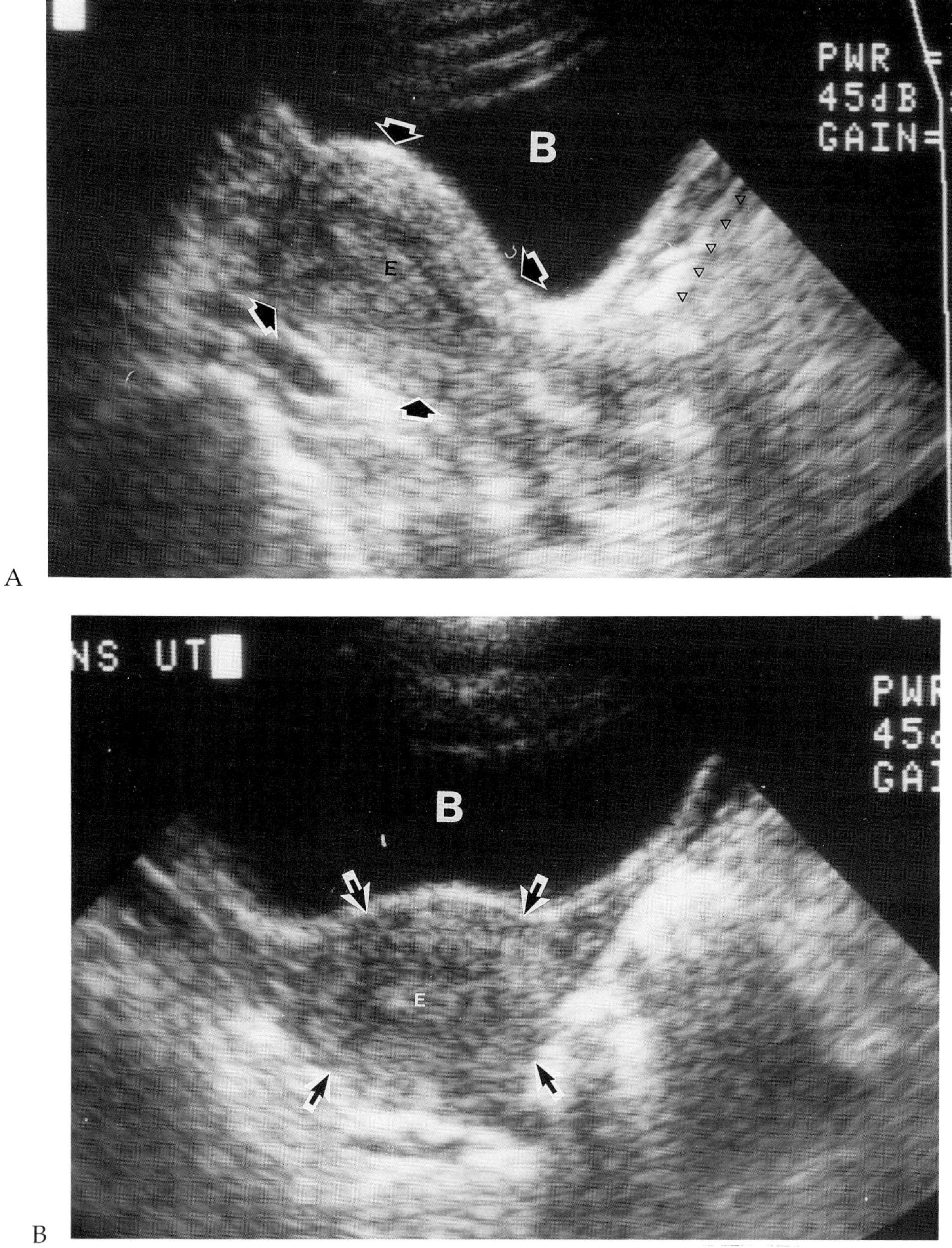

Figure 3.   Ultrasound scans of a normal uterus. Sagittal (A, top) and transverse (B, bottom) scans show the uterus (arrows) posterior to the bladder (B), vagina (open arrowheads), and endometrium (E).

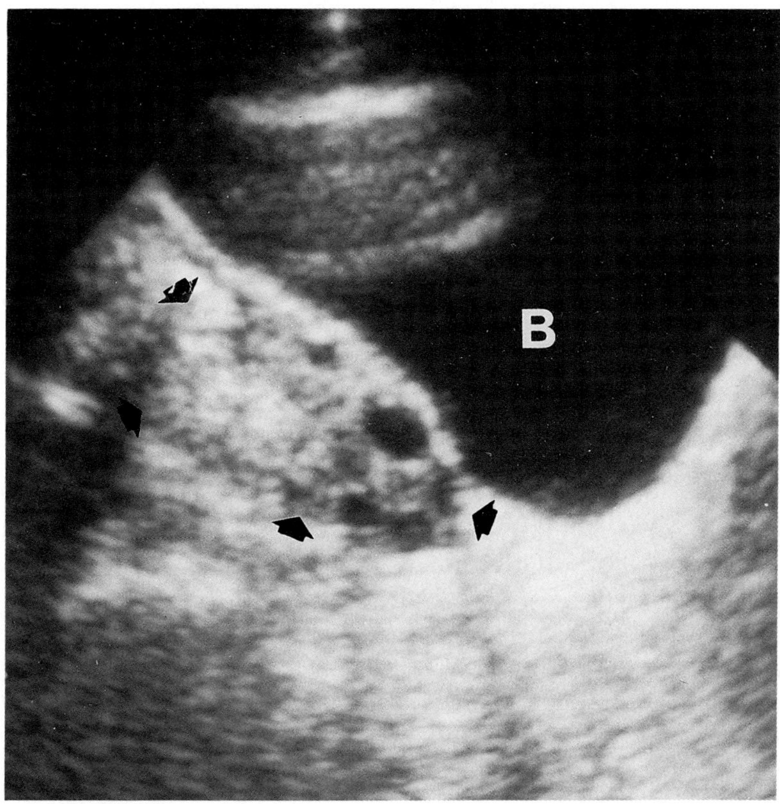

Figure 4.   Normal ovary. Sagittal scan of the pelvis shows ovary (arrows) posterior to the bladder (B) with multiple small follicles of various sizes.

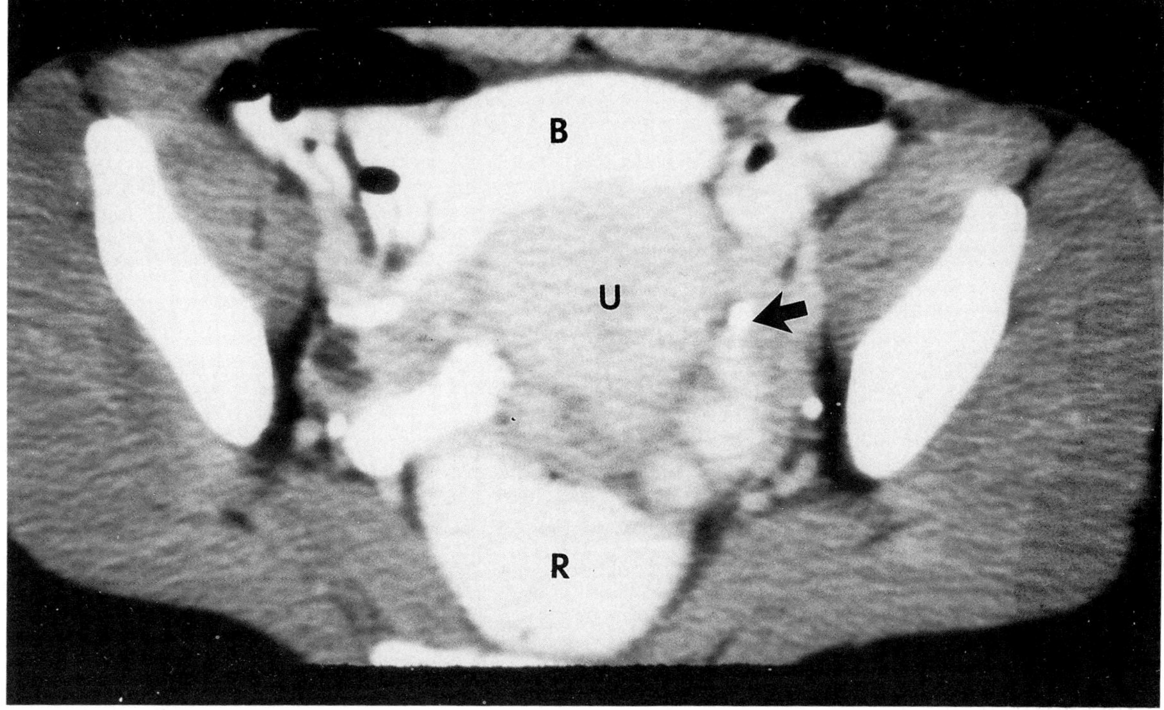

Figure 5.   A CT scan of a normal pelvis. The uterus (U) is seen posterior to the bladder (B) and anterior to the rectum (R). Left ureter (arrow) also is seen.

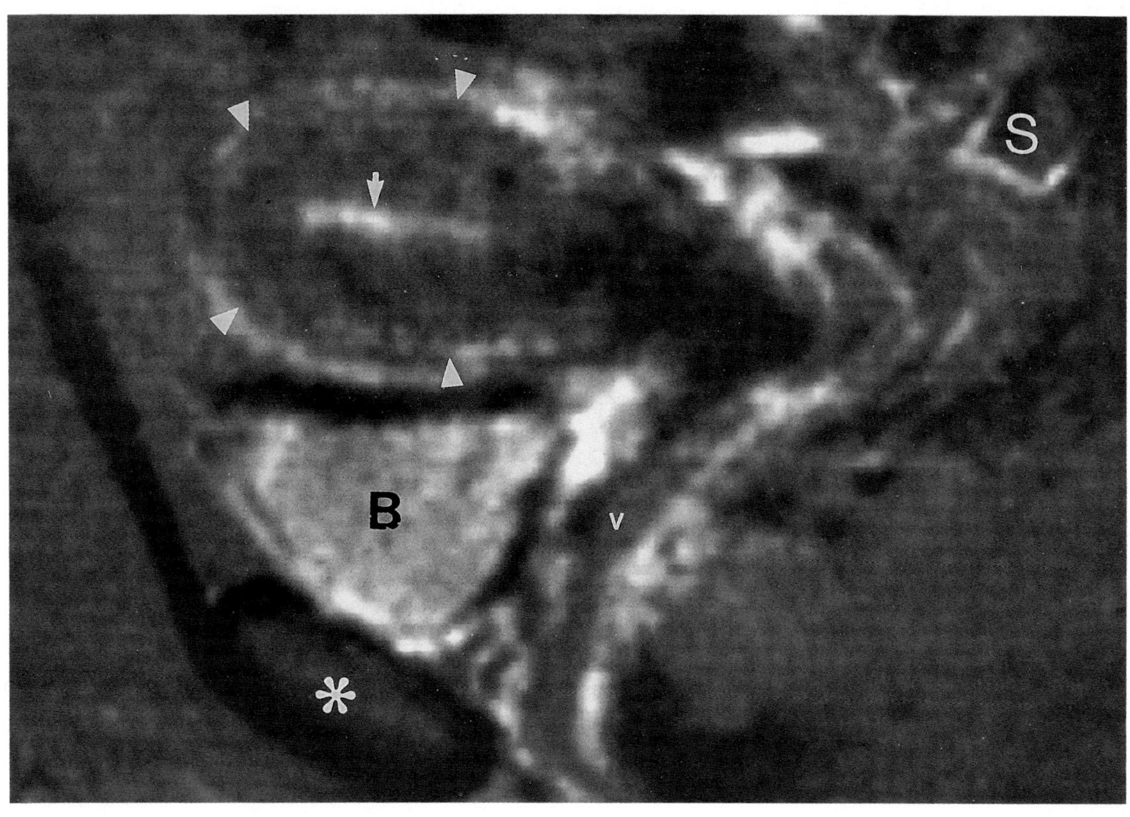

Figure 6.   MRI of the normal pelvis (sagittal T2-weighted). Vagina (v), uterus (arrowheads), endometrial cavity (small arrow), bladder (B), pubis (*), and sacrum (s) are apparent.

Gynecologic Problems Related to the Urinary Tract

Urinary Incontinence

Urinary incontinence is one of the most common female urologic complaints. The prevalence increases with aging and number of pregnancies, and is estimated to be 37% in women over 60 years of age.[1] The urologist's role is to diagnose the etiology of incontinence and recommend appropriate therapy. Radiographic imaging techniques remain useful in arriving at the appropriate diagnosis and plan.

Before discussing useful imaging modalities, it should be emphasized that no radiographic findings should take precedence over the findings of a careful urologic history and examination. A radiographic study suggesting cystocele would have little meaning if no cystocele were apparent at the time of pelvic examination. Likewise, radiographic findings associated with stress urinary incontinence will add little to benefit the patient if no incontinence is demonstrable by history or examination. The following imaging techniques are meant to assist with a workup of incontinence that has been documented.

Fluoroscopic Monitoring at Time of Urodynamic Studies

Contrast can be used as a filling medium during cystometry with fluoroscopic monitoring of the study. With appropriate catheters and transducers, subtracted bladder pressures (true detrusor pressure free of the intra-abdominal straining component) can be determined to differentiate stress from urge incontinence.

Depending on the sophistication of the fluoroscopic table, upright and oblique monitoring can be made to best view the vesical neck and the urethra. Contrast in the urethra is an abnormal finding if the patient is trying to maintain continence. It may represent either a deficient sphincteric mechanism, as in the case of stress urinary incontinence, or physiologic relaxation of the internal sphincter, which appears as funneling of the vesical neck during the uninhibited contraction associated with urge urinary incontinence (Fig. 7). The fluoroscopic image must be interpreted in association with the urodynamic findings in order to arrive at a correct diagnosis. Fluoroscopic imaging is not a prerequisite for appropriate workup in most cases of incontinence. Instead, it should be reserved for those patients whose incontinence requires complex urodynamic analysis.

Stress Cystogram

The workup of stress incontinence in the female patient is sometimes assisted by the resting and straining upright lateral cystogram. We refer to this study as the "stress cystogram," since its role is primarily for the study of stress urinary incontinence. These studies have been popular for at least the last four decades and were most commonly referred to as "bead chain cystography."

Normally, the urethrovesical neck, anterior vaginal wall, and cervix maintain relatively fixed relations to one another, being well suspended to the pubis, pelvic musculature, and fascia. As a result of aging, childbearing, and changes in the female hormonal milieu, these attachments weaken resulting in symptomatic lesions such as cystocele, uterine prolapse, and stress urinary incontinence. One objective way of measuring these changes is the stress cystogram. A 12-French radiopaque catheter is placed in the bladder, and the bladder is filled with 200 ml of contrast medium. Resting films are taken in the anteroposterior and true lateral views. The patient is then asked to perform a valsalva maneuver and the films are repeated. Using the true lateral view, lines are drawn as follows (Fig. 8). A "pelvic diaphragm" line is drawn from the inferior margin of the pubis to the junction between the sacrum and the coccyx. The urethral angle of inclination represents the angle of urethral axis rotation from the true vertical. The posterior urethrovesical angle is the angle formed by the urethral axis and the bladder base posteriorly.

In the normal female, the urethra and vesical neck are suspended behind the pubis, with the urethral axis or angle of inclination being less than 30° of posterior rotation from the vertical (Fig. 9). The posterior urethrovesical angle is less than 100°. The vesical neck position should be located above the line drawn to represent the pelvic diaphragm. Very little difference should be seen between the angles observed during rest or straining. As relaxation of supporting tissues occurs, the urethra will rotate posteriorly in the sagittal plane, increasing the urethral axis (angle of inclination). The posterior urethrovesical angle will become more obtuse, and the vesical neck will fall caudad below the imaginary line of the pelvic diaphragm. All of these changes can be associated with stress urinary incontinence and will be most pronounced during straining (Fig. 10). However, the presence of changes does not prove incontinence, as changes can occur in the absence of incontinence.

There have been numerous theories regarding the true mechanism of stress urinary incontinence. Most authors currently subscribe to the theory that "intra-abdominal positioning" of the vesical neck and proximal urethral sphincter is essential for normal continence. The sphincteric area will then be subjected to pressure increases similar to the bladder during strain or stress activities. Continence is maintained because the resting urethral pressure is normally greater than the resting bladder pressure. When the bladder neck and urethra drops, it may not be subjected to the same increased external pressures seen by the bladder during straining. Incontinence will then occur if the absolute pressure within the bladder is greater than that within the urethra. The stress cystogram therefore can objectively image changes in vesicourethral positioning as a result of weak supporting structures. When these changes are associated with true stress incontinence, restoring vesicourethral support with vesicopexy can cure incontinence. It must be emphasized, however, that even dramatic findings on the stress cystogram may not be associated with incontinence (Fig. 11).

In the past, the bead chain cystogram was extensively used. Green's discussion of patients with stress urinary incontinence based on the lateral straining cystogram is of historical significance. He suggested that procedures to correct stress urinary incontinence could be chosen on the basis of the type of findings seen on the study and he identified two types.

Type I was described as: "Complete or nearly complete loss of the posterior urethrovesical angle, but with the angle of inclination to the vertical of the urethral axis either normal (range, 10 to 30°) or at least less than 45°, as shown on the urethrocystogram in the lateral standing-straining view." Type II was described as: "Loss of the posterior urethrovesical angle and, in addition, a definitely abnormal angle of inclination to the vertical of the urethral axis, the latter being greater than 45° and often even completely reversed (greater than 90°)."[2] Green suggested that simple transvaginal repair or anterior colporrhaphy procedures could be sufficient to treat type I urinary incontinence. Formal urethral suspension procedures, such as the Marshall-Marchetti-Krantz, would be required for type II incontinence.

As procedures have been developed that are transvaginal and suspend the urethra (transvaginal needle suspension procedures), the differentiation between type I and type II incontinence has become less significant, as one procedure treats both in a relatively simple manner. As long as a true urethral suspension procedure (not a simple anterior colporrhaphy) is used to treat simple acquired urinary incontinence, a stress cystogram will seldom assist with decision making.

If a woman has undergone prior attempts at surgical correction or has been exposed to radiation or trauma, she may have stress urinary incontinence on the basis of urethral wall incompetence unrelated to urethral positioning. Neuropathic conditions of the urethra can also present this way. In this case, the urethra is unable to close sufficiently during stress and even under resting conditions. The lateral stress cystogram shows normal urethral positioning (Fig. 12). Examination and cystoscopy may show a scarred and fixed urethra. Stress incontinence of this sort is not related to pelvic relaxation and may be referred to as to type III urinary incontinence.[3] The artificial urinary sphincter or a fascial sling procedure may be required to correct this type of incontinence.

The stress cystogram has, therefore, found its principal utility in explaining failed surgical correction of stress urinary incontinence. If evidence of poor suspension is present by the stress cystogram and urologic examination, then a repeat suspension should be considered. If suspension appears adequate, type III incontinence may be present and require the artificial urinary sphincter or fascial sling procedure.

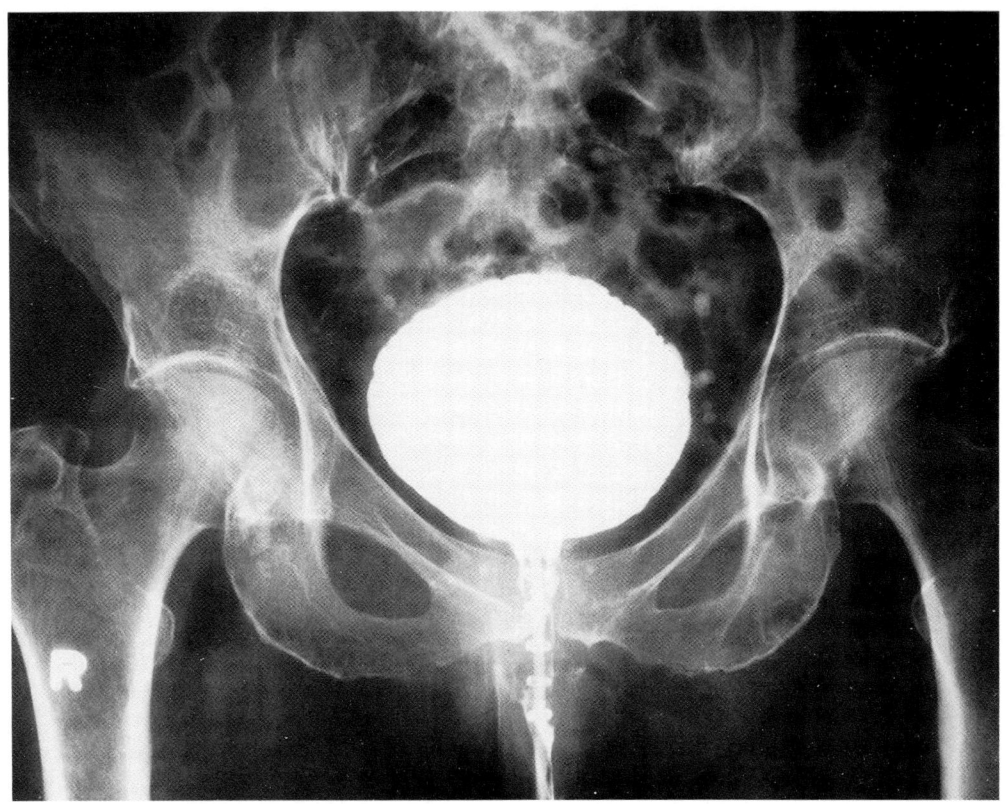

Figure 7.   Fluoroscopic monitoring during cystometry shows uninhibited contraction with wrinkling of the bladder mucosa and contrast seen in the proximal urethra as the vesical neck begins to funnel. Patient has a measuring urodynamic catheter in place.

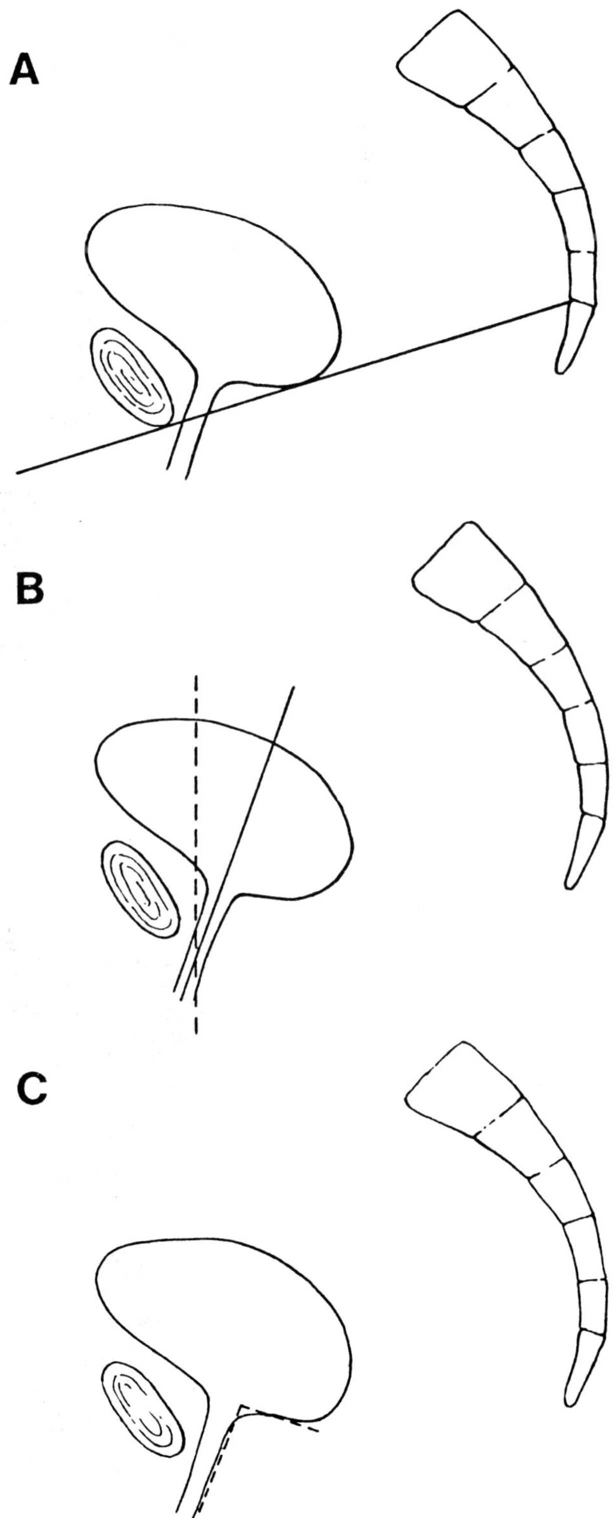

Figure 8. The stress cystogram. (A) Pelvic diaphragm line. Normally, the vesical neck is located above this. (B) Urethral angle of inclination (urethral axis). Normal angle is less than 30°. (C) Posterior urethrovesical angle; normal is less than 100°.

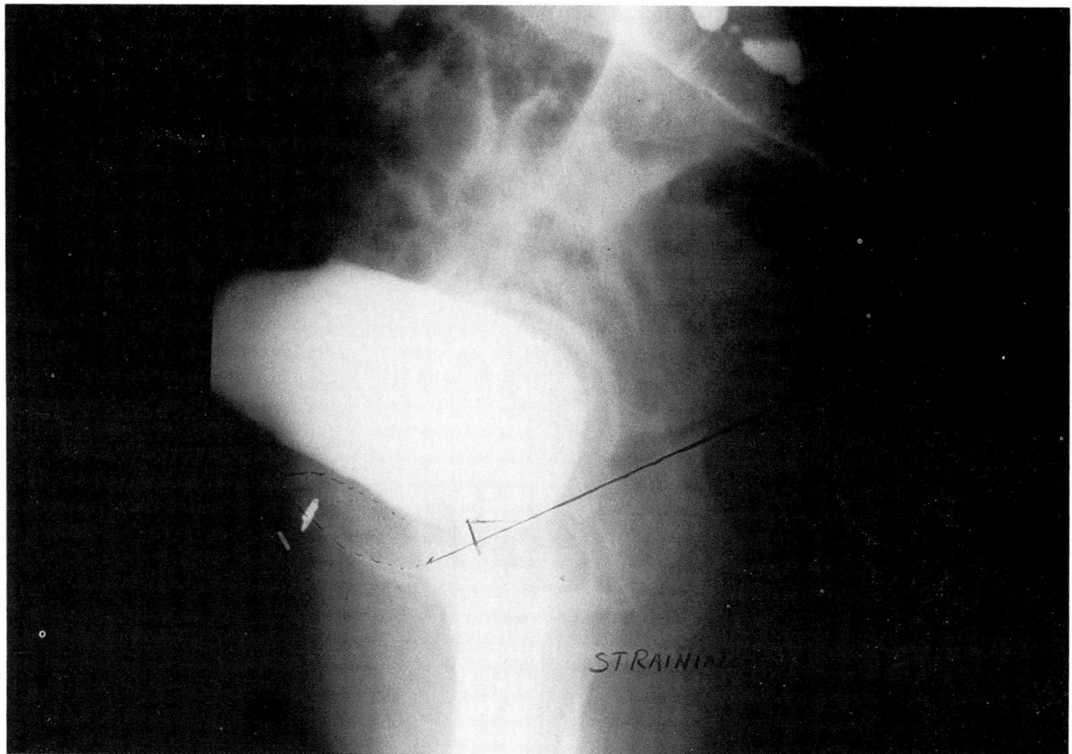

Figure 9.   Normal stress cystogram (lateral straining cystogram).

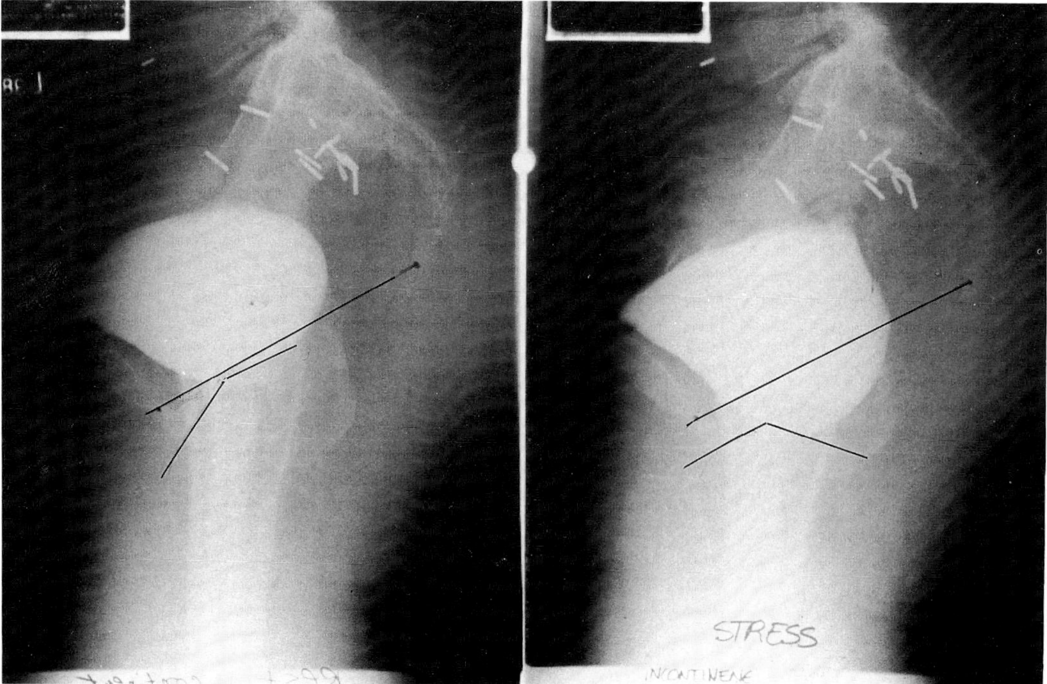

Figure 10.   Resting (left) and straining (right) lateral cystogram in a patient with significant stress urinary incontinence. The vesical neck is below the pelvic diaphragm line. The urethral axis and posterior urethrovesical angle abnormally increased. All changes are more pronounced with straining.

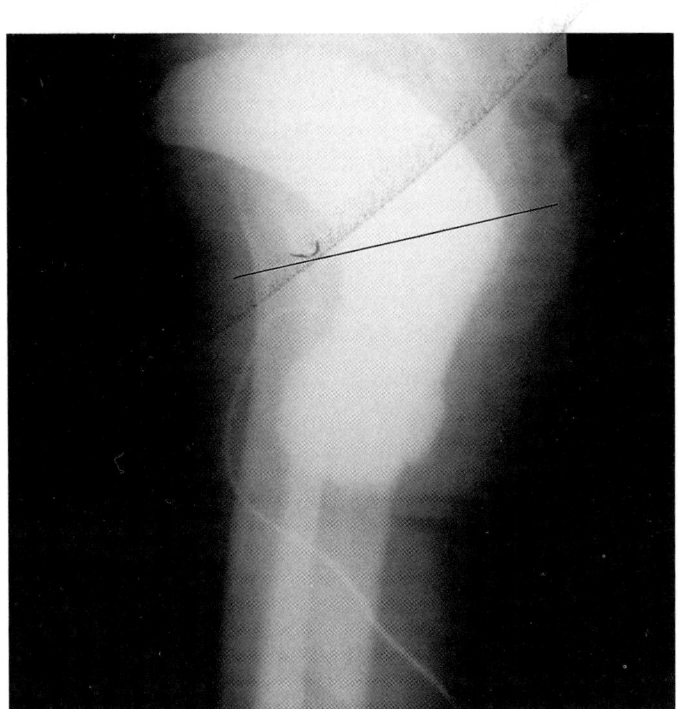

Figure 11. Huge cystocele on lateral cystogram. The patient had no incontinence.

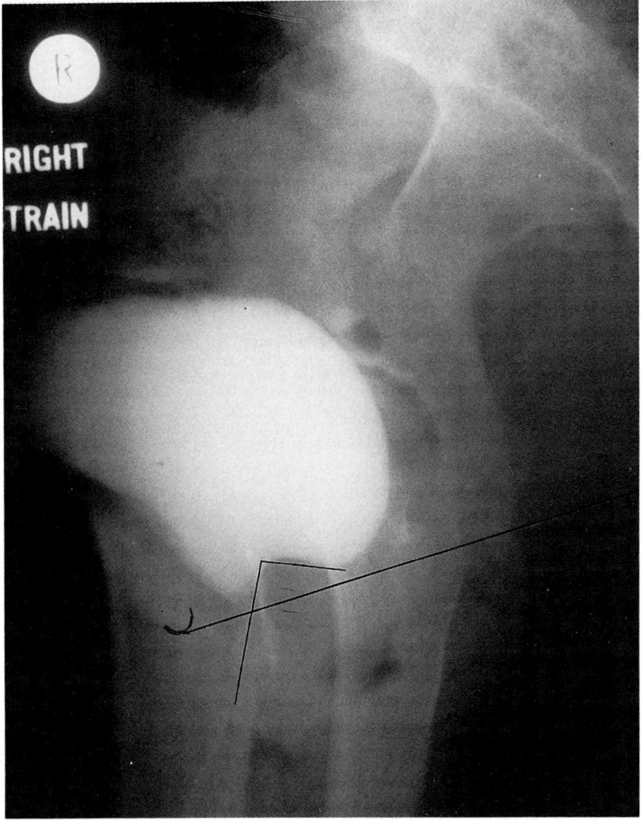

Figure 12. Type III incontinence. A patient with normal angles and vesical neck position, seen on lateral stress cystogram, after two vesicopexies. Contrast enters the proximal urethra because of scarring.

Prolapse

As mentioned in the preceding section, weakening of the female pelvic floor can result in loss of suspension of the urethra and vesical neck and result in stress incontinence. The same process can result in prolapsing of the pelvic structures such as the uterus, bladder, and rectum. The diagnosis is best made by physical examination, not radiographic studies. Complete uterine prolapse or procidentia can cause impressive hydronephrosis. The possibility of hydronephrosis should be entertained whenever high-grade vaginal or uterine prolapse is found on physical examination. The cause is caudal displacement of the ureteral orifices and trigone, which is involved with the prolapse (Fig. 13). Reduction of the prolapse with surgery or a pessary can relieve the urinary obstruction. The diagnosis is best made by IVU during prolapse.

Most commonly, a cystocele accompanies various degrees of uterine prolapse without any effect on the upper urinary tract. Radiographic imaging will add little to the diagnosis and management of prolapse in most cases.

Urethral Diverticula

Diverticula of the female urethra are rare. They can present as recurrent urinary tract infection, irritative or obstructive voiding symptoms, or dribbling incontinence. The diagnosis is frequently missed and is best made by keeping it in mind when evaluating a female patient with recurrent urinary tract infection or problematic dribbling incontinence. Occasionally, it can present as acute inflammation, in which case the lesion is more easily diagnosed.

Urethral diverticula are thought to be acquired from an infected or obstructed periurethral gland. These lesions are most often nontender and empty into the urethral lumen via a narrow neck. Urethroscopy will often fail to identify any opening unless simultaneous compression of the urethra is performed to express diverticular contents, which can be seen endoscopically. If the diverticular opening can be seen, endoscopic injection of contrast can be diagnostic. The diagnosis can be missed unless

urethrography is also performed. One should begin with simple voiding cystourethrography, as seen in Figure 14. Diverticula can fill dramatically during this study. Alternatively, retrograde urethrography can be performed.

Some radiology departments have special double-balloon catheters that can assist with these retrograde studies. A bladder balloon occludes the vesical neck, and a movable external balloon occludes the urethral meatus. Sideholes in the catheter, located between the balloons, allow for retrograde instillation of contrast and filling of diverticula. Such retrograde studies are seldom necessary.

The majority of diverticula is benign. Carcinomas can develop in female urethral diverticula, however, and should be suspected if an indurated mass is palpated or urethrography shows irregular filling defects within the diverticulum. Symptomatic urethral diverticula are treated surgically, and the radiographic studies can assist with the choice of procedure and preoperative planning.

Ectopic Ureteral Orifice

Ectopic ureteral orifices can present with symptoms similar to those of urethral diverticula. Unlike ectopic ureteral orifices in the male, female ectopic orifices can present with incontinence if they are located distal to the proximal sphincteric mechanism. In addition to the urethra, ectopic ureteral orifices may be located in the uterus, cervix, or vagina. Excretory urography and urethroscopy with retrograde pyelography (Fig. 15) are essential in making the diagnosis when the orifice is located in the urethra. When it is located in gynecologic tissues, the diagnosis can be difficult. Thorough examination, use of methylene blue or indigo carmine, vaginoscopy, upper tract radiographic imaging with contrast, and, occasionally, exploration are necessary to make a correct diagnosis.

Acquired Fistulae

A fistula can arise between the ureter, bladder, or urethra and the vagina as a result of surgical or obstetric injury, blunt or penetrating trauma, tumor, radiation, or severe inflammatory disorders. The most common origin is clearly iatrogenic associated with female pelvic surgery. Cystography or urethrography will occasionally make the diagnosis, in which case, the fistular tract is seen between the bladder or urethra and vagina (Fig. 16). In general, however, the diagnosis is best made by combining cystoscopy, vaginal examination, and bladder filling with colored solutions of methylene blue or indigo carmine.

Occasionally, a ureterovaginal fistula can develop. This is best diagnosed with an IVU or a fistulogram when the orifice is identified. Rarely, a vesicouterine fistula can occur especially after cesarean section delivery. This can present with hematuria during menstruation or incontinence. Contrast studies such as voiding cystourethrography (VCUG) can be very helpful to diagnose this unusual occurrence. (Fig. 17).

Whenever a urethrovaginal or vesicovaginal fistula is diagnosed, the upper urinary tract should be evaluated to rule out concomitant involvement prior to repair.

Iatrogenic Injury to Urinary Tract from Gynecologic Surgery

Injury to the urinary tract is one of the most common significant complications of gynecologic surgery. Unlike the vesicovaginal fistula, which is best diagnosed by clinical studies, injury to the bladder or ureter alone from gynecologic surgery is best identified by radiographic means. Excretory urography, retrograde pyelography, and cystography are usually diagnostic (Fig. 18). A plain film is essential in all 3 studies in addition to a complete emptying film after the cystogram. Failure to identify trauma to the urinary tract during gynecologic surgery is the most common cause of urinary fistulae to the reproductive organs.

Ovarian Vein Syndrome

Until the last two decades, many operations were performed for ovarian vein syndrome. Today, there are few indications for operating, since the syndrome itself rarely occurs. In the past, it was felt that the ovarian vein that crosses over the ureter could be responsible for hydronephrosis and pain of the partially obstructed ureter. The syndrome was described classically as right-sided pain, pyelonephritis, or recurrent urinary tract infection that developed after pregnancy. It was caused by a relative right hydronephrosis from a prominent crossing ovarian vein. The hydronephrosis was, in most cases, related to pregnancy itself as will be described later in this chapter. When hydronephrosis persisted after pregnancy, exploration frequently revealed fibrotic bands responsible for the extrinsic ureteral obstruction and not the ovarian vein itself. Furthermore, operations to resect the vein seldom resulted in resolution of symptoms. The impression of the ovarian vein on the ureter is still a very common radiographic finding (Fig. 19). The vascular impression itself is seldom of clinical significance.

Pelvic Masses

Benign or malignant pelvic tumors in female patients can result in ureteral obstruction through extrinsic compression or invasion of the ureter. The most common tumor to cause ureteral obstruction is carcinoma of the uterine cervix, followed by tumors of the uterus and ovaries. Pelvic inflammatory disease and endometriosis can cause similar obstruction and compression of the lower urinary tract. Radiographic studies with contrast, such as the IVU or retrograde pyelography, usually are nonspecific (Fig. 20).

Although ureteral obstruction by gynecologic tumor most often causes extrinsic compression, it can mimic primary ureteral tumors such as transitional cell lesions (Fig. 21). A CT scan can more specifically diagnose lesions in which a pelvic organ is the source of obstruction. Hydronephrosis can also be diagnosed, but the exact level of obstruction is less reliably delineated than with the IVU or retrograde pyelogram. Ultrasound, too, can diagnose hydronephrosis and image the pelvic mass but is very poor at imaging the ureter unless it is quite dilated. Obstruction is most often extrinsic unless the tumor has invaded the ureteral wall. A full discussion of imaging regarding the specific lesions is beyond the scope of this chapter.

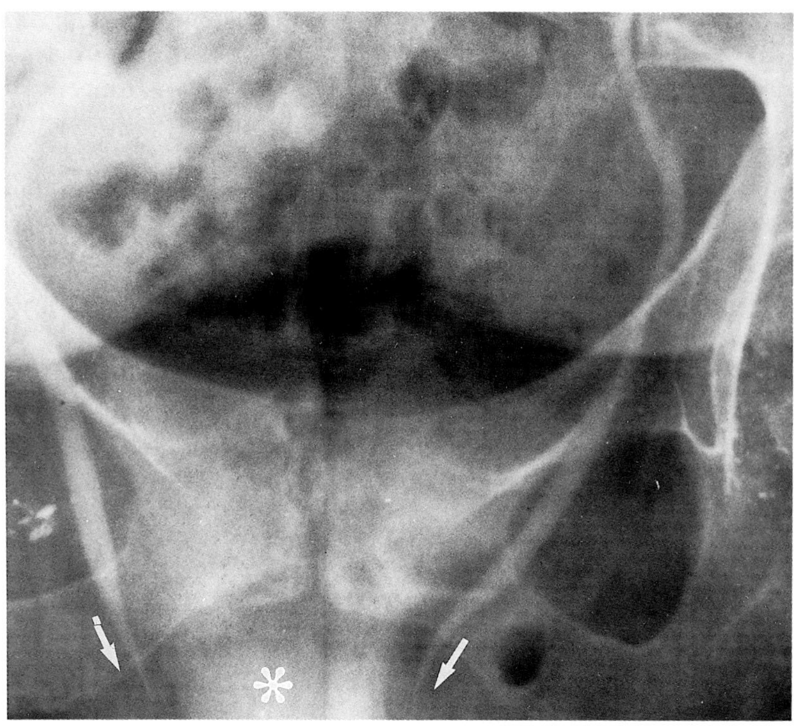

Figure 13.   Cystocele. Intravenous urogram showing pear-shaped bladder (*) prolapsing through the pelvic floor into the vagina. Note caudal displacement of the ureters (arrows).

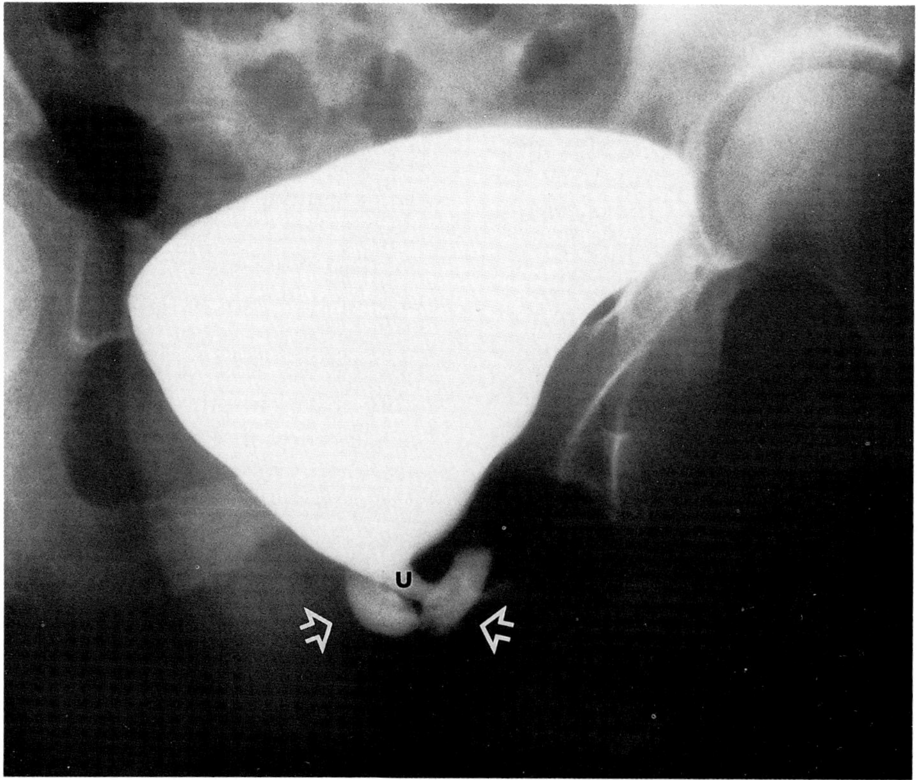

Figure 14.   Urethral diverticula. Opacification of diverticula (arrows) and the urethra (U) on the voiding urethrogram.

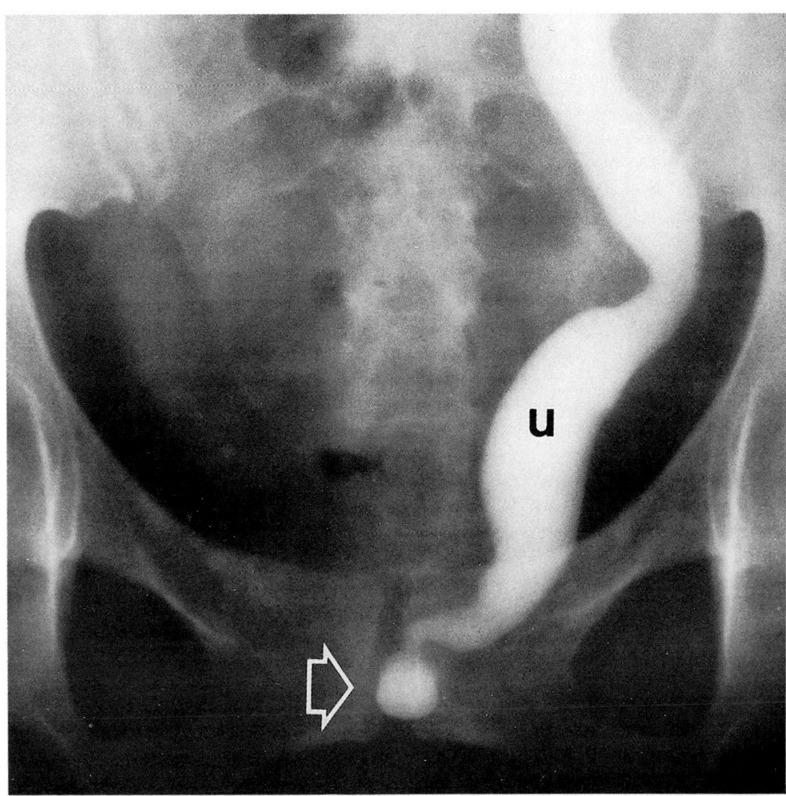

Figure 15.   Ectopic left ureter with ureterocele (open arrow). Stenotic orifice causing hydroureter (U), which empties into the urethra on retrograde study.

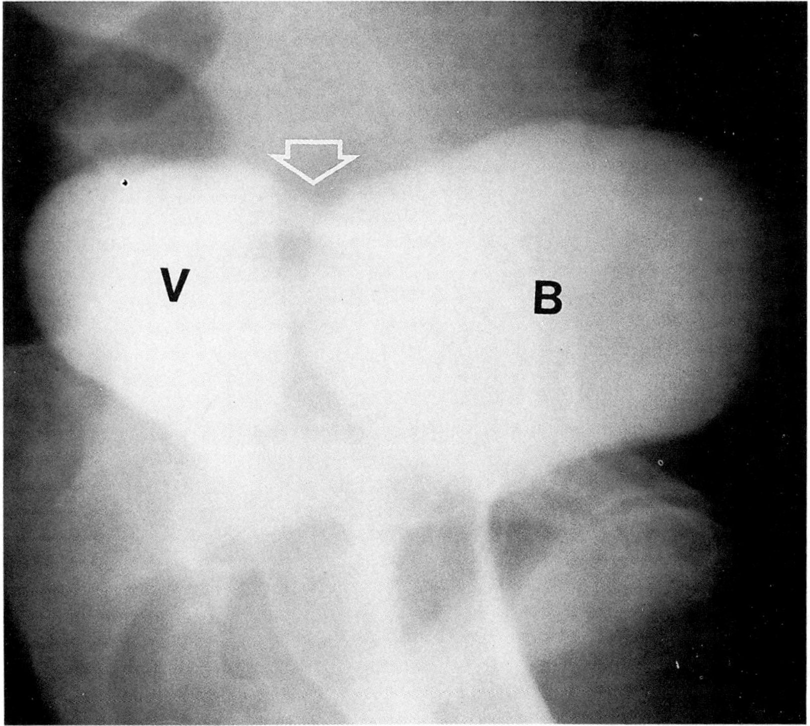

Figure 16.   Vesicovaginal fistula. Cystogram showing that contrast instilled in the bladder (B) has entered the vagina (V). Fistulous tract is marked by an open arrow.

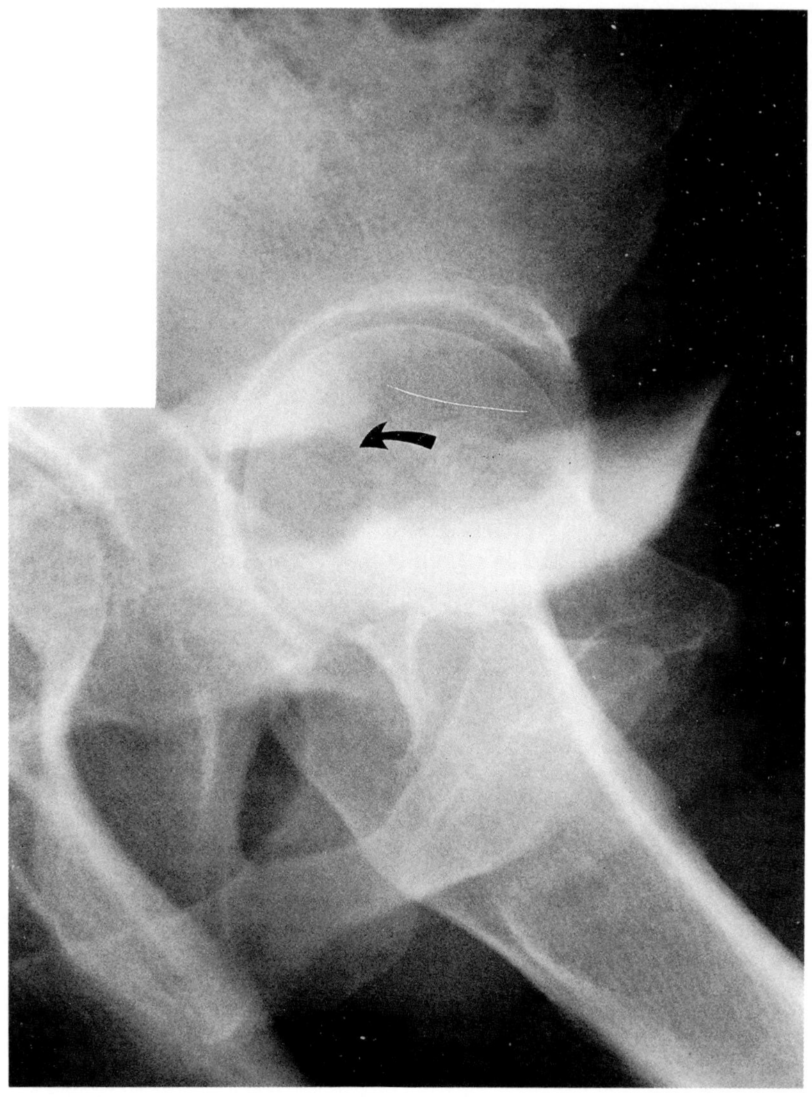

Figure 17. Vesicouterine fistula. Bladder fistula (arrows) to the uterine cavity seen on voiding cystourethrography.

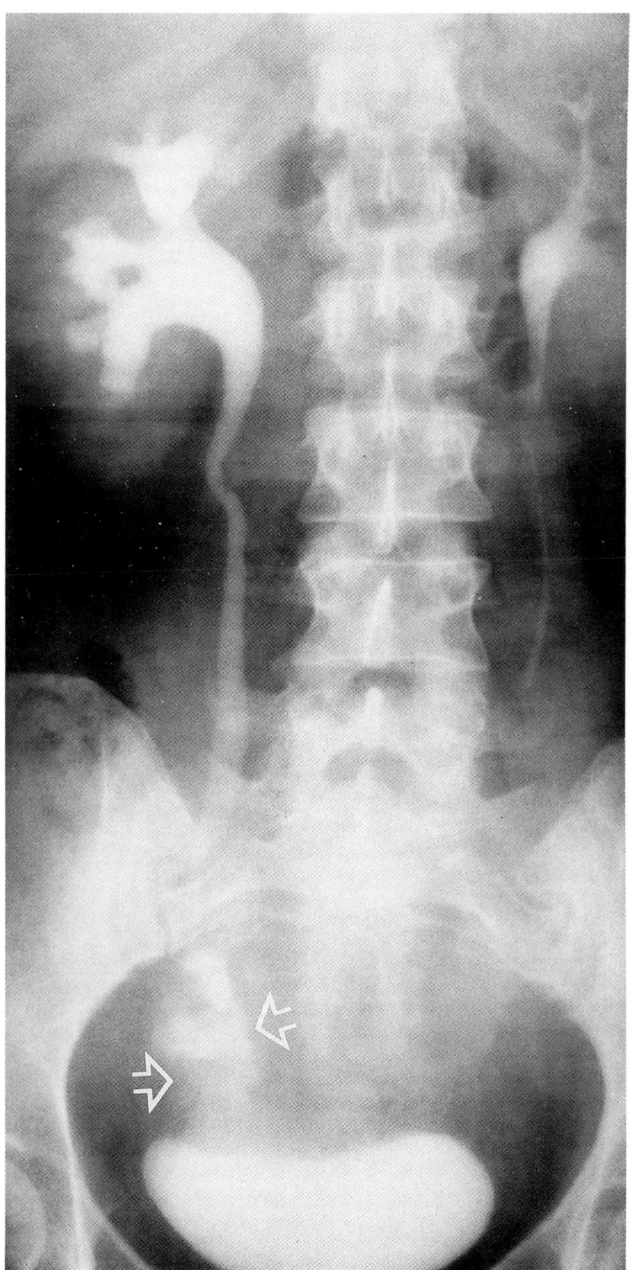

Figure 18. Ureteral trauma. Injury to the distal right ureter incident to a right salpingo-oophorectomy with extravasation of contrast (open arrows) from the site of the injury seen on intravenous urogram.

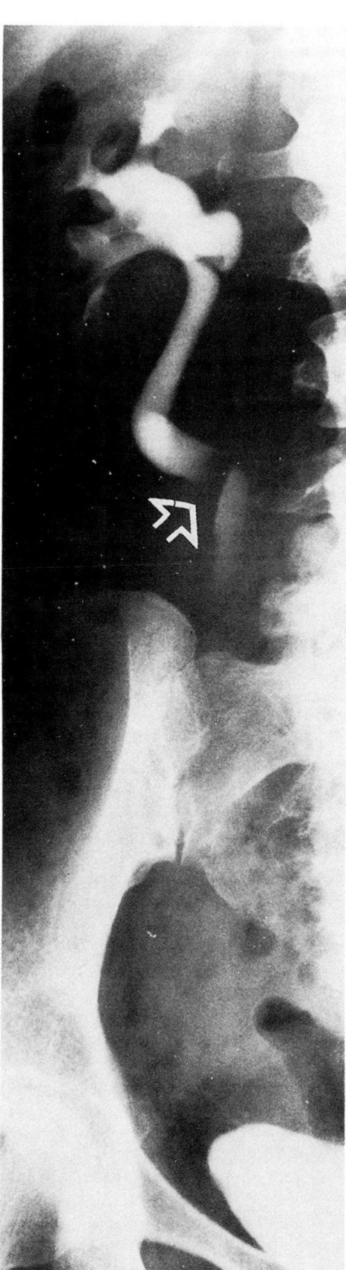

Figure 19. "Ovarian vein syndrome." Intravenous urogram showing a dilated ovarian vein causing vascular impression over the proximal ureter.

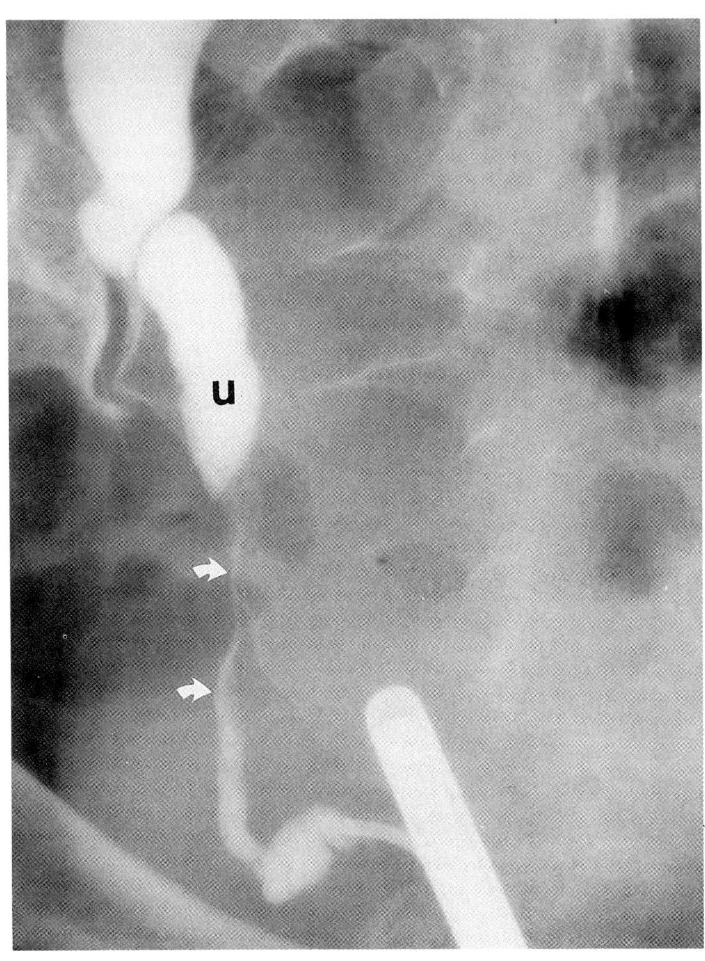
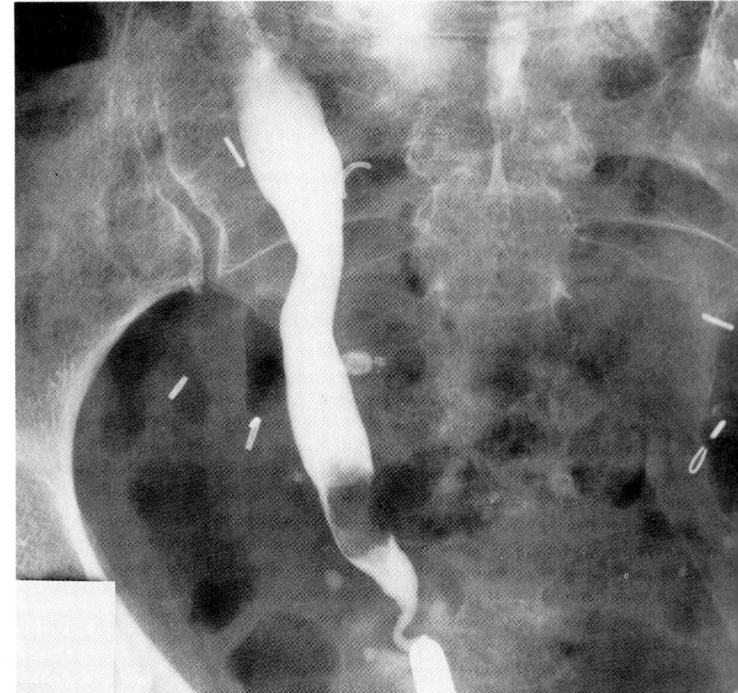

Figure 20.   Carcinoma of the cervix with extension of the tumor causing narrowing (curved arrows) and dilatation of the ureter (U) proximally. Appearance on retrograde pyelogram is nonspecific.

Figure 21.   Retrograde pyelogram suggests transitional cell tumor in a patient with uterine adenocarcinoma. Ureteroscopy and biopsy confirmed recurrent adenocarcinoma similar to the primary tumor.

Ovarian Remnant Syndrome

Ovarian pathology, both benign and malignant, can be a source of ureteral obstruction. The radiographic appearance of such obstruction is nonspecific on IVU or retrograde pyelography. Occasionally, a patient presents with ureteral obstruction with a history of either total abdominal hysterectomy and bilateral salpingo-oophorectomy or unilateral oophorectomy on the side of obstruction. These procedures may have been performed many years prior, but ovarian pathology can still be responsible for such obstruction even if the original pathology was entirely benign.

If the ovaries were not entirely removed at the time of oophorectomy, the small remnants can be a source of persistent symptoms and, rarely, ureteral obstruction. The ovary and ureter lie in close proximity near the pelvic sidewall and iliac vessels. When ovaries are removed for inflammatory processes or endometriosis, the dissection can be difficult, and ovarian remnants along with the pathological processes involved can obstruct the ureter with time. Symptoms of the original disease process usually cause presentation of the patient, and the ureteral obstruction may be silent. Renal ultrasound, IVU, and retrograde pyelography will define the ureteral involvement (Fig. 22).

Pelvic ultrasound and CT may identify the obstructing lesion extrinsic to the ureter where the ovaries normally lie (Fig. 23). The lesion can be as small as 1 cm and not be seen on imaging studies. Exploration is indicated if ureteral obstruction is diagnosed and ovarian remnant syndrome suspected. Premenopausal serum follicle-stimulating hormone (FSH) concentrations in a patient who has had bilateral oophorectomy and presents with ureteral obstruction is highly suggestive of ovarian remnant syndrome.[4]

Endometriosis

Endometriosis is a condition brought about by ectopic endometrial tissue. It is common, affecting 10% to 20% of women of childbearing age. The urinary tract may be involved. The most significant urologic sequela of endometriosis is ureteral obstruction. The mass effect, inflammation, or fibrosis associated with the disease can cause extrinsic compression of the ureter, resulting in hydronephrosis and even loss of kidney function. Endometrial implants can also be found in the wall of the ureter, causing intrinsic obstruction. Regardless of whether the lesion is intrinsic or extrinsic, the level of obstruction will almost always be below the pelvic rim.

Obstruction can be diagnosed by ultrasound or IVU, with the exact location and extent of obstruction best delineated by a retrograde pyelogram (Fig. 24). The radiographic appearance of endometriosis obstructing the ureter is nonspecific. The lesion should be suspected when cyclical flank pain occurs along with dysmenorrhea. Ultrasound or CT scan may show a pelvic mass (Fig. 25). The diagnosis can be made laparoscopically with biopsy, but open surgical intervention is frequently required to relieve ureteral obstruction and treat the primary disease. Fortunately, ureteral obstruction occurs in only 1% to 2% of patients with endometriosis.[5]

Hydrocolpos/Hematocolpos

Hydrocolpos is a fluid-filled mass caused by mucous secretions collecting in a vagina that has an obstructed introitus. Often, this will result in an associated uterine distention or hydrometrocolpos. The urologist is frequently involved in initial diagnosis and management of this rare condition. Congenital anomalies, including vaginal atresia, imperforate hymen, and vaginal septum can produce the condition. The presentation in these cases is usually in the neonatal period when a vulvar or midline pelvic mass is found. The mass can be imaged by ultrasound showing a fluid-filled structure between the bladder and the rectum (Fig. 26).

The condition can involve the urinary tract, causing urinary retention from urethral compression or hydronephrosis from ureteral compression. Congenital anomalies, including those of the urinary tract, may be associated. The treatment is surgical, and depends on the source of the vaginal occlusion and the associated anomalies.

Similar anatomic findings can be discovered

at menarche when the patient may present with pain, amenorrhea, and a midline pelvic mass associated with bulging of the vulva (Fig. 27). In this case, menses cannot drain producing distention of the vagina and the uterus. The fluid-filled mass contains blood from menstruation and is therefore termed "hematometrocolpos." The urinary tract may be secondarily affected.

With imaging such as pelvic ultrasound and CT scanning along with physical examination, the diagnosis should be made preoperatively so that adequate evaluation of the upper urinary tract, including IVU, can be performed. The surgical plan can then be more carefully designed.

Radiographic Exposure and Pregnancy

The urologist will not infrequently be confronted with urologic problems involving the pregnant woman. As discussed in the next section, the pregnant woman with urologic signs and symptoms may require workup with radiographic exposure. The urologist must be aware of the risks of radiation and weigh these against the benefits that the study will provide. Clearly, if the diagnosis and proper management can be achieved without radiographs, there is no indication for such studies. On the other hand, a condition may exist that can be dangerous to the patient if not diagnosed, and if the diagnosis is dependent on radiographs, the study should be obtained.

The potential consequences of ionizing radiation to the pregnant woman include spontaneous abortion, congenital anomalies, malignant disease, impaired growth and development, and mutations. However, the risks are negligible if the dose to the uterus or fetus is less than 10 rads.[6] A five-film IVU will result in a uterine (fetal) exposure of well under this dose. The American College of Radiology estimates the minimal effective dose for adverse affects to the fetus during the first trimester to be 10 rem. Above this dose, the risk might be 1 in 1000 per rad for the first 10 years of life. This, coupled with the 4% to 6% risk of congenital defects in normal pregnancies not exposed to radiation,

certainly minimizes the potential risks of ionizing radiation.[7]

Most diagnostic procedures ordered by the urologist should fall well below the 10-rad exposure limit already discussed. Regardless, if the patient is known to be pregnant, radiation should be avoided in elective imaging. Inquiries concerning possible pregnancy should be made in all potentially fertile women prior to any radiologic studies. Although the risks to the fetus may be small, the medicolegal issues may not be insubstantial if no attempt is made to obtain a history of possible pregnancy, particularly in view of the background rate of anomalies.

Hydronephrosis of Pregnancy

The upper urinary tract will show hydronephrotic changes in the majority of third-trimester women. One logical explanation is that the gravid uterus compresses the ureters between its posterior wall and the pelvic brim. Changes are often greater on the right than the left, with the left ureter thought to be buffered from compression by the sigmoid colon. Supporting this theory is the fact that hydronephrosis seldom occurs in the first trimester when the gravid uterus is still quite small. As the uterus enlarges during the second trimester and extends above the pelvic brim, ureteral dilatation begins to occur, starting at the level of the pelvic brim. Furthermore, after delivery, the ureteral dilatation tends to return toward normal within the first month.[8]

Another theory involves the changes in the hormonal milieu of the pregnant woman that may have a direct effect on the urinary collecting system. However, hormonal manipulation in the woman does not result in hydronephrosis. Regardless of the cause, the fact remains that hydronephrosis commonly occurs. Typical changes during pregnancy and the postpartum phase are seen in (Fig. 28). A diagnostic dilemma may arise when the pregnant woman presents with signs or symptoms referable to the upper urinary tract.

Asymptomatic bacturia and urinary tract infection are more common during pregnancy. Moreover, admissions to the hospital are not infrequent for flank pain, renal colic, and frank pyelonephritis. Diagnostic imaging is frequently limited by potential radiation risks to the fetus, and x-ray studies are seldom considered. Renal ultrasound poses no risk to the patient or fetus, however. The finding of hydronephrosis may be related to the pregnant state itself or to other conditions. If a stone is suspected, a delay in further diagnostic imaging because of the fear of irradiating the fetus may result in a delay of management that can pose a much greater risk to the patient and the fetus. This is especially so if infection is associated with the stone. As discussed earlier, the risk to the fetus from radiation is minimal for most diagnostic studies such as an IVU.

The decision to proceed with a radiograph in the urologic workup of the pregnant woman should be based on the diagnostic information the studies will yield. If the information that could be obtained would alter the treatment plan to manage the patient better, then the studies are probably indicated. Such is the case in the pregnant woman with ureteral colic from ureteral stone and infection. Ultrasound may not be able to image a ureteral stone, although endovaginal ultrasound is occasionally useful for distal stones (Fig. 29). If intervention would be considered should the diagnosis be ureteral stone and ultrasound cannot make the diagnosis, radiographic studies should be considered. A plain film (KUB) and a 10-minute film after contrast injection can usually yield significant information while limiting x-ray exposure. On the other hand, if the studies being considered would not alter the treatment plan, they probably are not indicated.

If a pregnant woman has persistent flank pain or infection associated with a hydronephrotic kidney, initial intervention will usually involve percutaneous nephrostomy or retrograde ureteral stent placement.[9] To proceed with either procedure without clearly establishing the diagnosis or confirming proper positioning with radiographs has its own attendant risks. The urologist should always be aware that contraindications to radiographs during pregnancy are relative and must be weighed against the risks of managing the patient without the assistance of radiographic knowledge.

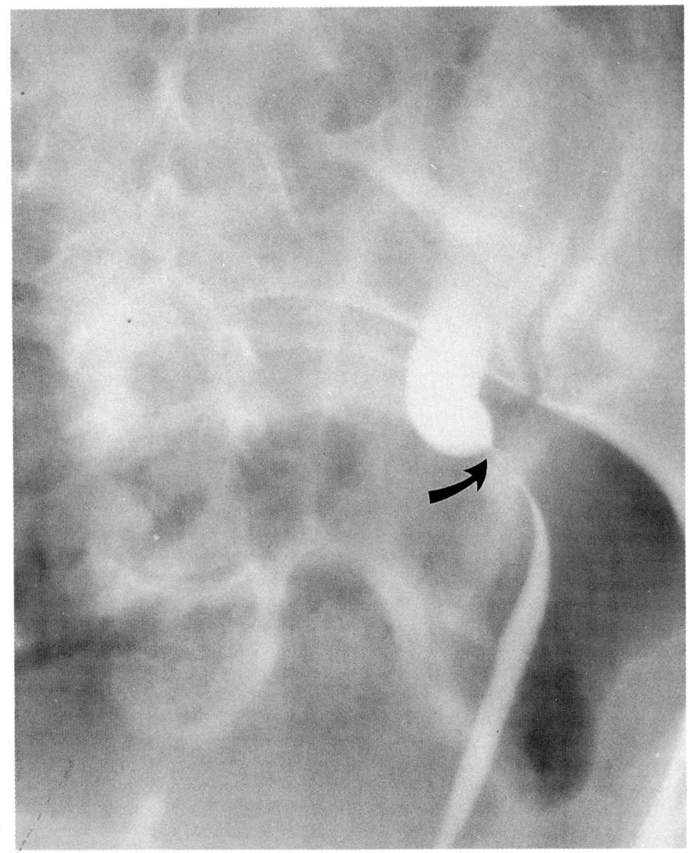

Figure 22.   Ovarian remnant has caused narrowing of the distal left ureter (curved arrow) demonstrated by retrograde pyelogram.

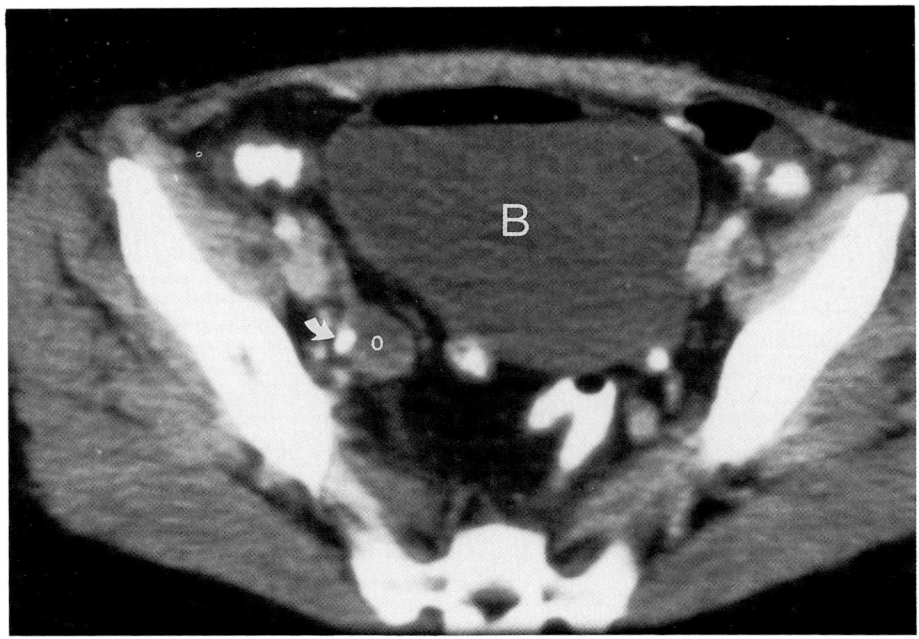

Figure 23.   CT scan of the pelvis shows ovarian remnant (o) adjacent to the right ureter (curved arrow), *B* = bladder.

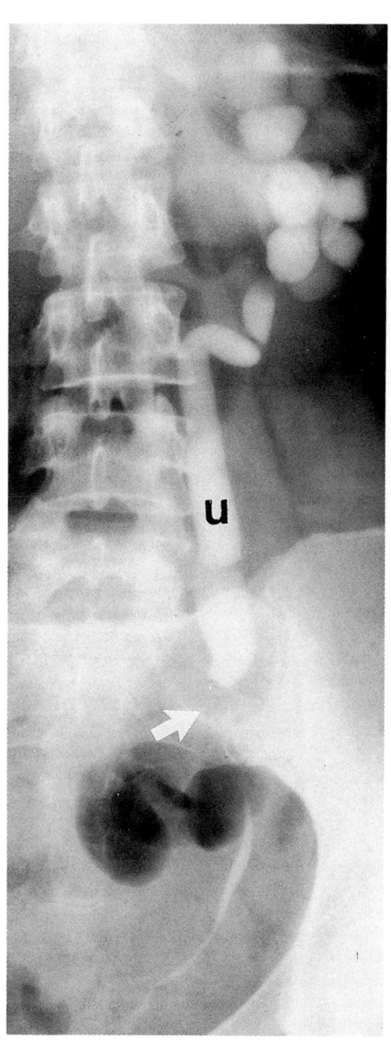

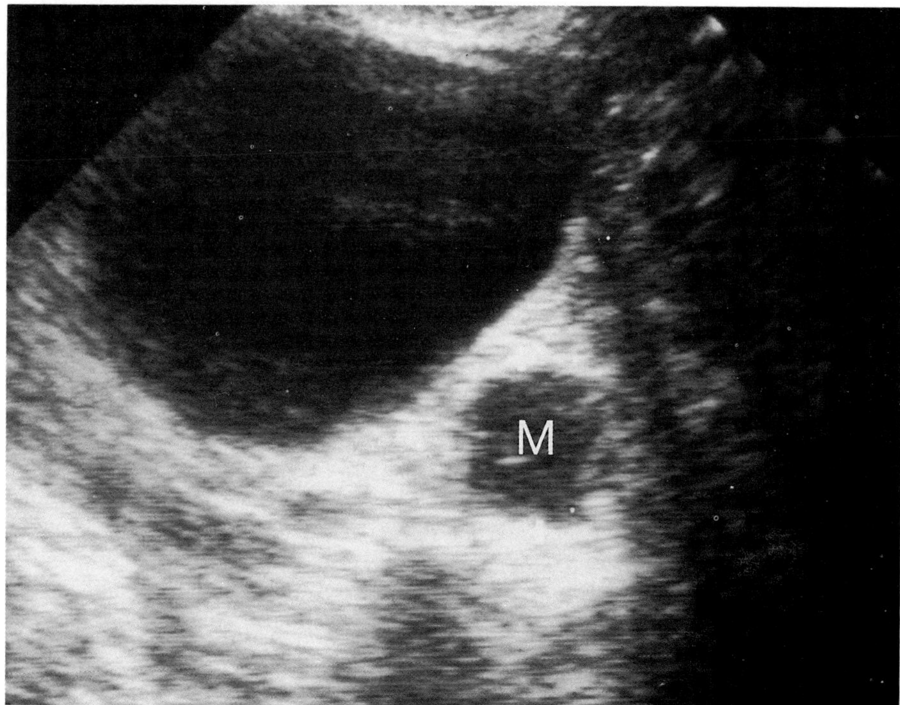

Figure 24. Endometriosis. Intravenous urogram showing a dilated ureter (U) caused by narrowing at the pelvic brim (arrow) as a result of invasion by endometrial tissue.

Figure 25. Endometriosis with obstruction of the ureter. Pelvic ultrasound scan shows a hypoechoic mass (M) in the left pelvis.

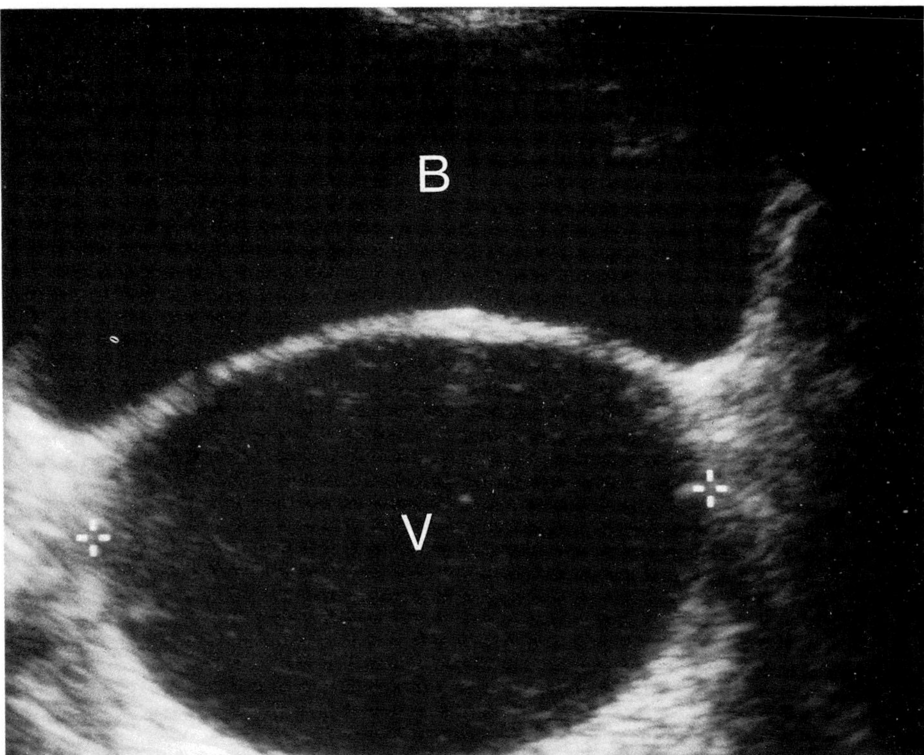

Figure 26. Hydrocolpos. Transverse ultrasound scan of the pelvis shows fluid within the vagina (V) posterior to the bladder (B).

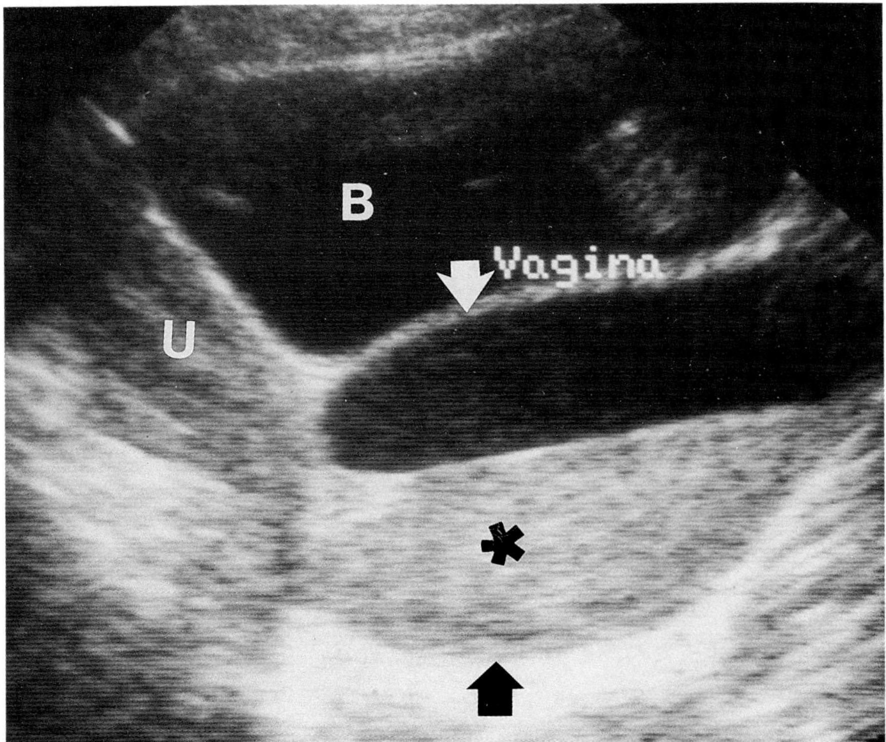

Figure 27. Hematocolpos. Sagittal scan of the pelvis demonstrates blood (*) layering dependently in a distended vagina. Anterior vaginal wall (white arrow), posterior vaginal wall (black arrow), uterus (u), and bladder (B) also are seen.

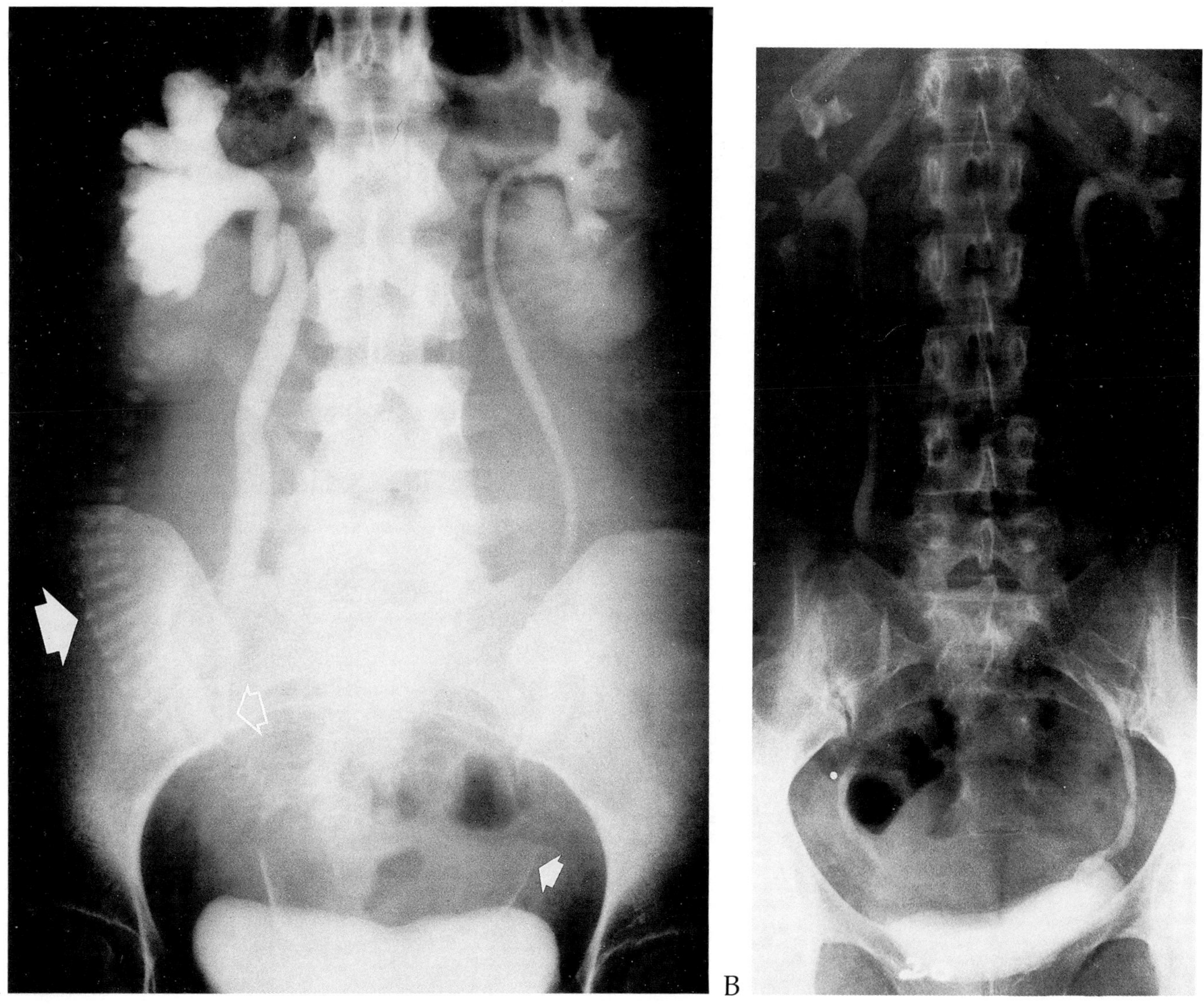

Figure 28. Hydroureter and hydronephrosis of pregnancy. Intravenous urograms (A, left) at-term fetus (arrow). Dilated right ureter above the pelvic brim (open arrow) and hydronephrosis. (B, right) Two months postpartum, the right upper tract has returned to normal.

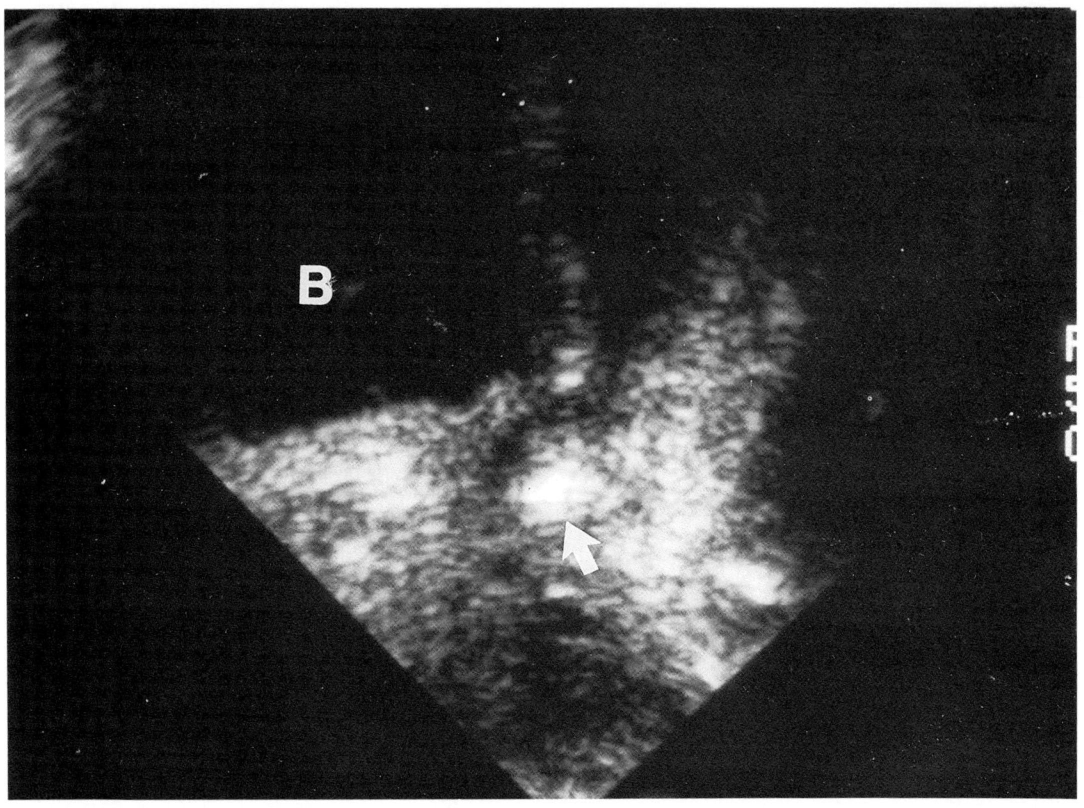

Figure 29. Distal left ureteral calculus. Transvaginal scan confirms a stone in the distal left ureter (arrow), B = bladder.

References

1. Diokno AC, Brock BM, Brown MB, et al: Prevalence of urinary incontinence and other urological symptoms in the noninstitutionalized elderly. J Urol 1986; 136:1022.
2. Buchsbaum HJ, Schmidt J: Gynecologic and Obstetric Urology. Philadelphia: WB Saunders, 1982.
3. Munday AR: The neuropathic urethra. In Munday, AR: Urodynamics: Principle, Practice and Application. Edinburgh: Churchill-Livingston, 1984; 288.
4. Steege JF: Ovarian remnant syndrome. Obstet Gynecol 1987; 70:64.
5. Mason W, Hill G, Herbert C, et al: Ureteral abnormalities in women with endometriosis. Fertil Steril 1986; 46:1159.
6. Bushong S: Late effects of radiation. In Bushong S.: Radiologic Science for Technologists. St. Louis: CV Mosby; 1988, p 513.
7. Whelan JG Jr: Diagnostic radiology in fertile or pregnant women. Kansas Med Assoc J 1988; 86:353.
8. Rasmussen PE, Nielsen FR: Hydronephrosis during pregnancy: a literature survey. Eur J Obstet Gynecol Reprod Biol 1988; 27:249.
9. Cass AS, Smith CS, Gleich P: Management of urinary calculi in pregnancy. Urology 1986; 28:370.

Index